Morning rounds were about to start in a patient lounge, and the staff filed down the hall with us following. In the lounge, we sat in a circle and went around introducing ourselves.

"I want to speak with the new residents right after this meeting is over," Greg Halper, the assistant unit chief, announced. It wasn't until several weeks later that I learned that an assistant unit chief is a fourth-year resident, not a member of the faculty. After the meeting, as the rest of the staff cleared out, we huddled in the middle. "Okay," Halper said after shutting the door behind the last of the staff. "You've probably heard that this is a very difficult floor to start out on. I'm here to run interference for you. I want to know about everything that goes on that doesn't seem right to you—anything funny with the staff, is that straight? Remember: this year can be very interesting for you, but you have to be careful and work hard to make it so."

"Looks pretty serious," I whispered to Anne as we straggled out of the room.

"I said that I wanted to be on any floor but this one," she responded. "When I was assigned here, I complained but couldn't change it. You know, this is called 'The Survival Ward.' If you can make it here, you can make it anywhere."

By Robert Klitzman, M.D.:

A YEAR-LONG NIGHT
IN A HOUSE OF DREAMS AND GLASS: Becoming a
  Psychiatrist*

*Published by Ivy Books

IN A HOUSE
OF DREAMS
AND GLASS

Becoming a Psychiatrist

Robert Klitzman, M.D.

IVY BOOKS • NEW YORK

Ivy Books
Published by Ballantine Books
Copyright © 1995 by Robert Klitzman, M.D.
Excerpt from *Behind the Scenes at ER* by Janine Pourroy copyright © 1995 by Warner Bros.

Note: All the details concerning staff, patients, and other people who appear in this book have been changed to protect confidentiality. None of the portraits of characters that appear here may be said to represent actual people. All are based on experiences I have had with many people in numerous hospitals located in different states and countries over many years.

http://www.randomhouse.com

Library of Congress Catalog Card Number: 95-95318

ISBN 0-8041-1436-6

This edition published by arrangement with Simon and Schuster, Inc.

Manufactured in the United States of America

First Ballantine Books Edition: July 1996

10 9 8 7 6 5 4 3 2 1

In memory of my father,
Joseph A. Klitzman

Contents

Acknowledgments   ix
Preface   xi

PART I

Nightwatch   3
Buds   13
The Survival Ward   23
Reversing the Current   26
No-no's   46
The Treatment of Choice   50
Roosters or Hens   73
What Is T?   76
Yellow Caps   84
Guests on Checks   97

PART II

House Wine   107
Home   115
Comrades   120
To Walk in the Valley   126
The Man in My Head   132
The Great Door Debate   138
Strings   147
Vows   157
Wire Glass   159
Talisman   167

Contents

PART III

The Other Side of the Couch   183
The Unopened Fanta   196
Chains   209
Heaven   . 215
Yellow and Red Balloons   228

PART IV

Cutbacks   237
No-goodniks   245
Harmony   282

PART V

Green   291
The Heat   297
Desserts   309
Follow-ups   331

Acknowledgments

I want to thank many people for their help with this book. First and foremost, I am enormously indebted to the patients whom I had the privilege of caring for and getting to know. Without them, I could not have become a psychiatrist, nor learned what I did, and certainly could not have written these chapters.

I also want to thank my colleagues—the other psychiatrists, residents, social workers, nurses, and staff members at the hospital where I trained—for their instruction and insight.

This book could not have been completed without the assistance of several people and organizations, notably the Robert Wood Johnson Foundation Clinical Scholars Program at the University of Pennsylvania, under whose auspices I wrote most of this book, and in particular, Sankey Williams, Samuel Martin, Beryl Miller, Rosemary Stevens for her initial encouragement, and especially Renée C. Fox for her friendship, unfailing generosity and support, and astute comments on this manuscript.

For reading portions of this text in this and other forms, I am grateful to Rebecca Stowe, Cheryl Sucher, Richard A. Friedman, Scott Clark, Royce Flippin, Deborah Hautzig, and Ellen Currie and her writing class at Columbia University. I also wish to thank William McFarlane, Jules Ranz, and Susan Deakins in the public psychiatry fellowship at the New York State Psychiatric Institute; the MacDowell Colony and its staff, where I worked on this manuscript; D. Carleton Gajdusek, Stacey Spence, and Mitchell Sally; and especially Philip Koether, who was there both during my residency and while writing about it. I owe enormous gratitude to my agent, Kris Dahl, for her continuing faith in this project, often when I needed it most. I also appreciated the help of her assistants, Gordon Kato and Dorothea Herrey. Finally, I am deeply indebted to my editor at Simon and Schuster, Robert Asahina, for his support, understanding, and insight through all the stages of this project, and to his assistant, Sarah Pinckney, for her many suggestions both large and small.

Preface

I wrote this book—on my experience of the process of becoming a psychiatrist—for several reasons.

My training often surprised and bewildered me, and I undertook this account, in large part, to try to make sense of it. Frequently as a resident, I found myself in utterly unexpected situations, in which my preconceived ideas about the profession proved incorrect. In the peculiar otherworld of a psychiatric hospital, ordinary rules of logic and behavior don't always apply. As residents, we were pressured to conform to an often very rigid model of how psychiatrists should talk and respond to people, and we had to change the way we acted and viewed ourselves. Some of my encounters—for example, when I failed to realize certain things about others and myself right away—embarrassed me when I initially reflected back on them, after my training was over. Yet my beginner's experiences taught me an enormous amount, marking the gap between my not being a psychiatrist and being one, and thus show how the profession "socializes" and transforms its members. How we as residents learn to think about ourselves and others shapes how we will approach patients for decades to come.

I also wrote this account after seeing that psychiatrists needed to become much more aware of the social, cultural, and human dimensions of their patients' lives. Compassion was too often in short supply. It was easy to pigeonhole patients into narrow categories, to prescribe drugs, and to blame patients for the failures when treatments didn't work. But a wider, more humanistic view seems critical, to strengthen the field.

This book can also help patients, their families, and friends, who often find psychiatrists perplexing or frustrating, yet can work with them more effectively if each side gains further insight into the other.

Finally, many people hold misconceptions about mental illness, as I did. This book, depicting a psychiatric hospital today and what goes on inside, illustrates specific issues and difficulties in treating mental disorders. The patients I got to know could benefit from less prejudice and from heightened appreciation of their specific situations and needs.

These areas are particularly important at the moment, as psychiatry becomes more and more biological and as managed care plays an expanding role, constricting treatment options. Increasingly, psychiatrists see the mind as nothing but an amalgam of chemical interactions and believe that drugs alone will cure almost all emotional problems. Amidst new medications heralded as "wonder drugs," such as Prozac, and fresh attacks on Freudian theories and mounting financial pressures, it is important to examine the profession and how psychiatrists handle clinical and moral issues. The treatment of mental illness requires more than narrow and unquestioned theories and approaches by themselves—whether biologic or psychoanalytic. Broader and more sensitive social and human perspectives, as invoked here, are needed as well.

These are the years and the walls and the door
that shut on a boy that pats the floor
to feel if the world is there and flat.

ELIZABETH BISHOP
"Visits to St. Elizabeths"

Human nature is the same in all professions.

LAURENCE STERNE
Tristram Shandy

PART I

Nightwatch

"You'd better hurry down to the twelfth floor right away," a woman said breathlessly on the other end of the phone. "Jimmy Lentz is revving up. It looks like he's about to blow."

I grabbed my clipboard and galloped down the stairs. I had just received my first page on my first night on call in a psychiatric hospital.

My shift had started earlier that evening. The light had been vanishing from the street, and the setting sun was casting long shadows as the other physicians all went home for the day, leaving me in charge of the hospital. I was unsure whether the night would be calm and quiet, with very little to do, or bristling with crises wholly new to me. I had stopped by each ward briefly to meet the nurses on duty for the shift and hear about potential problems with patients and various tasks to be completed before the rest of the staff returned in the morning. To remember everything the nurses said, I scribbled copious notes and tried to concentrate as hard as possible. As the only doctor in the entire hospital, I now had more responsibility over more patients than I ever had before and was the central authority in the building. I was excited to be there, and tried to look poised, confident, and professional in my long white coat. But inwardly, I was scared and kept praying that the night would go smoothly and easily and that none of the potential disasters mentioned by the nurses would come to pass. My lack of experience frightened me and left me shaky. The corridors outside the wards were deserted, all the social workers and other M.D.s and most of the nurses having gone home. An eerie hush hung over the dim and empty halls.

If the hospital was quiet, residents could stay in the on-call room and perhaps even sleep if there was nothing to do. I stopped by the room briefly and sat down on the edge of the mushy cot to try to organize a list of tasks awaiting me. The dark, narrow room served as a nursing office during the day, and contained only a desk, a chair, and a rickety metal cot squeezed into a corner. At the far end of the room, a dusty, dark green window shade hung down, completely covering a tiny window. Suddenly, a loud screeching noise pierced my ears. My beeper squealed and flashed a red four-digit number. I dialed the extension and was told to come to the twelfth floor to see Jimmy.

Down the stairs I scurried now, flipping frantically through my notes, trying to find some information about him. On the last page, a single sentence was scrawled: "Seventeen-year-old adolescent with schizophrenia, in tenuous control." Running down the stairwell, I tried to imagine what to expect and how to act. A reduced-size *Handbook of Psychiatry* bulged from my left-hand coat pocket and would presumably hold ready answers to problems that awaited. I hoped a rational, scientific approach would get me through the night.

On the twelfth-floor landing, I used my newly issued key—a four-and-one-half-inch metal rod with squared-off teeth at the base that looked as if it might unlock a jail cell. The heavy door groaned on its hinges and opened only with difficulty.

A nurse, Carol Walters, met me in the hall and escorted me to Jimmy's room.

"I don't want any medicine," Jimmy was telling his mother as they stood in the middle of his small room, their faces inches apart. She had apparently been allowed to stay long past official visiting hours because he was an adolescent and the understaffed nursing shift probably welcomed a little extra help in keeping an eye on him. He had long straight black hair. His baggy green sweatshirt read DON'T MESS WITH ME, and hung down over his loose, ripped blue jeans. The untied laces on his black high-top sneakers dangled down the sides of his feet. Behind him, on a small wooden table with a blue Formica top, lay a new, unused paintbrush beside a red, yellow, and blue box of watercolor paints—probably gifts, though unsuited to his present state of mind. In the corner of the room, a guitar in its black case leaned against the wall. I had played this instrument, too, when I was his age, and had a similar guitar case in the corner of my apartment.

"The medicine will be good for you," his mother was telling

him. She was a pale, older woman with steel gray hair pulled up tightly in a bun behind her head.

"I don't like it," he told her. He brought back to mind my own adolescence, that peculiar time in junior high school when my friends and I all had long hair, wore ripped jeans, and argued with our parents a lot.

"Take it for *me!*"

I didn't know how to react and decided, for the moment, to observe and try to understand what was happening.

"No way." He pulled back.

"You *need* that medication," she said. Her wrinkled white hand reached up and pressed his shoulder. He froze and suddenly glared at her, his eyes wide and bulging. He started breathing in and out heavily. He looked like he was about to erupt. I had never seen someone on the verge of exploding and had certainly never had to manage a patient in this state. He was straining to contain the tension boiling inside him. I felt danger, nervously stepped back and swallowed hard, but I had to do something.

"Excuse me," I interrupted, clearing my throat. "I'm Dr. Klitzman. The doctor on call here tonight." I tried to sound official and spoke in a deep voice. The words sounded odd, but Jimmy and his mother both stopped and looked at me, emboldening me further. "What's going on here?"

"I just want him to take his medicine," Mrs. Lentz said, turning to me. "But he won't listen."

Jimmy was still panting.

"I'd like to ask you to step out of the room for a moment," I said to his mother, thinking I could at least defuse the situation. She cocked her head, perplexed by my request, but when she saw I was serious, slowly retreated. The room simmered down.

"How are you doing?" I now asked Jimmy. He stared at the carpet. His ruminations were a mystery to me. "Jimmy?"

"I'm not too good."

"What's wrong?"

"Voices."

"What are they saying?"

He turned toward the wall. The single lightbulb in the room—low-wattage, bare, and hanging from the middle of the ceiling—emitted a dull yellow light. Jimmy's face was shaded, his eyes shadowed. Outside, night had engulfed the city.

Jimmy stood motionless, transfixed, helpless before his own

internal disturbance as if possessed. Hearing voices is a symptom of psychosis, often seen in schizophrenia, and horrifying to patients. I felt bad for him, as he seemed both sad and troubled before whatever he was feeling. He and I were both floundering before his ailment.

"Do you know what the voices are saying?" I asked gently. He hesitated. "It's time . . . to go."

"What does that mean?"

He still stared at the wall, his chest rising and falling. I was groping in some dark, labyrinthine cave, trying to gauge the obstacles before me. "To end my life," he finally whispered. My stomach twisted uncomfortably. Suicide and homicide are two potential results of mental illness for which psychiatrists are often held responsible and which I wanted to avoid here on my first night on call.

"Do you have a plan?" I didn't know if asking him would induce him to think of one, but it seemed important to know.

"Hang myself," he said quickly but solemnly. He had obviously given this question a lot of thought before I asked. He looked down at his lap. "With a curtain." He gestured vaguely at the drapes. "Even the sheets."

"Would you like to go to the Quiet Room?"—an empty room that, I had been told, patients often found calming.

Jimmy shook his head. "If I do I'll bang my head against the wall until I break it open. I have to stop the voices."

I didn't have many options. "I'd like you to take some medication to calm yourself down." I tried to sound as authoritative as I could.

"I don't want it."

"Why not?"

"I don't like the way it makes me feel—restless inside." The basic medications for psychosis can all have terrible side effects that, despite counteracting drugs, can even be disturbing enough to contribute to some patients' killing themselves. We psychiatrists get rid of symptoms that *we* don't like and give patients symptoms that *they* don't like. Jimmy and I were at an impasse. I felt trapped. The wooden edge of my clipboard felt rough in my sweaty palm.

I told Carol to sit with him and had his mother return to the room for the moment while I went to the nursing station to talk to the head nurse for the night, Donna Lambert, about what to do.

"Let's put him on MO," I told Donna, referring to maximal observation—a one-to-one companion.

"I don't think he needs it," Donna replied. She was in the middle of eating her dinner in the quiet, air-conditioned nursing station. "He'll come to us when he feels bad." She dipped a french fry into a pool of ketchup and popped it into her mouth. If he were on MO, a member of her staff—Carol or herself—would have to sit with him the whole night, which she didn't want to arrange. The other staff would have to do additional work on the floor. But she was not ultimately responsible, while I was, as the psychiatrist last seeing him. If a patient hurts himself, the hospital can lose millions in a malpractice suit.

My instinct told me that Jimmy's threat was real. "I'm very concerned about him," I said.

"We've seen him all night," Donna replied. "*You* just got here."

Suddenly, Carol came running down the hall. "He's just tried to hang himself!" she yelled. She didn't have to say whom she meant. "He jumped up on the table and started to tie the drapes around his neck."

We rushed back. "I'll call the aides," Donna said. I had Jimmy sit down, asked Carol to stay with him again for now, and requested Mrs. Lentz to wait in the patient lounge. Back in the nursing station, Donna phoned the male mental health aides from around the hospital. One or two of them were stationed on each ward. They now hurried to the nursing station and soon assembled into a small army. I described to them what had happened.

"Okay," Jack Sarvin, a tall aide from the ward, said. "Let's make a plan. Dr. Klitzman and I will offer Jimmy medication, and if he refuses, we'll put him into restraints. Tom," he said pointing to an aide with a pony tail from the floor below, "you grab the left arm. Doug," he said to another aide, "you take the right." He assigned Jimmy's legs to two other aides, and then turned to me. "You and I will first try to talk with Jimmy briefly. If he refuses the medication, we'll be ready. Donna, get the restraints." From a closet in the side of the nursing station she removed a stash of thick leather straps with heavy brass buckles which she draped over her arms. "How does that sound?" Jack asked me.

I had never witnessed a situation like this before. The brown leather straps looked like a horse's harness. This treatment sounded horribly crude. Whatever happened to talking with patients to ease their problems? "Are there any alternatives?" I asked. My mouth felt dry.

"No," Donna said quickly, jingling her keys in her hand and the buckles in her arms. Jack shifted his weight from one leg to the other.

I didn't want to look naive or ignorant about what to do, but I also didn't want to make a mistake, especially on my first night on call. I would be judged and evaluated in the morning, and aspired to do well here at the beginning of my new career. But I was about to give official approval for strapping a patient down and injecting him with drugs against his will. This prospect felt dark, cruel, and strange. The hospital workers were calling on me to execute a difficult task that I had never performed or even imagined performing. Tying patients down seemed part of the "old" psychiatry, of *One Flew Over the Cuckoo's Nest*.

"Trust us," Jack said. "We've been through this before."

There was no one else to turn to or ask. They had all worked here for years and looked like they knew what they were doing. My residency had started only three days earlier. This course of action, though unpleasant, seemed to follow from what had happened. Moreover, I didn't want to slow up this process or get the staff, with whom I'd have to work over the next three years, angry. Still, I was surprised that I was going along with it. The inevitability of this intervention astonished me. "I guess we don't have a choice," I sighed, though still holding out hope that some alternative solution might be found.

We filed out of the nursing station and to Jimmy's room.

"You really need to take your medicine," I said to him in my firmest, most adult-sounding voice, feeling as if at some high-level diplomatic peace negotiation.

His eyes narrowed.

"Why don't you want to take it?" Jack asked him.

"I want to see my mother first."

Perhaps if he saw her, he'd consent to the medicine. I asked Jack, who agreed, partly as a concession to me, that his mother could come back and say goodbye to him, but only for three minutes. "If he acts violently before that, he goes into restraints," Jack said. That part of the plan still dismayed me, but there seemed little choice

I went to the lounge to get Mrs. Lentz.

"I just don't see why he's like this," she sighed as we walked back to her son's room. "I've always tried to be good to him." Tears began to fill her eyes. I felt bad for her having to see Jimmy's disturbance and our response.

"We can talk about that later," I said. "But for the moment, let's just follow this plan."

She accompanied me back into Jimmy's narrow room. The other aides hovered in the hall on either side of the doorway, out of sight. Once inside, I stood behind his mother. "Why can't you calm down?" she asked Jimmy.

"I . . . can't."

"I didn't mean any harm when I told you to go get a job, you know."

They talked for a few more minutes, but he still refused the medication. "Your three minutes are up," Jack suddenly interrupted in what seemed like less time, but probably was the allotted amount.

"If she goes, I'm going to kill myself!" Jimmy declared.

Mrs. Lentz looked over at me, bewildered, as she hugged her son goodbye.

"You have to leave now," Jack said, stepping toward them to break their bond. She began to back toward me.

"No," Jimmy started. He looked at the door, sensing the troops gathered outside in the hall. "I'm going to take her hostage!" He suddenly lunged toward her and me, the two of us now standing together. He spread his arms wide. I jumped back, not completely sure whether he was going to attack her or me or both of us.

We escaped behind Jack.

"Grab him!" Jack yelled. The aides came storming in through the door, swarming past me and soon filling the room. Jimmy saw he was trapped. He stepped back toward the far wall in retreat. There, he arched his spine and pulled his arms up to brace himself. The four tall aides in T-shirts jumped him and quickly wrestled him to the floor. I stepped farther toward the door, glad I didn't have to take part in this physical process, but troubled that I had approved it.

"Let's lift him onto the bed," Jack called. "At the count of three." Jimmy squirmed in their arms but was no match for the athletic men.

"No," he whimpered. "I only want to see my mother."

"Soon enough," Jack told him, tightening his grip on Jimmy's calf.

"One . . ." Jack called out. Jimmy tried yanking an arm free, but Jack clamped Jimmy's wrist and pressed it to the cold gray linoleum floor. Jimmy kicked to free his legs, but Doug knelt on Jimmy's thighs for added leverage. I stepped farther back.

"Two . . ." Jack said. I cringed, unsure what was going to happen.

"Three!" Jack shouted. The aides elevated Jimmy's body into the air. Jimmy writhed as they carried him aloft, horizontally. I couldn't believe this was happening. They lowered him onto his wooden bed. Donna squatted down and slipped one of Jimmy's legs into a wide leather belt and tightened and buckled the strap, then knotted the belt's other end to the foot of the bed, below the mattress. She then proceeded to buckle his other leg and his two arms. Jimmy looked up, then shut his eyes.

Donna grabbed a syringe with a long silver needle, raised it into the air, and tapped the plastic vial of clear liquid to let out the bubbles. Then she pulled down Jimmy's pants and underwear, wiped his skin with a wet white alcohol swab, and shoved in the needle. Jimmy winced. She jabbed the plunger in, then jerked the needle out, and pressed a sterile cotton pad over the spot.

I felt aghast, uncomprehending. Treating Jimmy as if he were a captured animal mortified me, disturbing me both morally and emotionally. This procedure was completely different from the psychiatry I had envisioned and anticipated practicing. This event didn't fit with any of my experiences in medicine until now. In medical school, and thus far at this hospital, psychiatry had been presented as a fully modern science, with new medications and research advances. For Jimmy, it seemed that treatment today resembled that of two centuries ago. Nothing I had learned through years of classroom education had prepared me for this scene. Physical violence had always scared me. I had been mugged at age eleven, beaten up by a gang in a New York City subway station. Fights, with their danger and irrationality, chilled me.

This was brute management—"veterinary treatment" a professor would later term it—hardly scientific medicine. Was there no other way to help Jimmy? This hospital was prestigious, with noted psychiatrists on the faculty, and a list of famous people who had once been treated here. Was this the best the field had to offer? How little the profession seemed to understand about the brain to be treating schizophrenia, with which Jimmy had been diagnosed, in this manner.

No one had talked about this being part of the experience of being a psychiatrist, and no one questioned it now. Maybe I just didn't know enough. Maybe I was too squeamish, or there was something wrong with me because I didn't like this treatment and didn't immediately feel compelled by its logic. Maybe I should somehow be reacting to this task as merely "a job" and be less concerned with how Jimmy and his mother felt about it. After only three days of residency, I still expected to be helping the mentally ill by studying and understanding human nature, the mind, and the brain. I had come to this hospital filled with hope and expectation, having made it successfully through four years of college, four years of medical school, and a year of medical internship to get here.

A weight now sank into the pit of my stomach. I felt like the bottom was falling out of my dreams and plans. I didn't know how to deal with or process this experience. At the moment, I didn't have much of a choice and had to go on, but I felt alienated and somehow at odds with these events, as if stuck in another country where nothing made sense.

The aides filtered out of the room. Jack wiped his hands, one against the other. Jimmy was left sprawled and knotted to his bed.

The next morning, Jimmy was untied and allowed to go to breakfast. Afterward, he passed me in the hallway. He strode down the corridor staring at the carpet without looking where he was going, his head fixed down tensely, almost trembling, as if he were still carrying around a bomb inside him.

"That boy is escalating," Alice, the head nurse for the day shift, muttered in the nursing station. "He's cruisin' for seclusion." The Seclusion Room was the same as the Quiet Room, only the door was locked. Patients were kept there against their will to force them to calm down.

An hour later, Jimmy threatened his mother with his fist when she again begged him to take the medicine. Alice locked him in Seclusion. Through the ward, a harsh, insistent banging thundered. Jimmy kicked and punched the metal Seclusion Room door. "Let me out of here," he screamed. When I walked down the hall, he peered out through the small double plate glass window in the door. "Let me out!" He banged louder. Through the window he recognized me. His eyebrows pinched together, his face twisted with pain and rage. Our eyes met—his widening and pleading with me to let him free.

I hated seeing him there.

I hoped that, over time, residency would give me better ways of making sense of or dealing with this kind of situation, and that some good would come out of this episode. I would later see that the Seclusion Room could calm a patient down and keep other patients on the ward safe. But on this first post-call morning, I was left feeling uneasy. In the meantime, other tasks awaited me on other patients who could perhaps be helped more.

I was surprised to have been forced to be involved in a practice that seemed this shockingly crude and wasn't part of the view of psychiatry held by the profession or the public. Yet this experience with Jimmy made me realize that residency might be far more upsetting than I had imagined. I wondered how I'd manage to get through the next three years.

Up to this point, I hadn't anticipated undergoing much personal stress or transformation in becoming a psychiatrist. Some psychiatrists in medical school and in movies and novels such as *The Bell Jar* were cold, analytic "shrinks," who seemed part of a weird, warped world. That wasn't me. Presumably, I'd be different and be able to avoid that. These assumptions, which in retrospect had protected me, were now being challenged. Would I turn out to be a shrink like some others around me? How much did residents have to conform to this model? How much would I change or be able to stay myself? What would be the personal costs of entering this peculiar universe?

Jimmy followed my movements closely through the window of his cell. As I looked at him I shrugged to show my helplessness, and then averted my eyes—toward the ground. My heart bled for him. But I had to force myself to keep walking down the hall and hope to figure out a better way to respond to such a situation. In the background, his fierce pounding and muffled cries echoed in my ears.

Buds

The first time psychiatry ever occurred to me as a possible career was back in high school. In the spring of my senior year, while driving with some friends on a suburban street near my house, someone asked me what I wanted to be when I grew up. This question had always annoyed me. Back in elementary school, other boys had wanted to be firemen and policemen. Neither job appealed to me. But I didn't yet have any alternatives and usually pleaded ignorance. I had many hobbies and interests and didn't want to choose just one thing or, for that matter, know how to. But with only a few months left before going off to college, I decided to try to give the question some serious thought for once. Outside the car stretched rainy gray streets lined with neat manicured lawns and shrubs and aluminum mailboxes in Colonial motifs. A thick mist hung in the air. "A Supreme Court Justice," I finally stammered out. "Or a psychiatrist."

My answers surprised me. I didn't know any judges or psychiatrists. But at the age of seventeen both of these positions seemed to be ideals, addressing larger, important issues, enabling one to do something constructive or enlightened in the world, promoting civil rights or helping people to know themselves better.

I didn't dwell much on my answers and almost forgot about them when, a few months later, I left for college. There, I found myself liking courses in biology as well as the humanities, and was particularly inspired by the works of Freud, Jung, and Nietzsche. These writers seemed to raise the most moving and critical questions—how people experienced the world around them, interpreted their experiences, and made up myths and stories about their lives. These authors examined explicitly the issues that engaged me most in other writers' novels and poems.

Psychiatry seemed to follow from some of these interests and attracted me from the little I knew about it. I also thought I'd be good at what psychiatrists appeared to do: talk with people, find out about their lives and thoughts, and try to understand the mind and the brain. If the unexamined life was said not to be worth living, then examining lives was certainly a worthy pursuit.

Psychiatry also appeared to be in an exciting period, which continues today. These days, human beings view and define themselves in psychological terms. Mental disorders no longer involve gods, as in the past, but the mind and the brain. In the late twentieth century, psychological difficulties result not from demons, but from defenses, drives, dynamics, unconscious conflicts, and, more recently, from chemical imbalances and hormones. Psychiatry as a field would place me in a central position to fathom these issues.

At the time, my interest in psychiatry had other roots as well.

I am descended from a long line of rabbis. My grandfather, along with two great-grandfathers and at least two great-great-grandfathers, was a religious leader in Lithuania. An old black-and-white turn-of-the-century photograph of my great-grandfather rests on my bookshelf. He is seated in a high-backed wooden chair with carved flowers on the backboard, dressed in a black silk top hat and a long double-breasted coat. He has a long white beard, and round warm eyes just like those of one of my uncles. Beside him stands his wife—my great-grandmother—her hand on his shoulder. She wears a long silk gown and a vest with a long column of close, tiny buttons. Her hair folds inward neatly—probably a wig, as was the custom.

A story is told about him in the family. When they had a daughter who had reached marriageable age, he took her one day to his class of rabbinic students. He looked down the rows of young men, selected the one whom he thought the most promising, and decided that this student would marry his daughter. The newlywed couple became my grandparents.

I never met them. My grandfather died a few months after my birth. But he appears in a home movie taken shortly before my arrival: tall, in black with a black hat and a long white beard, a commanding, haunting figure from a lost world.

My father rebelled against this background. He hated going to synagogue, got into fights about it with his father, and went into business instead. But, perhaps through some quirk, an interest in studying and reflecting on more scholarly ultimate questions about man and human nature seemed to have been passed on to me. Business for its own sake turned me off, just as my father had been repulsed by *his* father's profession. Perhaps I was unintentionally following some larger pattern: a grandson pursuing the values of his grandfather. In any case, I felt some connection to this heritage.

I was born and raised for several years on the Upper West Side of Manhattan, where I was exposed to a variety of cultures. Initially, I went to a public school where my class included kids of many ethnic backgrounds, representative of the community in the 1960s. In addition, many classmates' parents were artists and writers. My Cub Scout den mother was Sigmund Freud's granddaughter. She was warm, fed us bountiful after-school snacks, and engaged us in activities that were often more cultural than sporting. Her son, Freud's great-grandson, was a friend in my scout troop as well.

On weekends, my parents took my sisters and me throughout the city to parks, museums, zoos, and botanical gardens.

When I was eleven my family moved to suburbia, but I kept my interest in different cultures and experiences. The town where we now lived on Long Island, however, had been entirely rural until the recent encroachment of small suburban pockets. I was teased for having long hair and bell-bottom jeans, which wouldn't reach this area for another two or three years.

To pay all the bills, both my parents worked long hours in the garment district of New York and commuted, which meant they weren't around much. There was no day of the week on which the whole family was home for the entire day, and my three sisters and I were often left on our own.

I was the only boy in the family. Two of my sisters were identical twins and were each other's best friend. Strangers and even some acquaintances couldn't tell them apart. Our family still disputes over who is shown in some baby pictures. But I saw differences. One was also born five minutes before the other, which had a big impact on them psychologically. The younger adopted the role of the "youngest child," and was more conciliatory in the family. The other became more outspoken and assertive. Though their physical features remained uncannily similar, as they got older the differences in their personalities became more distinct.

Over time, their interests diversified. Their responses to various choices and decisions became increasingly unique. Though identical genetically, the increasing contrasts in their personalities astonished me as we grew up, marking how far biology determined someone's personality, and the extent to which environment and social situations played a role. I watched this "natural experiment"—though never thinking of it in these terms—observing how personalities blossomed in different ways.

My older sister hung out with them as well, and I followed my own pursuits. I liked nature and science and, as a boy, grew plants from seeds, at first on the windowsill of our New York City apartment. I placed carrot tops in tin pie pans and potatoes in jars of water to watch tiny buds sprout and leaf. Later, in junior high school, I built a shortwave radio and listened to stations from all over the continent. Reading books and writing attracted me as well, as did political issues, and in our suburban town I worked as a volunteer for local progressive causes and candidates. I was drawn to activities that in some way engaged what I felt at the time to be ultimate issues.

As I got older, my curiosity grew about how various people thought and worked. I liked meeting and getting to know others, and learning how they experienced the world and approached the dilemmas of life. This inquisitiveness resulted in part from my feeling somewhat different and something of an outsider in my family, not part of the inner group of my sisters and my mother—my father was always very busy and tended to be much more distant and removed. At the same time, I also became increasingly self-examining and self-reflective.

In my suburban high school, most of the brighter kids had firmly decided they wanted to be doctors and talked about it frequently. Though toying with the idea at the end of my senior year, I was far from being sold on it. Not until college, when psychiatry began to appeal to me for clear and specific reasons, did I seriously consider medical school. Psychiatry seemed to follow from interests in nature and science, in literature, and in social issues; it offered a means of combining them and was a way of coming to know and understand other people.

Within psychiatry, I was drawn to the psychological questions of how individuals view and define themselves, as well as to biological issues. Most psychiatrists are more geared to one approach or the other as the field as a whole undergoes a transition. Some have said that psychiatry used to be "brainless"—ignoring the brain and dealing almost entirely with the mind—and is now becoming "mindless"—focusing almost exclusively on the brain and virtually forgetting the mind.

Though at the end of college other careers tempted me, such as going to graduate school in the humanities or being a freelance writer, I continued on my path and applied to medical school. At the time, in the late 1970s and early 1980s, through recurring recessions, the security of a profession also had some allure, though it was not a deciding factor. My parents liked the idea of my going to medical school. It made them proud, as I would be the first doctor in either of their extended families. My father had never finished college and had always encouraged my sisters and me to pursue our educations as much as we could. Yet their preferences about my career weren't enough to sway me—at least not consciously.

Before starting medical school, I had an experience that was to have an enormous impact on me. To explore my interest in medicine, I had worked in a laboratory at the National Institutes of Health during a summer vacation, investigating the slow virus disease kuru. After I graduated from college, the opportunity arose to study this disease in Papua New Guinea, where kuru had spread as an epidemic for several decades among a group of peoples in the eastern highlands, at one point wiping out ninety percent of the women in the Fore linguistic and cultural group (anthropologists increasingly avoid using the term "tribe") and sixty-five percent of that group's total population. I arranged to postpone medical school for a year to study the disease and its incubation periods, tracing back recent clusters of cases to particular cannibalistic feasts, in the context of which the virus had been transmitted. When a member of the group died, his or her loved ones would eat the body as part of an act of mourning, spreading the kuru virus in the process.

Of many experiences there, one stayed with me the longest. Before leaving, my guides introduced me to Satuma, a local witch doctor who claimed to cure the disease.

I was astonished. The virus causes similar neurological diseases in the West, including Creutzfeldt-Jakob disease, and is believed to have no treatment. How could a barefoot Fore villager, raised in the Stone Age, have a cure?

He listed his patients, almost all of whom had gotten better. Those who didn't I had met and diagnosed with the disease. I knew that anyone who developed even a headache or a hurt back now thought he or she had kuru. These psychosomatic cases apparently constituted his cures.

He told me his treatment. He first administered several herbs that I knew had been tested at the NIH and found to be ineffective against the virus. He uttered an incantation and prescribed several behavioral changes. For one week, the patient was not to drink water, eat any salt, or touch a member of the opposite sex.

"Why do some people still get sick?" I asked.

"They didn't follow my advice. They drank water or ate salt or touched a member of the opposite sex." Failures in treatment weren't blamed on the treatment, which was wholly ineffective against the virus, but on the patient. His definition of kuru allowed him to feel that he was usually successful against the virus. Clearly, in the midst of this epidemic, villagers were glad to have a doctor who, they believed, offered some control and provided some hope over the illness and reduced their sense of utter helplessness and vulnerability.

I told Satuma that the disease was spread by a virus transmitted at the cannibalistic feasts.

"No," he replied. "Kuru is caused by sorcerers."

"Then how come the number of kuru patients is decreasing?" The feasts had stopped a few years ago. The virus's incubation period can be decades, and cases were still occurring, though much less frequently.

"That's because the sorcerers finally heard our pleas to stop their evil magic." The tribe's treatments and interventions were credited with the decreased rate of kuru that had, in fact, resulted from ending the feasts. Moreover, the New Guineans argued that their theory—and not mine—was correct, because they had cured the disease and white men hadn't.

I saw the need to be wary of claims of cures that, though strongly believed, may not be accurate. Diagnoses, though citing empirical data, might also be relative ways of organizing experiences, and not reflect anything absolute or a priori about patients' complaints.

I assumed that in medical school and residency these observations would be distant and irrelevant. But that would turn out not to be the case.

My experience in New Guinea also furthered my dedication to medical science and to testing rigorously and discovering the truth—whether about human nature, the mind, or the brain—to avoid being misguided and misled. I saw, too, how important it was to observe and comprehend the social and cultural contexts of medical care.

A few weeks after I returned from my trip to New Guinea, medical school began. During this training, other specialties besides psychiatry soon intrigued me. Neurology seemed the field that would have the most exciting discoveries in the future—about how the brain worked—though possibly not for decades or even in my lifetime. Pediatricians seemed the nicest specialists as a group, choosing their specialty because they loved children. But the residents and faculty in psychiatry seemed the most interesting. These residents were the only ones who still talked about going to films and reading books, both activities I enjoyed. Psychiatry also seemed likely to permit me to be more engaged with patients' lives and with issues that had appealed to me until now.

Some friends were wary of my choice. "Psychiatry today is like internal medicine in the last century," a medical school classmate who planned to enter neurology told me one day. "The field is just beginning to move away from witchcraft and is slowly modernizing with the introduction of effective drugs and more scientific approaches. But it still has a long way to go." In other words, now that psychiatry was becoming less concerned with the mind and more tightly focused on chemicals in the brain, it was becoming more acceptable. Psychiatry was also, along with pediatrics, the lowest paid of medical specialties.

"You really want to become a psychiatrist?" a writer I knew asked. "But you seem too normal to be a shrink."

"Aren't psychiatrists more screwed up than their patients?" my sister Lisa, one of the twins, asked.

"No, not necessarily." Though some of the psychiatrists I met in medical school seemed highly neurotic, many others exuded warmth and compassion, and lacked any obvious traces of mental illness.

"Won't it get to be too much after a while," my mother asked, "talking to crazy people all day?"

"I think it would be interesting."

"Well, I suppose if that's what you want to do ..." She sighed. Some fellow medical students who gravitated toward psychiatry were pressured by their parents to pursue other fields instead. The stigma faced by the mentally ill seemed to be applied to those who cared for them, as well. Some of these classmates started in other specialties and switched to psychiatry later.

In the spring of my third year of medical school, "Psych Night" was held. Graduating fourth-year medical students who would be starting internships in the fall talked to us about the process of applying to and interviewing with hospitals for spots as interns and residents. After graduating from four years of medical school (which had followed four years of college), we would begin our first postgraduate, or PGY-I year— internship—during which we would rotate onto different medical wards. The following year would be our second postgraduate year. We would be called PGY-IIs or "Twos" and most of us would then specialize, by doing a residency in a particular field. Residencies vary in length, extending two years after internship for internal medicine and pediatrics, to three years for psychiatry, and four to six years for surgery. During those years, residents work in a variety of settings in which their specialty is practiced, from inpatient wards to outpatient clinics.

Admission to internships and residencies was highly competitive at better programs. Students could apply to hospitals in those areas of the country in which they wanted to live, and usually submitted applications to five to ten programs. Each psychiatry program required three to four intensive interviews of forty-five minutes to an hour each.

"Interviews can be tough," one student said. "Speaking to one psychiatrist after another—often to psychoanalysts trained to pick apart your defenses. They'll want to know all kinds of deeply personal things about you that aren't in any way relevant. But the interviewers want to see how you deal with emotional issues. Unfortunately, it doesn't look too good to say, 'That's none of your business'—even though it's often the case. It'll seem you have something to hide. So choose some area of your personal life that you're willing to discuss— preferably some area of conflict, something you're unsure about or haven't completely figured out—and be prepared to talk about it. They'll ask you about your relationships, your feelings about your parents, and any deaths or divorces in your family." He also told us about an applicant who decided to reveal his homosexuality if personal questions were asked. Yet everywhere the applicant discussed it, he was uniformly rejected. Surprisingly, the field was much less open-minded than I would have thought, which disheartened me.

"Also, since psychiatry is outside the computerized match process that other fields of medicine participate in," our speaker continued, "you may be unfairly asked to commit yourself to a program before they officially offer you a position. Be careful or you can be put in a difficult spot and get screwed."

Letters of recommendation were needed from people in other branches of medicine. One professor of internal medicine looked disappointed when I told him of my choice of specialty. "I've seen a lot of fine fellows go into psych," he said. "But it does something to them. They change."

I went on interviews anyway.

At one, after discussing my interests, accomplishments, and career goals, the interviewer leaned forward in his chair. "Well, I've heard and learned about all these other things," he said, dismissing them as if bored, "but I haven't heard about *you*! Do you have parents, for instance?"

"Yes, I have parents."

"Well, what are your relationships with them like? What was it like for you growing up?" I didn't think this was relevant to my qualifications as a resident at his hospital, but I proceeded to tell him, though shaken and hearing my voice wobble. My conversation earlier in the interview had been devalued and disregarded.

At another interview, a white-haired psychiatrist in a blue sport coat with white stitching and white slacks sat me down in an empty conference room. "I like to treat these," meaning interviews for residency, "as if I were meeting a patient for the first time," he said. "I follow an evaluation format as I would with a patient. Okay?"

"Sure."

"Name?" I told him. "Age?" I answered. "Where do you now live? Whom do you live with? . . . Are you married or single? Why are you applying to this program? . . ." The standard first line of any medical history on a patient is, for example, "Mr. X is a thirty-three-year-old single white male living alone, now coming in with a chief complaint of . . ." A chief complaint is what the patient answers verbatim to the question

"What brings you to the hospital?" and reflects the patient's understanding of his situation, which may or may not be the same as the doctor's. I liked this interviewer's refreshingly straightforward style at the time. In contrast, other interviews sought much more subjective and diffuse replies. Only in retrospect do I see in this interviewer's approach the beginning of a process of equating residents with patients that would come to shadow much of my training.

One senior psychoanalyst asked me what personal problems in my life I would like to work on. I said I noticed that I often sounded mopey on the phone when I spoke with my parents and wasn't sure why. I hadn't planned this to be an area of emotional conflict to discuss but it seemed to fit the bill. He nodded and continued on.

I was accepted to several programs and chose one at a major university teaching hospital that had researchers and clinicians at the cutting edge of scientific knowledge about the human mind. I arrived eager to begin, filled with idealistic notions about entering a field that was exploring and explaining uncharted domains of the brain, dealing with questions that had been addressed by poets, philosophers, theologians, and scientists for centuries.

I moved into an apartment a few blocks from the hospital. I had always had roommates in college and medical school and now for the first time had my own apartment, with my own kitchen and living room.

I started my internship and, as the end of that year drew near, couldn't wait to enter my new specialty. Residency would be the longest job I had ever had; I looked forward to entering a new world.

The Survival Ward

The first day, I reported for orientation to the psychiatric hospital, part of a sprawling university medical center. En route, I walked through the marble lobby of the main building. The shiny modern glass-and-stone entrance made me feel part of something important and special. I quickened my pace.

That morning, I sat through a long series of introductory lectures. The director of the psychiatric hospital, Dr. Abraham Farb, joined us at noon and introduced himself. "We're good here," he said. "And we know we're good because you all chose us as the place to do your residency." After all our interviews and decisions about programs, my fellow new residents and I would have liked a little more affirmation of our choice than the mere fact that we had chosen them, thus making them a good program. His comment seemed peculiar, the value of the program based, in his mind, on nothing more than our subjective decisions.

At noon, an older resident, Judy Van Meter, was assigned to take me out to lunch. We went to a health food restaurant near the hospital.

"So you've been put on the twelfth floor," she said when we sat down. She smiled to herself. "Well, good luck."

"What does that mean?"

"You'll see. I'm just finishing there. And I'm glad it's over. It's the toughest ward in the hospital, you know." My heart started beating faster. "It's infamous. But it's also where you learn the most."

"What makes it so hard?"

"The personalities. The unit chief, Dr. Steve Kasdin, is a psychoanalyst. He's brilliant. But be careful. He'll want to know all about your personal life. Whatever you do, don't tell

23

him anything. I made that mistake. These psychoanalysts," she said, referring to other faculty members and him, "can figure out a lot about you, but they shouldn't be using their clinical skills on co-workers. He's there as your supervisor, not your analyst. But don't get on his bad side either.

"Then there's Henry Nolan, the associate unit chief, a psychopharmacologist. The two of them disagree all the time. Just don't get caught between them. The most important thing," she said, leaning forward over her plate of pasta, "is that you learn to treat everyone there, including the staff, like patients."

"What do you mean?" I was perplexed.

She chuckled. "You'll find out. But you can't treat them like normal people. You have to be careful and on your guard at all times. Remember: it may not seem it when you're inside, but it's really a nuthouse. The year is very tough. It's like doing your medical internship"—which I had just completed—"all over. Only worse. You know nothing, and you get treated like shit. You'll get a great education. But you'll never be the same person again. I guarantee."

We got up from the table and walked back down the street toward the hospital. I felt anxious and apprehensive about what I was getting myself into.

At the corner, a homeless man in tattered brown clothes with a bottle of liquor tucked in his pants swayed, mumbling to himself and looking searchingly at passersby. He resembled patients I had cared for on medical wards in the past and re-oriented me reassuringly. Despite the "weirdness" of the hospital and the staff, patients like this needed basic kinds of help and constituted an unambiguous goal. Pedestrians out for lunch breaks or shopping flowed past him, keeping their distance as he stood speaking to the air. I wondered how bad the twelfth-floor ward could be.

The next morning I started. Over the three years of residency, I would be assigned a series of six-month rotations—first with inpatients and then with outpatients. If I made it through all these stages, I would be a psychiatrist. Each rotation would require different skills, pose different problems, and teach me new aspects of the field.

Three other residents and I were assigned to the twelfth floor. The four of us decided to arrive there together on our first day. One of them, Anne Simmons, had done an elective there as a medical student and knew her way around. She led us to the right elevator. She was a tall, thin woman with shoulder-length blond hair that swayed as she walked quickly.

When we got off on the floor, we faced a small alcove with several unmarked doors—two in front of us and one on each side. Anne pressed a small button beside one of them. Straight in front of us, at eye level as we exited the elevator, was the lock—much higher than usual on a door. Thumbtacked to the door was an index card with letters in blue magic marker. "BEWARE," the sign said. "Elopement Risk. Keep Door Locked At All Times." I wasn't sure what an "elopement risk" was. But I vaguely remembered that in psychiatric hospitals, patients who run away are said to "elope," as if leaving the hospital was analogous to running away from one's family and home.

"Get away from that door!" we heard a voice bark from inside the ward. We looked at each other, confused, and stepped back. Then a key grated, a bolt clanked, and the door moaned low and painfully on its hinges. A tall man in a red T-shirt and blue jeans, who I later learned was Jack Sarvin, a mental health aide, held the door open for us as he continued a discussion with someone down the hall—presumably a patient who had been standing by the door. Jack didn't even glance at us but kept talking to the person, ignoring us as we entered. He slammed and relatched the door behind us.

We followed Anne down the hall. Jack quickly passed us on the side, never uttering a single word to us or showing any recognition of our arrival. I didn't feel very welcome.

The walls were covered with layer upon layer of thick glossy yellow paint. The carpeting, originally red-brown, was worn to gray. We passed a lounge where several patients sat, some in hospital pajamas, staring off into space. Two sat at a table playing Trivial Pursuit.

Anne led us to the nursing station. On the wall, the head nurse had posted an organizational chart of the ward. She had placed Dr. Kasdin and herself on top and the four new residents on the bottom.

Morning rounds were about to start in a patient lounge, and the staff filed down the hall with us following. In the lounge, we sat in a circle and went around introducing ourselves.

"I want to speak with the new residents right after this meeting is over," Greg Halper, the assistant unit chief, announced. It wasn't until several weeks later that I learned that an assistant unit chief is a fourth-year resident, not a member of the faculty. After the meeting, as the rest of the staff cleared out, we huddled in the middle. "Okay," Halper said after shutting the door behind the last staff member. "You've probably heard that this is a very difficult floor to start out on. I'm here to run interference for you. I want to know about anything that goes on that doesn't seem right to you—anything funny with the staff, is that straight? Remember: this year can be very interesting for you, but you have to be very careful and work hard to make it so."

"Looks pretty serious," I whispered to Anne as we straggled out of the room.

"I said that I wanted to be on any floor but this one," she said. "When I was assigned here, I complained but couldn't change it. You know, this is called 'The Survival Ward.' If you can make it here, you can make it anywhere."

Reversing the Current

As I had suspected as a medical student and intern, compared to the rest of medicine, the treatment of psychiatric patients involves many specific difficulties. Knowledge about the mind and the brain is still limited in many ways and knowing the inner life of another person is virtually impossible. On the twelfth floor I would now see firsthand and closer than ever before how effective or wanting psychiatric interventions were and how clear or unknown were their mechanisms of actions. Internal medicine generally has more definitive methods of diagnosis and better-understood treatments. It could be disconcerting to follow approaches that didn't have as established a scientific explanation or base. Yet, against these odds, and despite these obstacles, I sensed that treatments could sometimes work.

The first patient assigned to me on the ward was Helen

Beckett. I glanced at her chart quickly, straightened my tie, and marched down the hall to meet her. I was excited, as well as nervous.

"So young?" she asked when I introduced myself. She pulled her head back and scanned me up and down, skeptical. "I'm old enough to be your grandmother." She turned away as if to dismiss me. I was taken aback. I hadn't anticipated being immediately rebuked.

She was sixty-eight, had frizzy white hair, and wore black spectacles with pointy corners. As she sat at the edge of her bed, she even looked like my grandmother, whom my mother had recently put into a nursing home. I was used to deferring to people Helen's age and showing respect.

"How do you feel about having a younger doctor?" I fumbled, unsure what else to say.

"I don't like it," she snapped. "I'm ready to go and get out of here." Her chart had said she was depressed.

"But we're very concerned about you." I didn't know who the "we" was, but it sounded right to say.

"If you're really concerned about me, you'll let me go." I could understand her antipathy toward the hospital. The ward felt uncomfortable to me, too. But more experienced psychiatrists had thought she needed to be here. An older resident in the emergency room and a psychiatrist on the outside had arranged for her to be admitted.

"But you've been having problems, and we'd like to try to help you."

"My only problem right now is that I'm stuck here."

I was stumped as to how to convince her to change her mind. "Why do you think you're here?" I hoped she'd have some insight.

"My brother brought me."

"Why was that?"

"Ask him." I wasn't getting very far.

"Did you think there was anything wrong?"

She paused. "My vision."

"Your vision?" I asked, surprised, having thought she'd talk about her mental problems.

"Yes. My brother took me to a doctor who gave me drugs to poison me. They destroyed my vision." According to her chart she became depressed a month ago, and stopped leaving her apartment or eating. She lost a lot of weight, though she was slim and frail to start. She was afraid that the superintendent in her building was spying on her and contaminating her water. Her brother had taken her to a psychiatrist who started her on medications that she refused to take. That's when her brother brought her here. "I refuse to take any more of your poison," she told me now. "This is my body," she said, her forefinger beating on her chest. "And I do what I want with it." I agreed philosophically with her position, but she had put herself in a dangerous situation. I felt like I was facing a brick wall.

"It seems you have a hard time trusting doctors," I said.

"Oh, I trust you, Doctor. I trust you, I trust you, I trust you, I trust you."

Already I felt there was no way I could win with her. She had a view of the world that was completely coherent, a way of interpreting anything I said or did as being against her, and it was impossible to get her to see things any other way. I suddenly realized that I was confronting psychosis. That term is bandied about in everyday life. But it wasn't until now, meeting her, that I felt what it meant. In everyday life, people say, "So-and-so is psychotic" or "delusional." But I had never had to oppose an actually psychotic person before. A particular vehemence with which she defended her arguments separated us. It is difficult to describe many mental states. They don't lend themselves to words easily. A medical school professor had once told me, "You know you're talking to a schizophrenic when you feel you're communicating with a person through a pane of glass." In the 1950s and 1960s, critics of psychiatry argued that severe mental illness didn't exist a priori but was simply the result of people being labeled with such terms and put into large institutions that in turn shaped behavior.

Deinstitutionalization occurred—tens of thousands of the mentally ill were discharged from large state mental hospitals—and many eventually ended up homeless in the street. It became only too clear that severe mental illness did exist and wasn't simply a product of individuals being forced to fit into the institution of the hospital. Yet the definitions of psychiatric disorders were still being revised and refined. Nonetheless, Helen's logic clearly differed from mine.

"I think you're making me a guinea pig," she told me now.

"No we're not."

"Then how come the doctor on the outside kept changing the medications I was on?"

"That's because everybody needs a different amount or

combination. People's bodies vary." She stared at me, still suspicious. I thought there must be something I could say to convince her, but I didn't know what. I glanced at my watch. Our time was up.

That afternoon, I had supervision with Dr. Henry Nolan, the associate unit chief. His office was located on a narrow hallway off the ward. I had to unlock the door of the ward to get there.

"Have a seat," he told me, pointing to a blue plastic chair by his desk. His desk was empty, not a paper clip or a piece of paper present. The walls were barren. In the corner stood a fish tank, the filter bubbling. I didn't see any fish swimming in the clear water. It was as if they had died and he had never replaced them.

"Why don't you go through your patients and tell me about each?"

I started with Helen. I began to tell him about my meeting with her, when he suddenly shot his forefinger vertically up in the air to above his head, then turned it upside down and nosedived, landing his finger, tip first, onto his hard wooden desk.

Was he showing me that her course was up-and-down? "I'm not sure what you're saying," I stammered out.

"Shock her."

"Shock her?"

"Yes. Give her ECT." I hadn't considered it as an option before. ECT was how the staff referred to electroconvulsive therapy, known as "shock treatment" among patients. ECT must have been presented in medical school lectures at some point but it made no impression on me at the time. At the end of medical school I was left thinking that ECT was mostly a historical phenomenon. The little sense I had of it from the popular media had been negative. It sounded unnecessarily severe. Through med school and during my internship, I had never seen a patient receiving it.

Helen would undergo general anesthesia, with all of its possible complications, and her brain would be electrified, all because she had symptoms such as being afraid of her landlord. Shock treatment, along with lobotomies, seemed an embarrassing folly from the past, far from my realm as a psychiatrist today. I recalled what a neurologist once said to me in medical school. "Our fields do opposite things," he had told me shortly before I graduated. "I try to prevent seizures; your field induces them through ECT. We both apply scalp electrodes. But I use them to detect electrical activity," as in diagnosing epilepsy. "You just reverse the current, flipping the voltage," causing an epileptic fit. He chuckled, rotating his wrist in the air as if spinning a knob. I was horrified, feeling I was supporting the wrong side. Hardly thinking of ECT as a part of modern psychiatry, I was surprised that he saw it as a defining activity. Neurologists, though, spending all their time on the mechanics of the brain, are closely aware of anything relevant to their field.

"Why ECT?" I asked Nolan now.

"It's the best treatment available for delusional depression. Patients also recover more rapidly than with medication."

"For how long would she get it?"

"Give her six to twelve treatments—three a week—until she improves. Then I like to give them two extras. Just for good luck. Hopefully, she won't relapse and get depressed again immediately afterward. No one knows for sure if the additional treatments really help, but it's a little bit of insurance." He sounded almost nonchalant. "I have some papers on ECT I'll give you. Read up on it tonight. After she agrees, give her a week to clear her body of any drugs. Then we can begin. Also make sure that she has enough medical insurance to cover her for the duration of the treatment."

I left his office and proceeded slowly down the hall, feeling slightly shaken by his brusqueness. My mind was spinning. I grasped a wooden handrail that ran against the wall, used by patients who wanted to hold on to something steady as they walked.

Helen was napping on an orange sofa in the patient lounge, her head resting on the back of the couch. Entwined and knotted in her two frail hands were the straps of her large navy blue pocketbook. She appeared tranquil, neither bothering anyone nor complaining of any psychiatric symptoms. I would now shoot electric current in her brain in the name of curing her.

The next day, I sat down with Helen and told her about ECT.

"See, I told you so," she said, glaring at me. "You're making me a guinea pig."

"No we're not. ECT is the most effective remedy for you."

"Are you sure?" She looked me in the eye. "Have you used it on other people?"

What would I say, never having done so? Henry Nolan's articles said that ECT was more effective than drugs or psychotherapy for a certain type of depression in which delusions are also present. Helen had delusions and symptoms of depression and thus seemed to fall into this category. Placebos had a thirty-three percent success rate, drugs helped sixty-six percent of patients. ECT reportedly cured ninety percent, but I was still a little wary.

Once, ECT had been widely used on other diseases—everything from schizophrenia to personality disorders—until it was found not to meet its initial promise. These disorders are now generally treated more successfully by other means. ECT remains controversial with the public, banned in one city in the country and opposed by several groups and much public sentiment.

Psychiatry has enthusiastically supported many treatments in the past that have later been found to be ineffective. The field's history is filled with claims of cures that eventually failed to be substantiated. In the name of curing their mental problems, patients have been lobotomized, sterilized, injected with insulin, induced to vomit, and bled to reduce the volume of blood in their bodies. Thorazine and other neuroleptics are now used much more cautiously because of long-term irreversible side effects. Almost every treatment offered in psychiatry was initially oversold: enthusiastically used on a much wider group of patients than it would later be found to be effective for. The pressure to treat problems immediately has frequently been stronger than the scientific knowledge available at any point in time. But psychiatrists have never been good at recognizing their own hubris.

Helen would serve as my test case concerning the effectiveness and dangers of ECT.

During my internship in medicine, I occasionally had to convince patients to undergo therapies that I had been taught would be best for them, though patients initially opposed them. In Nolan's articles I learned that ECT had potential side effects, cracking teeth and causing myocardial infarctions, or heart attacks, though these complications were rare. At the moment, I was representing the profession and was charged with supporting what was best for her, even if she disagreed. I was suddenly in the position of authority and had to fill my new role, and support what was said to be best for her, despite my personal doubts.

"Several studies have shown it to be the best way to treat the type of problem you're having," I said in my most professional voice.

"What problem? My only problem is that I'm cooped up here."

"You're depressed."

"I'm not so sure." If she didn't want the treatment, she had the right to refuse. But her reluctance seemed related to her paranoia and delusionality.

"Would you be willing to think about it at least?" She squinted suspiciously, trying to size me up.

The next afternoon, I met with her again. She still rejected ECT. Her paranoia was deeply rooted. Nothing I said changed her mind. "Would you talk to your brother about it?" He was her only living relative.

"Maybe."

I called him up, explained the problem, and arranged a meeting.

He arrived on the ward the next day. He was an elderly white-haired man with the same round-shaped nose as his sister. "Sign the form, Helen," he told her. His voice sounded tired, probably from similar battles with her.

"I don't want to. I want to go home."

"But you know that things were no better at home."

"I don't like it here."

"It'll help you," I said.

"I don't want your help."

"Well, I don't want you coming home," her brother finally told her, "if you don't have this treatment done." She studied him for a long time, working her mouth. She saw he was resolved. She looked back down at the consent form on a clipboard in her lap, and hunched over the paper. "Just do it!" he said. She sighed, and sank in her seat. Then her hand slowly jittered on the page as she signed her name in a gentle flowery script. Surprisingly, her signature had been preserved despite her illness, providing a glimmer of her former self.

I felt bad that she was being implicitly coerced, but she needed the treatment. I let out a breath and eased back into my seat.

She dropped her hand and slouched back as well. Looking up at me, she noticed my name tag. "Your name is Robert," she observed.

"Yes," I said.

"That was my ex-husband's name, too. I wish he were still here now. May he rest in peace."

Residents take turns delivering ECT. I had been surprised to receive in my mailbox on the first day a memo listing the dates of our respective rotations in the ECT suite. It turned out that mine would begin the following week.

The night before, I scrutinized an instruction manual issued by the hospital on delivering ECT. ECT began before morning rounds, so I would have to get to the hospital earlier than usual. I didn't sleep too well that night, worried about over-sleeping and apprehensive about using what felt like potentially risky machines.

The next morning, I rose at dawn and headed to report to the ECT suite. I had planned a little extra time to find it and be ready. When I arrived, the set of pale green cinder-block rooms was empty. The center treatment room was lit by dust-coated fluorescent bulbs, one of which flickered on and off from the ceiling. The stark light stung my eyes at that hour. Machines and equipment were stored on carts along the walls. The middle of the room was bare.

A nurse, Mary O'Connell, arrived a few moments later. After a cursory "good morning," she arranged IV lines on chrome hooks dangling down from long tracks on the ceiling. She rolled a metal cart, its red paint chipped, to the middle of the room. This crash cart, as it was called, was filled with vials of drugs and respirator equipment used both in procedures that required general anesthesia (in which someone is put to sleep) and in cardiopulmonary arrests, in which the heart or lungs have ceased to function and emergency efforts are made to re-suscitate the patient. Both uses might be called on here.

Tremulously, I opened the ECT manual to commit it further to memory, and to try to make it second-nature, but I was almost unable to concentrate.

An old medical adage concerning complicated procedures is "See one, do one, teach one." Mike Patterson, another resident on the twelfth floor, had just completed his ECT rotation and would be instructing me. A few minutes later he breezed in and set down his coffee on top of a metal box that sat on a shelf. He was tall, with wavy red hair, and hailed from Colorado. "This," he said, pointing to the box, "is the regular ECT machine. All you really have to do is press the button here."

He pointed to a small red plastic square. "Hold it down until you hear a click. Then let go."

"That's it?"

"That's all you have to do to zap them. And this," he said, laying his arm across the top of an adjacent electronic apparatus with fewer gadgets, housed in a square black plastic suitcase, "is the Black Box."

"The Black Box?"

"Yes. Use it when the standard machine won't deliver enough volts. For the regular machine, you look up on the chart how much to buzz the patient and then set the dials. But with the Black Box, you never know exactly how much current you're actually giving. The patient receives a shock for as long as your finger stays on the button." This procedure sounded imprecise and risky, even more frightening than the other ECT machine, which would at least tell me how *much* current was jolting her. Both these machines resembled nothing so much as instruments of torture. Yet Mike seemed to feel none of my skepticism or sense of oddity.

Mike turned around. "Where's the first patient?" he yelled.

A rust-colored curtain hung along one wall. Mary slid the drapery aside to reveal a small waiting room separated from the rest of the suite. On the wall hung a framed poster of a forest waterfall. A table lamp cast a golden circle onto a wooden desk. The little room seemed cozier than the rest of the suite. Mary wheeled a stretcher out of the antechamber. She stopped as she entered the treatment room and tucked her auburn hair into the sterile blue paper bonnet.

"Who's this?" Mike asked.

"Carmen García." Mary rolled her into the middle of the room. The patient, on hearing her name, propped herself up on her elbows.

"Please don't hurt me," Carmen pleaded in a Spanish accent. She was a buxom woman, nude except for a hospital gown that was snapped around her neck but flopped open in front to reveal her breasts. Mike motioned in the air for her to lie flat. "Don't," she cried. "Don't do this to me."

"Just lie down." She eased down onto the thin black cushion covering the stretcher. There was no pillow.

"Please!" she whimpered.

"The treatment's meant to help you," he assured her. "You signed the consent form last week agreeing to have it done." She peered up at him with big eyes, her eyebrows raised. I wondered if we would cancel the procedure. A central tenet of the Hippocratic Oath was "First, do no harm." This intervention seemed at least potentially harmful.

"You've been very depressed," Mike said, standing over her as he tilted his head to one side and raised one of his eyebrows to appeal to her. "This procedure is going to help you." He crossed his arms. She faced a room of health professionals, in whose hospital she was a patient. All of them spoke English better than she did.

Carmen's eyes moistened. She nodded slowly, then closed her eyes.

Dr. Samuel Dixon, the anesthesiologist, pierced her brown skin with an IV needle. "I'm just starting an IV to give you some fluid," he said, working quickly before she could change her mind. He turned to me. "We put patients to sleep," he explained as he injected a syringe of anesthetic into the IV tubing. "She also got Valium on the ward before being wheeled down here."

"Here's her chart," Mike called out, dropping a metal-bound loose-leaf notebook onto the windowsill. The dusty sill and the top of the standard ECT machine formed our desk area. A transistor radio on the shelf played a Top 40 FM station. Beside the radio stood an empty Almaden wine bottle serving as a vase. Two stalks of dried leaves, now sooty, tilted against the inside of the bottle's neck. Furry gray dust coated the brown glass. Behind the shelf a dirty window overlooked the hospital parking lot. Employees were beginning to drift into the building for the day. The sky looked overcast and chilly.

We were about to flick a switch, sending current into Carmen's brain, to force her to conform to our beliefs about how she should think and behave. It felt spooky just going along and not questioning this procedure. Yet, there had been no discussion of doing anything differently. No one had even said that this procedure might be disturbing. Often in my medical training thus far, I had had to do things that were unpleasant or frightening, like assisting at my first operation, opening up a patient's abdomen, or injecting toxic experimental chemotherapies into patients. But those activities were easier. Their mechanisms of action were better known. Even experimental chemotherapies were still "medicine." Electrical cardioversion—shooting a bolt of current through the heart to alter an irregular rhythm—also troubled me the first time I performed it, but it, too, made sense. Medical school had taught me how the heart muscle tensed and relaxed as a result of electrical charges, and thus pumped blood through the body.

But electrifying the brain felt different. Massive trauma to the brain appeared to erase certain beliefs and behaviors. In the past, insulin had been injected into patients to induce convulsions and coma, to try to relieve depression and delusions. But this practice was dangerous and eventually abandoned.

Electroshock probably worked in a similar manner, traumatizing the whole brain rather than localizing its effects more finely or precisely. The brain was both less mechanical and less replaceable than other organs. Although electrical activity sped through the brain and was detected on electroencephalograms—or EEGs—the function of this activity wasn't clear and was probably a by-product of small electrical discharges produced by individual cells. These charges, cumulatively producing wavelets, essentially constituted background noise, probably serving no other purpose in the nervous system as a whole. ECT, affecting the whole brain, seemed nonspecific and crude.

The human brain is a vastly complex machine. Every brain contains several billion neurons. Each neuron, or nerve cell, branches into thousands of dendrites, connecting to about one hundred thousand other neurons at individual synapses. At each synapse, thousands of receptors confront one other, sending and receiving chemical signals. What makes receptors produce delusions or pearls of wisdom is virtually unknown. Interventions in this system could be hazardous. There are as many neurons in one person's brain as there are people in the world and far more than there are telephones around the globe. To describe the daily events in one brain is in some ways analogous to deciphering everything that happens over the world's telephone lines in a twenty-four-hour period—understanding every phone call, all of the words spoken, all of the information passed, the decisions made, the arguments and agreements that occur in different voices and tongues—a massive cumulative amount of information or data in languages we don't always comprehend. Psychiatrists' claims to know the full effects of electrifying the whole brain seemed as precarious as predicting the results of knocking out the world's telephone lines for a day. Much would happen, but it would be hard to predict exactly what beforehand.

I thought back to slices of a brain I had seen in a medical school neuroanatomy class. To transform thought into matter seemed counterintuitive to me. Something as ephemeral, magical, and invisible as my very being, dreams, imagination, and experience of sublime moments was buried in these dappled gray lumps. In class, the brain—firm and weighty—had settled into my hand lifelessly. It resembled nothing so much as uncooked meat. The closest visual analogy to the human brain in daily life was probably a three-pound package of ground beef. Yet just as we don't imagine a live animal when we look at steak, I had difficulty conceiving of myself somehow being encoded in a pile of flesh such as that in my hand during the class. I resented the notion, though intellectually feeling it to be true. Posited at the core of all religions is something omnipresent, transcendent beyond our flesh, separating the soul from the body. The ability or inability to embrace something more than mere physical matter distinguishes believers from nonbelievers, atheists from the faithful—these differences all stemming from the disconnection between that mound of flesh in my hand and the notion of mind.

I wouldn't ever want my brain "buzzed," as Mike called the process. It represents an ultimate loss of control. ECT resets the brain to erase behavior and speech that a patient, a family member, or a psychiatrist deems undesirable. The brain coordinates many functions. My hand now scrawls across a page, jiggling a pen in my fingers and producing words recognized by the eyes and brains of readers. I was wary of electrically resetting the brain of another person through a procedure that remains poorly understood.

Damage to the brain is more troubling than damage to the liver, for example. Killing a few extra liver cells by accident doesn't matter as much. Some organs are more homogenous and now even transplantable, replaceable. But not the brain.

Mike flipped through Carmen García's chart. "You look up how much of a shock she got last time," he said. Her chart was a fat loose-leaf notebook containing all of the hospital's information about her in notes scrawled in different handwritings, some more legible than others. As Mike flipped through these fragmentary descriptions, a portrait of Carmen García emerged. Her husband had brought her into the hospital three weeks before, after she was still depressed and delusional despite treatment with medications. She had trouble eating and sleeping.

"Last time she had a good seizure," Mike concluded, "receiving one point five volts"—actually millivolts, but in the ECT suite we called them volts—"for a duration of one point

two five seconds. We'll just repeat those settings." He fiddled
with the dials on the box. "Put a blood pressure cuff around
her right calf," he ordered, "and check her Babinskis." I
wrapped the cuff around her leg and pulled a reflex hammer
from the pocket of my white coat. When I scratched the metal
point on the bottom of her right foot, along the outside of her
sole, her toes crunched downward, away from her head, meaning that her Babinski reflexes were normal, that her foot and
leg weren't paralyzed. Later, if her toes didn't move, it would
indicate that her leg was sufficiently paralyzed from anesthetic.

Mary squeezed a toothpaste tube, forcing a swirl of oyster-
white cream to snake out. She smeared this paste on the sides
of the patient's skull, coating her temples. By now Carmen was
drowsy from the drugs. Mary wiped off her fingers on a Kleenex and then swung a rubber headband around Carmen's scalp,
wrapping the strap around Carmen's trimmed hair. Adhered to
the rubber strip were two metal discs that Mary positioned
over the patches of paste.

Mary stuck electrodes into the two discs on either side. The
metal plugs looked as though they were being inserted into
Carmen's temples, as if the stainless steel nubs were being fit-
ted into sockets buried in her brain. Sam pushed on a second
syringe marked with a pink sticker that read "Succinylcholine," a muscle relaxant. Carmen's eyes shut. Her muscles
shivered a few times, wavering like the fine movements of a
bird, then flopped flaccidly. She was unconscious. I retested
her reflexes. On the left, her toes were indeed paralyzed. On
the right, where the blood pressure cuff had cut off her circu-
lation and occluded the drug from flowing down her leg, her
toes still flexed, unaffected by the muscle relaxant. Her body
was anesthetized, except for her right foot and calf. During the
seizure induced by ECT, her body would be motionless except
for her right foot, which, undulled by the drugs, would respond
to the current by vibrating—the only visible sign of the electricity blasting through her skull.

Sam nuzzled a tube down her mouth. Though unconscious,
she rocked her head back and forth to resist being muzzled by
the oxygen mask, as if shaking her head to say no.

"Nice deep breaths now," he said to her, though she was
somnolent. He looked up at us and nodded. The transistor radio played in the background.

Mike pushed the button.

A few moments later, Carmen's right toes crunched up, the

big one squeezing down on her tensed foot, in so-called tonic rigidity. Then her foot began to shake, entering a period of clonic jerking. This rhythm spread, her entire right leg soon rattling back and forth—almost in time to the music on the radio. Her foot fanned the air, flapping from side to side. My gaze was fixed intently on her helpless, rocking appendage.

Gradually, her limb beat more slowly. Her foot stilled. Her ankle quivered and twitched a few final times. Her foot then stopped and plopped, exhausted, to one side.

"Not bad!" Mike announced, interrupting my train of thought. "Twenty-six seconds." He had timed the seizure on his plastic digital watch. He pressed another, smaller lever on the machine, and a narrow strip of graph paper automatically spewed out of the contraption with a hum. He ripped the paper off its spool. "The bumpy line here means she's having an electrical seizure," he said pointing to the paper, etched with a green grid. "First you add up the number of boxes. Each box is one second of an electrical seizure." He reeled the strip of paper through his fingers, tabulating the number of squares. "Twenty-nine seconds recorded. Not bad at all. We won't have to zap her again. Sometimes the motor seizure—what you see in her foot—and the electrical seizure—what the machine measures—vary." The electrical waves in her head may begin or end a little before or after the movement in her foot. The electrical seizure lasts as long as the recorded electrical waves, the motor seizure continues for however long her foot actually shakes. "Sometimes neither is long enough."

"What do you mean, long enough?" I asked, disturbed by his matter-of-factness.

"Oh, at least twenty seconds. Twenty to twenty-five. If it's much less than that, it doesn't count and you have to do it again."

He picked up a wide rubber stamp, pounded it against a dried ink pad, and thumped it onto Carmen's chart. He filled in the blanks now printed—the settings of the electricity and, most important for treatment, the length of her electrical and motor seizures. Her experience was essentially recorded in those two numbers: 26 and 29. As a result of them, she would be zonked out for several days, too forgetful for anyone to talk to her about her problems.

"What do you think of this?" I asked Mike.

"How do you mean?"

"It isn't very . . . pleasant," I mumbled quietly, while Sam was busy adjusting the oxygen tank.

"The hospital calls it a service responsibility," he said. "You know what that means, don't you? We're basically cheap labor."

"But this seems pretty barbaric."

"It's a crude science, but hey, it works." He appeared fully prepared to follow the profession's dictates. This procedure was just a job to him, simple and straightforward, something to get through. He avoided troubling questions raised along the way. I was astonished that neither he nor other residents had expressed any doubts. I couldn't quite shake the sensation that this procedure was reminiscent of those that took place in the dark cellars of eighteenth-century insane asylums. I would soon hear residents occasionally complain, "I have to do ECT this week." The common objection, however, was that they had to perform the procedure in addition to, and not instead of, their other clinical duties, lengthening their workday by several hours. Other tasks still had to be performed; meetings still had to be attended. In short, the common complaint about ECT was that it meant extra work. But the emotional burden was never publicly admitted or discussed. No one had even suggested, "You may find this upsetting," or that it was odd that we administered a treatment that had been so controversial in the past.

The procedure forced us to take a more hardened stance toward our work. My job was now only to press a button and then observe how many seconds a seizure lasted, as measured both by the rocking of a foot and by the number of boxes the machine's inked needle zigzagged across. These tasks could be performed by a trained nurse but were assigned legally only to a physician. Before starting residency I hadn't envisioned my job as using potentially dangerous treatments on patients whom I had never before met. I trusted the treatment, to the degree that I did, because of Henry Nolan's sheaf of academic papers and his recommendation. But I felt distanced from the experience, going through the motions like an automaton. Residents who requested in previous years that the hospital hire a faculty member to perform this task had been turned down repeatedly, purportedly because the hospital wanted to provide trainees with the opportunity to perform the procedure, though residents insisted it was merely to save money.

Carmen began to rouse. Still unconscious, she thrashed

about. Her body started to flop toward the edge of the narrow portable stretcher.

"Get back in bed," Mike scolded, though she was still stuporous. "Come on now." He heaved her back onto the stretcher and hoisted up the guardrail. Mike motioned for Mary and me to help hold her down. I pressed against her soft, slender arm. My other hand held her warm leg through the rough bed sheets.

"Don't worry," Mike said, his muscular arms straining to press Carmen's limbs onto the stretcher. "They're not all this bad."

Eventually Carmen calmed down. I wandered over to her a few minutes later. "How are you doing?" I asked, trying to smile.

She nodded and tried to smile back. I patted her arm. Then she was wheeled away.

"You do the next one," Mike told me. "Roll her in," he shouted to Mary.

Mary flung aside the waiting-room curtain and pushed a stretcher toward the middle of the room. On it lay Helen Beckett. Mary rolled her into the ECT suite. "My God, Doctor, it's you," Helen declared. "Dr. Shock!"

"Hello." My throat was suddenly dry.

"How long is this going to take?" she asked me. "It better not be long."

"Just a few minutes." Sam pricked her skin to start an IV line.

"Ooh! You hurt me," she said, swinging her head around. "It's already starting. Is that the beginning of my treatment?"

"No, we're just setting things up," I said. I placed the blood pressure cuff on her leg, and pumped up the rubber ball, the size of a plum tomato, in my sweaty palm.

"Ouch! So tight?" Helen raised her head to look down at it.

"I'm sorry. I have to." I was surprised how little air flowed through my mouth.

"You *shockiatrists* better know what you're doing!"

Mary quickly applied the pearly paste to Helen's temples, swung the rubber strap over the cream, and inserted the electrodes. Sam injected the first anesthetic into Helen's IV tube. "You're going to be going for a nice plane ride now," he told her. "If you want more, come back Wednesday." Her eyes fluttered shut.

"What are you giving her?"

"A little sodium Nembutal. She may need something longer-acting though. We'll see."

"EEE ..." Helen moaned. "OOOO ... AHHHHGGG ..." Her head writhed back and forth.

"I guess she wants more," he muttered to himself.

He pierced the IV tubing with a second syringe and squirted in another medication. She stilled. He shoved a special straw up her nostril. She wrestled, though drugged. She now resembled a surgical patient on whom we were about to operate. Her body lay before us as we poked and injected it. Her personality had been cleared away. Only the automatic, so-called lower regions of her brain functioned. We were acting on her body but not on "her."

"You have to figure out how much current to give," Mike said. I looked on a Xeroxed table Scotch-taped to the wall, listing the appropriate settings for patients' weights and genders. I flipped the two dials counterclockwise as far as they would go to the zero or off positions. I pushed them hard into these notches. The voltage knob didn't align precisely with the calibrations on the box but sat to the right of each printed number. The machine had probably been repaired once, the cover removed and then replaced, shifting it over by one-half centimeter in the process. Though it didn't make much of a difference overall, the dial now sat between individual calibrations rather than pointing exactly at any one marking on the box. I carefully counted the number of notches the knob had to turn, and flicked it, listening carefully for each click. Carmen García had been easier to treat since I had never met her before. I was much more connected to Helen and knew her as a person—afraid and here partly as a result of coercion. I knew intellectually that this procedure was supposed to benefit her, but I was still scared.

Helen Beckett had refused to give up her beliefs. I was electrically taking them away. The notion haunted me that in a few decades ECT might be remembered as a peculiar and primitive relic. When I worked in Papua New Guinea, several people, called "longlong," were psychotic. Men who were longlong violated taboos, picking and eating crops that ordinarily only women were allowed to touch and dressing as only women were permitted. The tribe used neither drugs nor ECT. Extended families cared for these tribesmen. In that culture, the "mad" were allowed to be free.

Sam injected the succinylcholine. When Helen's left foot

was paralyzed, his large gloved hand covered her nose and mouth with a black oxygen mask. "Looks like she's ready," he announced. "Are you guys all set?" Helen appeared asleep.

"Okay, press the button," Mike said to me.

"I do it?" I asked, surprised. "Already?" I glanced at the knobs to make sure they were correctly set.

"Hurry up. Push it," Mike urged beside me. "The drugs might start to wear off."

I reached up toward the machine, aiming at the small red button. My finger squeezed the smooth, well-worn plastic square. "Chugachugachugaclick," the machine rumbled. I let go, too stunned and uncertain to move. The cinder-block room suddenly seemed colder. The equipment and other people in the suite seemed far outside me. My heart pounded. I didn't know what would happen next, but there was no way to turn back. I felt at a loss, watching. Seconds passed that dragged on like minutes. The second hand on my wristwatch ticked, but everything else remained quiet, motionless.

Then, her big toe curled. Her right ankle bent toward her left, stiffly, and then started vibrating. The seizure had started. Her foot rocked, then gradually stilled. The hand on my wristwatch had pushed through twenty-five seconds. I tore off the long strip of graph paper from the machine and tallied the number of boxes.

"Mrs. Beckett?" Sam shouted. Her head lolled from side to side. She didn't respond. "Helen, Helen . . ." he repeated.

"What?" she finally replied. She was still alive. He exhaled in relief and smiled but didn't speak. I sighed as well.

Mary placed her hand on Helen's forehead. "Helen, do you know where you are?"

"What?"

"Do you remember my name?"

"No."

"I'm Mary," she said softly, leaning over and brushing away Helen's bangs.

"Mary," Helen whispered back weakly. Mary squeezed her hand gently, and Helen tightened her fingers around Mary's. Mary unhooked the IV and trundled Helen out of the room, back to the twelfth floor.

I administered ECT to three more patients, then wandered back up to the floor myself to start my day on the ward.

Over the ensuing weeks, Helen received a total of nine additional treatments—three a week. On those days she was tired and subdued, slept until the early afternoon, and spent much of her time in bed. She became mildly forgetful, too—an expected, short-lived side effect—but also less tense, suspicious, and depressed.

Slowly, her amnesia resolved. She began to attend senior adult group, life skills group, and dancercize. She wrote out a list of errands she had to do before going home. I was amazed. Despite my initial qualms, ECT had dramatically helped her, with no residual side effects. I now appreciated the treatment's potential power and saw that I had been holding the prejudices of a layman, and had a lot of practical knowledge and experience to gain.

A few days later, on a sunny afternoon, Carol took Helen on a stroll to a small park across the street from the hospital. "It's the best thing I've done since being here," Helen told me afterward. Helen hadn't been outside in weeks but was still only able to leave the hospital under someone else's care because her gait was still precarious from the ECT. Carol and the other nurses were usually busy, however.

I mentioned to Steve Kasdin that I thought of taking Helen out for a walk as well, during one of our sessions.

He peered at me askance. "I suppose that would be all right," he said, with hesitation. "Provided she doesn't see it as constituting a date."

"A date?"

"Yes. You're a younger man. She's an older woman. Even geriatric patients have sexual fantasies, and she might interpret your invitation romantically."

"But all I want to do is take her for a walk. She's been cooped up here for weeks."

"Well, with patients it could upset the relationship, the transference," he said. "But I suppose you can risk it if you want." Transference was the Freudian notion that a patient transfers feelings about parents and other significant figures in his life onto his therapist. Transference occurred, and needed to be noted, and was used extensively in certain types of treatment, notably psychoanalysis, where it was a central aspect of the therapy. But Kasdin's application here of this psychoanalytic principle seemed extreme. I was doing something humane for her. She had been confined in the building and prior to that hadn't left her apartment for weeks. Yet to Kasdin nothing was innocent or straightforward. He followed his theories, while I felt most concerned about her at a basic human level. His comment seemed even more inappropriate, as her problem had most recently been basic cognitive and motor difficulties impairing her ability to walk by herself, not emotional issues.

The next day she and I stepped outside into a pool of sunlight. We walked to the edge of the hospital driveway and back. "I'm so happy you took me outside, Dr. Klitzman," she said as we got out of the elevator and back onto the ward. "It makes me feel like a normal human being again."

Later that day she telephoned a woman from her neighborhood beauty parlor who came to visit her and did her hair and nails.

A few days later when I walked into Helen's room, instead of lying in bed she was standing up before the small green ceramic sink in her room, combing her recently dyed chestnut hair in the mirror. Decorating her room now were silver-framed photos of her late husband and herself that her brother had recently brought from home.

"Do you remember those thoughts you had in the past about being poisoned?" I asked her.

"Being poisoned . . ." she repeated vaguely, as if questioning herself, trying to recollect. "Not really. I think I was pretty confused when I came in here." She seemed a different person. Her depression and suspicion had astonishingly vanished. The fact that ECT's mechanism was still largely unknown left me apprehensive, but I was nevertheless grateful and relieved. Though I had to force myself to give her ECT and overcome my reluctance to do what was unpleasant and potentially harmful to her, she had benefited from the treatment. Until then, I had assumed that the act of helping patients would in itself feel positive and affirming. But now I realized that treatment could require blind leaps of faith and be painful to both patients and me. Biological treatments might work despite how little we knew about the brain, how disturbing they could be to administer, and how much they distanced me from the patient. ECT forced me to treat patients as less than individual human beings, and more mechanistically, as if they were purely biological entities, lacking choice or free will, and were almost animal or machinelike. But the treatment could work. My personal expectations about a treatment could prove wrong, and the results of psychiatric interventions would not always be easy to predict.

Helen placed her hairbrush down on her bureau. "I don't remember what came over me there or what happened," she said. "But I feel like a different girl."

"You look much better."

She smiled. "Thank you," she said proudly, taking my comment as a compliment, as if for her own role in her improvement. She glanced at herself in the mirror. Her smile widened. "Thank you."

No-no's

With Helen I saw that biological interventions could work, but I was soon learning about psychological approaches to mental illness, as well. The field of psychiatry consisted of two major areas. Biological psychiatry focused on understandings of biological processes in the brain and the use of biological treatments such as drugs and ECT. Alternatively, psychological approaches concentrated on the mind, and the use of treatments such as psychoanalysis and other types of psychotherapy. Each of these two camps within the profession was represented by faculty members who taught us their respective areas of specialty, with no faculty member having equal expertise in both. To sort through and integrate these often contrasting viewpoints, we would in many ways be left on our own.

Initially, psychological tools and strategies were taught in lectures and seminars. The first such seminar was from the unit chief, Steve Kasdin, who as a psychoanalyst was an expert in psychological approaches and in conducting psychotherapy.

"How," Kasdin asked, standing in front of the room at the end of a long conference table one day over lunch, "should you start a session with a patient?"

I looked at Anne, who didn't know how to respond either. I had assumed you just began and got the information you needed, or said things you had to say. In my initial interactions with Helen, for example, we had just started talking. I already had been told to go conduct psychotherapy with patients, and it was assumed that I would know how to. This class, now starting, would meet once a week for an hour and teach specific principles and techniques. In medical school, psychotherapy had been discussed very cursorily, and we had not used it there in any ongoing way. I had never been in psychotherapy myself, and though I had seen my share of Woody Allen films and *New Yorker* cartoons, I didn't know how to effect transformation on the deepest levels. For me, therapy was still shrouded in mystery. I hadn't thought much about how the specific mechanics of psychotherapy actually worked.

No one in the class responded to Kasdin's question. A few moments passed.

"Don't you start by asking them their name?" Mike finally blurted out, easing the tension.

"Presumably you know that already. You've been assigned the person as a patient. You've gone out to the lounge to bring them into your office and you've probably asked, 'Mr. Smith?' Now you have the patient in your office. What do you say to start the session?"

"How about asking them how they're doing today?" Anne suggested.

Kasdin shook his head. "That's okay if you're at a country club or a social gathering. That's what you'd say to a friend. But what you say now is going to set the tone for the therapy. The patient hasn't come to your office for a social occasion. He or she expects more from you. If he wanted a polite conversation, he would have gone elsewhere and not come here, having to pay you."

"How about letting the patient start?" Sarah Gould, another resident on my floor, asked.

"That can be awkward. The patient's looking to you to say something."

"We give up," I said. "What should we say?"

"I like to start by saying, 'So . . .' " He gestured, spreading out his hand toward the chair across from him where Anne was sitting. "That way you let them start where they want, and you can hear what they're thinking or feeling without prejudicing them or framing their comments too much." We all nodded, surprised but impressed by the simplicity of his comment.

"A second major issue you will face," Kasdin continued, "is what to call patients. Any ideas?"

"By their names?" Mike suggested jokingly. We all laughed, relieving more of the pressure in the room.

"By their first names or their last names?" None of us answered. Whatever we said would probably be wrong. "What do you do with a patient who says, 'Call me Joe—everybody calls me Joe'?"

No one spoke. "Go ahead," Mike suggested, "and call him Joe?"

"But it might be his wish not to be a patient," Kasdin explained.

Sarah Gould twisted in her seat. "But I may feel more comfortable calling some patients—especially kids—by their first names." She was planning to enter child psychiatry. "No one may have ever called them Miss or Mr."

"You have to make a decision," Kasdin replied. "But you must preserve the most professional dignity and distance you can! That's what's critical. You can call a patient by their first name, but you should consciously decide that's what you want to do. It can be good or destructive for the transference. What patients call you is important. You have to refer to them the same way they refer to you. If you expect them to call you Doctor, you should show them similar respect and call them Mr., Mrs., or Ms. If you call them by their first names," he said, shaking his head as if disapproving of the idea, "they can call you by your first name back." As medical interns, we had treated patients more informally. We had often called patients by their first names, while patients had called us Doctor.

"But what if the patient is our own age?" Sarah asked. "Some could be our friends if we met them on the outside."

"You have to decide. I would still have them call you Doctor and you call them Mr. or Ms."

"But that feels so strained and shrinky." She scrunched up her nose.

"It doesn't matter. You'll always have patients who are your own age, even when you're in your fifties as I am. You have to get used to being separated by a professional distance from your contemporaries. That's part of learning to be a psychiatrist—realizing that you're different from other people in other fields." Sitting there, I didn't like the implication that we needed somehow to separate ourselves.

"I also have a policy about shaking hands," he continued. "I do it at the first session as a peace gesture. But not after that."

"What do you do if a patient wants to shake your hand at

another time?" Mike asked. "And he thinks you're being rude if you don't."

"I point out to him, 'So, you seem to want to shake my hand a lot.' You try to understand why he does it. Everything you do with a patient has meaning and will be interpreted by them on all kinds of levels. Remember: the relationship that they build with you in their heads—the transference—can be very powerful. Never underestimate it. Patients fantasize all kinds of crazy notions about you. You'd be surprised."

"But people shake hands all the time outside the hospital," Mike said.

"You can do that here, too," Kasdin went on. "But don't miss its significance. That's the important thing." I was not used to being this self-conscious and scrutinizing of my inter-actions. I preferred being more spontaneous with people and expressing what felt right, based on my experience and general intuition. It seemed that I would have to change how I acted with people, that in basic fundamental ways I couldn't just be myself.

"What about if a patient wants to have sex with you?" Kasdin continued. Anne chuckled softly. "What's so funny?" he asked her.

"I know someone who just started on the borderline person-ality disorder unit at another hospital," she said. "When he mentioned to the unit chief that he was a little nervous, he was told, 'Don't worry, if you can keep your bottom on your chair, keep your clothes on, and keep your hands to yourself, you're doing better than ninety percent of your colleagues.' "

"This is the one no-no," Kasdin said. "You can shake hands if you have to and call patients by their first name, but don't get involved with them. It'll get you into real trouble.

"When you start treating a patient," he continued, "use the model of a blind date and try to find out as much as you can about the person. Chances are that will not be easy. The patient will try to conceal his symptoms and minimize his patholo-gy—that's his job. Your job is to uncover what's wrong with him. Things will get sticky as you encounter resistance and as transference develops. Patients will try to entangle you in all kinds of things. It's important to stay light on your feet.

"In talking to patients, you need to bear in mind several things. You need to pay attention not only to the content of what patients say but to the process as well. When patients talk about the past, you need to think about the present. When patients focus on the present, you need to think about the past."

Psychiatry, and particularly the practice of psychotherapy, seemed to offer new insights and ways of thinking about and interpreting interactions with people. My intuitive sense seemed correct that this field would be interesting. The kinds of questions that had drawn me into this career were, in fact, studied, and would be important.

But I would have to develop a different way of interacting with people, avoiding some approaches and learning others, almost as if playing a role on a stage.

"None of your interactions," Kasdin concluded, "can be taken for granted. You can't treat patients as you would other people. At all times you have to watch what you say and do."

The Treatment of Choice

Though I had seen how biological treatments could be effective, despite my initial doubts, and was now learning more about psychological approaches, the path to take with patients still wasn't always clear. Different supervisors sometimes offered conflicting strategies for a particular patient, and I would have to figure out which approach to adopt. Patients benefited to varying degrees and often in unexpected ways.

Nancy Steele was admitted late one afternoon in early August, shortly after Helen Beckett went home.

"This morning I woke up jittery," she told me when we met in my office. "I don't know why. But today's when I usually go see George—that's my shrink. Dr. George Cameron. He went away for the rest of the month. Before he left, he made me talk about his vacation till I was blue in the face, and I thought I'd be fine. But this morning, I don't know what came over me. It just hit me. My mind was all jumbled, and I couldn't control myself. That's when I did it."

"Did what?"

"I took some pills. Aspirin. Then I called my internist and he had me come here." She glanced around my office. "I just couldn't control myself and fucked up again. I can't believe it." She started to cry.

After drying her eyes she told me about her past. She had grown up in Cleveland as an only child. Her mother had died of cancer when Nancy was eight, and her father remarried, though Nancy never got along with her stepmother. "My dad's a radiologist, and I think he's an alcoholic, though he says he's only a social drinker."

Nancy had finished two years at a community college in Southern California and had worked for a while in different jobs to support herself—as a graphic artist, a makeup artist, a freelance fashion designer, a waitress. "But my real love is painting. Mostly watercolors, but some oils. I like painting flowers and birds. I would love to support myself doing that but I can't. As it is, my father has had to bail me out financially a couple of times." Still, she had managed to exhibit her work several times at a gallery downtown.

I liked the arts, and several of my friends were artists and writers. I knew how hard it was to support oneself in these endeavors—the sacrifice required and the elusiveness of success. "We artists are a depressed bunch," Nancy went on. She told me about her favorite artists, some of whom I liked as well.

"I started seeing George Cameron several years ago," she said. "He helped me put my life back together. I had just broken up with my last boyfriend; George got me to stop drinking and using drugs. I was in pretty bad shape in the past. I even had a few ODs back then. But George helped me. Only now, every time he goes away, I fall apart again. Last year the same thing happened, and I got admitted to the hospital then, too. This time we talked about it for months. But look what happened! Doctor," she said, sniffling, leaning forward in her seat, "please try to help me."

Nancy was tall and attractive, with long black hair and bright green eyes, and she spoke with a quick, crisp voice. She wore a black cotton blouse with a pair of blue jeans and white tennis shoes. I could imagine seeing her in a downtown club or at an art opening. She seemed brighter, more articulate and thoughtful, and less disturbed in some ways than my other patients, and interested in exploring and trying to understand her life and the problems she faced. She was closer to the kind of patient I imagined treating in psychiatry, someone whom talking and verbal skills could help. It was exciting to have a patient who seemed similar in some ways to friends and acquaintances, and I looked forward to working with her.

I glanced at my watch and realized that I had another meeting. "We're going to have to stop in a moment," I said cautiously. "But I'll come back and talk to you later."

"You're not going to leave me too now, are you?"

I could stay with her longer and miss my meeting—which had started a few minutes ago, anyway. But Kasdin had told me that an important principle was sticking to time limits and not extending them. I needed to bring closure to the session now. Another forty-five minutes might not alter her situation very much. "I think it's a good idea that you came here. We can see what we can do to help." My voice sounded distanced and professional, but I had to leave. "Don't worry," I added. "I'll be back soon."

Later that day, Kasdin met with me for supervision. His office was a long narrow room furnished in various shades of beige—light beige walls, a tan sofa, café-au-lait leather chairs in the corners, and matching lampshades. The lamps, set on low tables in all four corners, cast dim yellow light. Higher up, the room was dark. When I stood up, I was out of the lit area and plunged into shadows, which disconcerted me. The monochrome felt confining, like being stuck in a cave. Above his sofa hung a huge framed poster of a chess game in progress. The board was shown set up before a half-opened window. On the left side, a woman's arm stretched out toward one of the pieces. I couldn't tell if she was about to move the piece or had just done so. On the right side, a cat sat watching, brooding. The woman's opponent was unseen. Along the wall were old photos, the figures grainy.

"What do you make of your new patient?" he asked me.

"I just met her. Let me get out my notes," I said, reaching for my clipboard.

"No." He smiled. "Don't. I don't want you to."

"What?" I then had five patients, including two new ones admitted in the past twenty-four hours. Fragments and details of what they each said had blended together in my mind. I had made notes to myself to keep them all organized and distinct.

"I want to hear whatever comes into your head spontaneously about her," he said. "Tell me your immediate impressions. Don't read from your notes."

"I might leave things out."

"But your impressions and what you remember or forget are all significant data. That's what's important." This approach seemed at odds with a scientific method, but I went ahead anyway.

"She seems very upset about what's happened," I began.

"Go on."

"She's had it hard for several years," I relayed some of what she told me.

He was silent. I tried to see his eyes, to read them as I spoke to see if I was on the right track, but he sat stone-faced, his large round glasses reflecting back the few dim lights in the room and obscuring his eyes. His silence unsettled me, compelling me to keep chatting away to fill the void. I would have appreciated his feedback as to whether my impressions were appropriate or relevant, but I realized that his technique was psychoanalytically based.

"Right," I said. "Well, she's pretty upset about his leaving. I kind of felt bad for her." That sounded too personal and unprofessional—too revealing of my own feelings toward her. He twirled a lock of hair that protruded from the back of his head as I spoke but said nothing. "She seems likable," I added.

"Be careful!" he suddenly proclaimed. He pointed his finger at my chest. "She *wants* you to like her. Remember that you're entering a unique phase of therapy right now: the honeymoon phase. You want to engage her in treatment; she wants you to help her. You should show her that you're interested in exploring her life with her. When she opens something up, you can say, 'Tell me more about that.' " He lifted his hand and held it out. "Or, 'How do you understand that?' " He glided his other hand to the left. "Make her curious about how and why she does things." He made it sound easy and leisurely. "But watch out."

"How come?"

"She may try to seduce you." I looked at his sixty-year-old balding head. The gray hair on the sides was long and a few strands were brushed over the top of his scalp. His comment surprised me.

"Seduce me?"

"She's going to try to hook on to you and to get under your skin. I once had a supervisor who used to say that 'Everything in therapy is really about sex except sex, which is about aggression.' " I smiled but was puzzled. I couldn't tell how wholeheartedly he accepted this proposition. He didn't give any indication as to how much he believed it, but I suspected he thought there was some truth to it and that he was being at least partly serious. Yet his comment sounded too pat, as well as overly reductionistic—almost a parody of a psychoanalyst. I assumed Nancy Steele was primarily seeking help, as medical patients had the previous year during my medical internship. She presumably saw me as her physician, not as a potential sexual partner. I didn't think of my treatment of patients as based on sexual thoughts.

"She's probably a borderline," he continued, meaning that she had a borderline personality disorder. This term refers to a pattern in which the patient often feels empty and bored, confused about his or her identity, acts impulsively, and makes recurrent suicidal gestures.

The category is a murky one. For years, it was thought that there were patients who were on the borderline between psychosis and neurosis, who responded with irrational and impulsive behavior to stresses around them, but who generally did not have a thought disorder (e.g., with delusions or loosening of associations—symptoms found in schizophrenia). Researchers have more recently redefined the diagnosis of borderline personality disorder by the series of symptoms displayed. Psychoanalysts have tried conceptualizing borderline personality in their own terms, emphasizing the emotional emptiness felt by these patients. The patients themselves are overwhelmingly women being treated by male psychiatrists, and the treatments available have always been, at best, of only minimal efficacy. The treatments provided should theoretically work, but often have problems. Feminists have questioned whether the category represents, at least in part, an aspect of female psychology and behavior exacerbated and pathologized by the male-dominated medical world.

"We used to admit patients like this to the hospital automatically whenever their therapists went away for a month of vacation in August," Kasdin now told me. "Today, we don't do that, but she probably would have fit into that category." He smiled. His thin lips stretched briefly, their edges pulled apart, a polite but ingenuous smile, as if to indicate that he recognized that this practice of confining people in hospitals was now widely seen as an inefficient use of medical resources, and perhaps as unnecessarily restrictive. Yet he appeared to miss that lost time from the past, when higher-functioning patients were treated here in the hospital. He seemed to feel that nothing was wrong with it. Though psychiatry continually altered its practices, he maintained an air of confidence about his current opinions. He seemed to believe that his approaches at any one time were correct.

"Managing a borderline patient is still difficult though," he added. His term, "managing," sounded more applicable to a business than to a patient. "With borderlines it's important to start and stop exactly on time. If you begin late or cut them short you'll never hear the end of it. They'll look for things to be mad at you about. Don't give them any ammunition. Don't give them anything about which they can complain or feel gypped."

He suddenly peered over my head. I turned around and saw a large clock hanging over my chair: visible to him but not to the sitter, presumably usually a patient. "Our time is up," he announced. "But be on the lookout." I wandered out of his office, alone.

That afternoon, I met with Nancy again and heard more about her life. She still seemed reasonably pleasant and not as threatening as Dr. Kasdin had implied.

The next day, I met with Henry Nolan in his stark white office. While Kasdin was a psychoanalyst, Nolan, a psychopharmacologist, specialized in psychiatric drugs. "Interesting new patient you've got there," he said when we sat down. "What do you think of her?"

"She seems borderline and depressed."

"Does she meet the necessary five out of nine criteria needed to make a diagnosis of depression?" He bounced the tips of his fingers together.

"I'm not sure."

"Let's see," he said. He pulled out the top drawer of his desk. The wooden drawer was barren except for a single, well-worn paperback book and a sharpened yellow pencil with a squared, unused eraser. He removed the book, the *Diagnostic and Statistical Manual III—Revised*. "She needs to meet five of the following criteria to be diagnosed with major depression. Has she felt depressed most days, most of the time on those days, for a period of fourteen or more days?"

"I think so." I didn't know exactly how many days it had been.

He then asked separately about her appetite, her weight, her energy, her sleep patterns, her concentration, her thoughts about death, and whether she had apathy, or feelings of worthlessness or guilt almost daily.

"I'll have to check," I answered to several of these questions.

He snapped the book shut and held it aloft between us. "We do not yet have the data we need," he declared, emphasizing each word, one at a time, by shaking the book up and down as he said them. "She is required to have five of these nine criteria to be diagnosed as depressed."

"She says she's depressed."

"That's not enough for a diagnosis."

"She looks kind of depressed, too."

"Lots of people say they're depressed, but if she doesn't meet these criteria, we don't have target symptoms to follow for marking her progress. And if we don't, it's not worth treating her." I assumed he meant with medications. "Remember always to DSM-III-R your patients in the beginning," that is, to diagnose them according to the categories in this manual.

His stance toward Nancy seemed mechanical and not very compassionate or sympathetic. His checklists of symptoms and categories seemed too rigid, simple, and reductive, and much different from Kasdin's approach. The contents of her thoughts and feelings, and the details of her life didn't seem to matter to Nolan. It wasn't critical what she was depressed *about*. The mere fact of her being depressed was what concerned him. He was an expert, though. Maybe I was naive in thinking that other aspects in her life were important besides the answers to the yes-or-no questions on his list.

The next day I asked her about these various symptoms. She did not meet the criteria for major depression, though she met the milder criteria for chronic depression or dysthymia. "How are things on the ward going?" I asked her.

"Okay. I've been hanging out with other patients. Last night a bunch of us were bored so we sat around and talked about each other's suicide attempts."

"You talked about each other's suicide attempts?" I asked, amazed.

"Sure. All you doctors had gone home, and there was nothing else to do. What were we going to talk about? We don't have much else in common."

Afterward I ran into Nolan and told him what I had found out about Nancy's symptoms. "An antidepressant trial might benefit her dysthymia," he said, "though the research on this is new and hasn't yet been put into wide practice. I'd treat her, though. She probably has an underlying biological diathesis."

"What does that mean?"

"There's probably a biological origin to her problem. We don't know what exactly. We can only guess; probably a deficiency of serotonin receptors." Our knowledge was scant, yet he attributed her malaise to a tangible, biological cause. He might, in the end, be right. But he was merely speculating. Still, I prescribed nortriptyline, a standard antidepressant.

For my next meeting with Nancy, I was unavoidably delayed by several minutes. "I'm sorry, I had to take care of a problem that came up," I told her.

"Are we going to have less time now?" I was surprised that it meant so much to her. It was only a few minutes, and we were meeting three times a week.

"We'll be able to make it up." We began to talk when my telephone started ringing. "Just a moment," I said, reaching for the receiver.

"Don't you have an answering machine? Do you have to answer it? I see you so rarely and I need your help." I took a deep breath. The ringing continued noisily, disturbing me. Finally, I picked up the receiver and spoke briefly. She looked peeved.

"That seemed to bother you a lot," I said after hanging up, sounding like a shrink.

"You're my doctor. I don't want you tending to other people's business when you're supposed to be helping me. I need your help!"

"I have other patients, too, though." I felt she had put me on the defensive.

"But right now I'm here in your office, and you're supposed to be helping me. I don't even know if there's anything you can do for me here. Maybe it was a mistake coming here. Nothing's ever going to help me."

"People often get hopeless when they're depressed." I had once heard Kasdin make this comment. It sounded accurate, but came out as formulaic.

She shook her head. "It would be better if I just ended it all."

"How come?"

"I feel shitty all the time."

"Do you think you might do anything?" This was a standard question that had to be asked in these situations.

"I have razors."

"What does that mean?"

"Maybe I'll use them. I'm so unhappy."

I didn't like this suddenly dark situation. Suicide attempts are difficult to predict. Lawyers and the press act as though psychiatrists can accurately foresee suicide and homicide—a belief that has given the profession a niche in the legal system. But psychiatrists have no sure formula for divining people's future actions. I can make educated guesses, based on a patient's history and on common sense. But often, the only evidence available is what patients are willing to admit. A patient may state that he wants to hurt himself or someone else. The risks of predicting incorrectly and not intervening with a patient who then injures himself weighed heavily on my mind.

"Do you think you will do anything?"

"I just get so confused." She looked down at her lap. She seemed genuinely distressed and had said she had attempted to harm herself recently at home.

"Would you be able to come to the staff if you felt that way, though?"

She looked away. "It feels like a prison here." I wondered whether to confiscate the razors. I might be overreacting and too controlling and parental. But if she kept the blades, she might cut herself. I wasn't sure what to do. My brow sweat, and I clenched my fist in my lap under my desk. In retrospect, she was being somewhat provocative, and I was angry at her for putting the burden on me. I was having to deal with her inability to say she would control these thoughts on her own. But at the time I just felt nervous and weighed down by being accountable and implicitly responsible for the outcomes of her actions.

I phoned Dr. Kasdin when she left my office. "Nancy Steele has razors and says she might use them!" I said breathlessly. He said nothing. A few moments passed. "Ah . . . What should I do?"

"If you take them away, you may infantalize her. She'll regress." Some patients regress in hospitals and stop trying to tackle their problems on their own, relying too much on the staff to take control and make decisions for them instead. "Appeal to her healthier side. Tell her that if she thinks she's going to use the razors, she has to hand them over. Until then, I wouldn't penalize her. Encourage her to come to the staff; try to make her understand her behavior. There is a syndrome of delicate cutting in which patients, usually women, occasionally scratch their wrists when they feel empty. The pain helps them organize themselves and feel real. She might fit into that category." The concept was counterintuitive, but I accepted his comments.

I wandered back to the nursing station to let the nurses know about the situation. Henry Nolan was standing there and listened, too.

"My God," he said, folding his arms across his chest, "if she says she's going to hurt herself, stick her in the Seclusion Room or put her on MO," maximal observation. "And snatch the razors," he continued. "You have to be direct with her. You can't make her understand. Get her to cooperate. That's enough. An insight-oriented approach won't work with her."

"But won't that make her more dependent on us, more regressed?"

"Is she that advanced, that we need to worry about regressing her?" He had a point, though it conflicted with Kasdin's approach. He suddenly looked at his watch and left.

I sat down at the counter where Mike was writing some notes. "How are things going?" he asked me.

"I'm not sure what to do with Steele," I said, shaking my head. I told him the story.

"You have to do what you feel most comfortable with. Whatever you decide, don't end up with a sleepless night over it." I was surprised but relieved that the criteria other residents used was whether they would be comfortable. That wasn't necessarily in the patient's best interests. The two might be the same, but not always.

"It sounds like she's a bad borderline," he said. "I hate patients like this. They're the worst."

I chose not to act strict with her and to try to work with her.

I departed for home but found myself still concerned. Might she injure herself overnight? Was it possible she might not be alive in the morning? I felt others escaped responsibility, leaving me accountable and besieged. That night, I had trouble sleeping.

* * *

In the morning, she was still alive. Nothing had happened, and I felt relieved.

Later that day she approached me in the main corridor. "Doctor, please help me. I bumped my head last night, and I feel dizzy now. Will you examine me?" I examined her briefly. She was fine.

The following evening, she again came up to me as I was about to leave. "My stomach aches," she said. "And pains are shooting up one side of my head." Some patients complain about bodily discomforts when they're depressed. Nortriptyline also has side effects. But she might just be seeking some extra attention. She insisted the pain was sharp, though she looked comfortable.

My duty was to be available to help her, and I didn't want to shirk it or overlook a possible problem. I was just starting in the hospital, and she was one of my first patients. Throughout medical school and internship, instructors had taught me to try to fulfill patients' requests concerning treatment and to put the patient first. But now I was antsy to go home and was irritated that she was catching me at the last minute. I could ignore her and leave or take a few minutes to assess her and end the issue. Otherwise, she might bother the nurses and the doctor on call at night. "Okay, let's go to the treatment room, and I'll examine you quickly." My voice betrayed my annoyance. She could have brought up these problems earlier. I'm sure she realized that after a long day, I'd feel less eager to help her.

Her physical exam found nothing wrong, and her pain then disappeared.

The next morning when I arrived, Nancy was waiting for me in the hallway. "Just the man I want to see," she declared.

I heard the heavy door to the ward slam and latch shut behind me. "Shit," I thought to myself.

"I want a pass this weekend!"

"You haven't·been here very long yet. Patients usually get passes as part of their treatment, when they're getting ready to leave the hospital."

"But I feel cooped up."

"You have to be here for now."

"I have to get out. If you don't give it to me, I'll have to put in a sign-out letter." In a sign-out letter, a patient writes that he or she wishes to leave the hospital. The doctor then has seventy-two hours to decide whether he should discharge the patient or go to court to ask that the patient be hospitalized involuntarily.

She didn't seem ready to be discharged yet. But a pass might calm her. This wasn't a prison, after all.

"That lady is sick!" Henry Nolan declared when I mentioned the possibility of a pass. "You need to be tough with her. Just tell her she has a disease that requires treatment. She needs to be in the hospital for that. If you approve her pass, you're being bullied."

"Ugh," I thought. "I'm giving in to her."

"Henry," Alice, the head nurse, said, overhearing our conversation. "Don't tell the man that. Let her go on a pass. Otherwise she'll be locked up here all weekend and will be hell for us nurses to deal with."

Nancy was standing at the doorway. "Well?" she asked when I left the nursing station. "Do I have a pass?"

"You need to be here for now. We're still getting to know you," I said, sensing that she wouldn't like this. "Patients usually go to occupational therapy activities first, before going out on passes." As I had explained to her, passes are used, in part, for mobilizing toward discharge.

"Then the only way I can leave is by putting in a sign-out letter!"

"Why not wait and see? I'm sure you'll be able to go on a pass sometime soon."

"I'm sick of always waiting for other people. I want to go now. Hand me a sheet of paper," she demanded from Alice.

"What are you doing?" I asked in astonishment.

"This is the only way I'm going to be able to get what I want. Where's a pen? Here," she said, reaching up to the breast pocket of my white coat, grabbing a black felt marker, and yanking it out. She dated the letter.

She had stolen my pen! I felt my personal space had been intruded upon and violated. I had other tasks to finish and was standing next to her, waiting for my pen, which she was using to oppose treatment I was trying to provide.

"To whom it may concern," she wrote neatly in a floral script.

I felt rage boiling up inside me. "Hold on a minute," I finally said. "I need my pen back. Give it back to me." I felt like I was in elementary school. To my surprise, however, she immediately lifted her arm and placed the instrument in my fingers. She folded up the piece of paper, pocketed it, and sauntered off.

I retreated to my tiny office, slammed the door, collapsed in a chair, and sighed, frustrated. The room was quiet and soothing. Outside, the sun sparkled. In the far distance a car honked. A dog barked. I had expected to be learning how to help patients by working together with them, and had assumed that patients would be interested, eager, and cooperative, as they generally were in the rest of medicine. But I had been mistaken. Psychiatrists got paid to deal with difficult people and situations.

Nancy was fed up with Dr. Cameron, her parents, her stepmother, and now the hospital. She felt wronged by them, and was now channeling her resentment toward me.

She was getting me angrier than any patients in medicine ever had. I had been raised to respect and try to work with other people, and had become good at finding and reaching consensus when disagreements arose. I had felt obliged when working in internal medicine to act like a doctor, to follow the Hippocratic Oath and help patients as much as I could, and not to be fed up, which would be selfish on my part. I wasn't used to refusing patients' pleas totally. But I was now being torn between Nancy's wants, my supervisors' conflicting approaches, and my own frustration, and I felt yanked apart as a result. I felt tense in ways that were new to me—helpless and alone.

I was seeing how medical patients had been easier to treat in many ways. They might be seriously ill and could even die. But tangible laboratory tests could assess their daily fluctuations. Psychiatry lacked such indices. Assessments for treatments now were still far less clear, hinging on my emotional responses and subjective impressions, on what patients uttered—often in asides, or in rage—and on thoughts that they withheld or were unable to express. No longer were objective laboratory tests precisely printed on computer printouts, marked with asterisks to be rechecked if they weren't within normal limits. Now, my actions were guided by what patients chose to confide in me and how I interpreted what they said. I would have to learn to trust my own intuition and gut reactions more.

Nothing I provided entirely erased Nancy's sense of having been wronged and abandoned in her life. Yet it was difficult to say to myself, "This is only a job, I can simply perform the required tasks and not become too personally involved." Nancy kept asking for more, threatening me, exasperating me, and refusing to cooperate. It seemed that the field didn't have a good treatment for her. But patients with borderline personality disorder came to psychiatrists. We didn't turn them away but accepted them for treatment and tried our best.

I saw that I would have to force myself to become more distanced, and not be as involved emotionally. It became clear to me why the profession fostered a sense that patients weren't like "us" and couldn't be treated as friends or acquaintances.

The next day, Nancy plopped into the chair in my office. "I'm still getting these horrible thoughts inside of me," she told me. "My life's going nowhere. Here I am spending a month in a mental hospital. What's the use of living? Why shouldn't someone be allowed to kill themselves if they want to? That's what I want to know. It's my only way out."

Kasdin had suggested that I attempt to predict her feelings to her. "You probably will have thoughts of wanting to injure yourself," I said, "but it would be a mistake to act on them." She sat stunned for a moment, blinking her eyes, trying to think what to say next. My comments had made a small impression on her. I spoke with her further, but she remained sullen when she left my office.

As I was getting ready to leave the ward, Nancy cornered me. "I forgot to mention," she said, "that I've been having trouble sleeping. Can I get a tranquilizer?" The nurses had reported that she had been resting well. One feature of depression is that patients often feel they aren't sleeping, even though they are. Insomnia, if she had it, needed to be observed by the staff to determine whether it was a sign of increasing depression. Priority was placed on evaluating the larger, overriding disease, not just treating individual symptoms. In the meantime, while this assessment was being made, treatment for her sleeplessness would have to be withheld. This tactic of holding back remedies felt awkward. But I understood it as part of my new job, placing my perceptions of patients' long-term benefits over their immediate short-term relief, even if they preferred otherwise.

"The nurses will have to observe if you aren't sleeping before I can prescribe anything," I told her.

"But I hate being up all night. You have no idea what it's like. It isn't fair. If I can't sleep at three A.M., why should you? I should call you up at home to tell you about it. Then you'd believe me."

"I'm trying to help you, Ms. Steele. That wouldn't be smart."

That night at home I read a novel to relax and then climbed into bed.

At 3:30 A.M., my telephone rang.

My eyes slowly searched in the dark of my apartment for the phone. "It's me!" A voice squawked through the receiver. "It's Nancy Steele. I can't sleep!"

My eyes focused. "Ms. Steele, you are not allowed to call me up at home."

"But Doctor—"

"You should speak to the nurse on duty." My hand fumbled to hang up the phone. No patient had ever called me up at home. The light from a street lamp shot through the blinds on my bedroom window. I lay awake, angry and helpless. What could I do? I dialed the nursing station, unsure what the night staff could do, either. But no one else would be awake at that hour to call about it. Carol Walters, who was on duty, placed Nancy on "telephone restriction" until the morning. I had never heard of that status, but at least Nancy wouldn't be able to phone me again.

My heart pounded. Every ten minutes, I glanced at the red digits of the clock radio, agitated. A colon flashed the seconds. Finally, I dozed off.

She had crossed the line.

"What else could I be doing with Steele?" I asked Kasdin the next day. I told him about her call.

"What you're doing is fine."

"I get a headache when I talk to her."

"That alone should tell you her diagnosis. Your reactions to her are important pieces of data. What she's doing to you is a sign of her psychopathology. It means that whatever else, she's borderline. After a day of seeing patients like her, I feel like a used dishtowel, discarded by patients who get to walk away. She wants to see that you can handle her anger when it overwhelms her. She wants you to draw limits and take control, even when she fights you about it. I don't even take on patients like this in my private practice anymore. They're like sea urchins. They look nice from a distance. But get too close and they sting. Just don't let her get to you."

"Sounds simple."

"You're more involved with her than I am. The further one gets from a patient, the easier he or she is to treat. She's just in a rage at Cameron for leaving. How are your other folks doing?"

I told him briefly about my other patients, and our session ended.

My interventions were the best that could be reasonably offered. The field didn't have techniques that would help Nancy dramatically over a short period of time. During this brief hospitalization, psychiatric treatment wouldn't be able to change the impact that decades of relationships had had on her. The most I could do would be to get her to recognize this situation—but even that seemed almost impossible here. The initial expectation was that we would help her. As a result, I was trying my hardest, though unprovided with tools to do what was being demanded of me and feeling distressed as a consequence. My attempted interventions might not be capable of making her significantly better, of getting her to control her impulses.

"Tell her that she has to be here for now and has to cut out all this nonsense," Henry Nolan said the next time I saw him. "Just read her the riot act." I wasn't completely sure what he meant—presumably that she had to behave or else—though it sounded more punitive and parental than psychiatric. But with that, he stomped away.

"The hospital's just making me worse," she complained at our next appointment. "Don't they teach you anything useful in medical school or residency?" The clock on my desk ticked loudly. A fragile hand paused between every second as it slowly crept through its small increments.

I was annoyed, and decided to use my own responses in this interchange. "Do you know how mad you sound?"

"No."

"How do you expect I'm going to feel after hearing all this?"

"I don't know."

I said what I felt and made an interpretation. "I think you're trying to make it difficult for me to help you."

"Everybody's just letting me down." Her eyes began to moisten.

"But this feeling of being abandoned is important to try to understand. You have to realize that sometimes you're going to be alone. Your psychiatrist is not going to be there all of the time for you. He can't be." She removed a Kleenex from a box of them on my desk and dried her tears.

* * *

"How is Steele doing?" Henry Nolan asked at the next team meeting, where the staff responsible for each patient—the faculty, nurses, social workers, occupational therapists, and treating resident—all got together once a week to discuss the patient and to agree on a plan for the week. Donna Lambert and the other nurses and I sat around a small table in the lounge as we discussed each of my patients. "Is she still depressed?"

"She seems to be." I told him about my recent interactions with her.

"What's her antidepressant level?"

"It's therapeutic," meaning it was in the range that had been found to be effective for most patients.

"Then let's try adding lithium to see if it helps her. Talking with this lady further isn't going to be very helpful."

"She's also suicidal sometimes."

"Well, she probably will kill herself one day," Nolan said. He lifted his hands up halfway in the air, opened his fingers, shrugged, and then let his arms drop, as if to say, "That's that—what can you do about it?" "Hopefully it won't happen while she's here," he added.

Were there, in fact, people who were destined to kill themselves? I thought a psychiatrist's job was to prevent them. "Why do you say she'll probably kill herself?" I asked, amazed at his assertion. I was shocked at his distance and seeming unconcern.

"Look at her history. Look at her life."

He said the words calmly and they fell into the still air. Everyone else at the meeting nodded quietly. Donna strained not to appear bewildered or surprised and to accept what had been said as obviously true.

The following Monday, Dr. Cameron returned from vacation. Nancy went on a pass to visit him in his office. She reported feeling better. The lithium might have benefited her a little, too, though that wasn't clear. She told Alice that she thought it did help but told me it didn't.

"If Cameron accepts her back into treatment," Kasdin told me, "send her home and have her continue with him. In the long run, their relationship may not be good for her. Her hospitalization may be related to her work with him. Psychotherapy may be too stimulating for her. For some patients, no treatment is the treatment of choice. But in the short run, he's one of her only supports, and we should take advantage of that. Have her continue with him. You can't restructure her personality here in thirty days. If you had more time you could try."

The twelfth floor was an acute ward; patients stayed an average of one month. Rooms cost six hundred dollars a day.

I explained the plan to her.

"But I don't want to go back to Cameron. I don't ever want to see him again."

"But he knows you best."

"I just want to go home."

"You can't unless you see him."

She pouted and left my office.

The day before her scheduled discharge, she put in a pass and filled out a personal goals-setting form, routinely completed by patients prior to their discharge. Patients were asked to list their main goal. Nancy wrote: "to kill myself." The form then read, "List at least four steps that will be necessary to achieve this goal." In the left-hand margin were numbers one through four, with a blank line beside each for the patient's response. Nancy had written: "One: to get discharged. Two: to fire my outpatient psychiatrist. Three: to stop my medications. Four: to kill myself."

I was astounded. Nothing was straightforward with her.

"Try to keep her mobilized," Kasdin said, "if we can"—that is, continue to allow her to leave the ward by herself to go elsewhere in the hospital, encouraging her to be as functioning and as little regressed as possible.

"You didn't approve my pass today!" she said when I sat down with her.

"I understand you handed in a treatment goal form."

"I'm sick of this whole thing. I don't want to see Cameron or any other psychiatrist. You don't know how humiliating it is to have to go from one of you guys to the other, and to have to see him again. Enough is enough."

"I think it's best if you see him."

"Forget it. For all these months—first with him, then with you—I've been beholden to someone else, and I resent it. It's my life, not yours and not Cameron's, and I want to do what I want with it. I want to go home and not have any therapy."

"Why don't you think it over?"

That night, she walked up to Carol in the hallway. "Can I speak with you a moment? Nobody wants to give me what I want. Everyone tells me what I have to do, I'm a piece of garbage. I feel like hurting myself again." Carol spoke with her and invited her to come to the nursing station to talk further if she wished.

Nancy returned to her room, shattered a framed picture against the wall, picked up one of the jagged edges from the floor, and scratched her wrist. Blood welled up into the bruise.

The next morning, she wore a wide bandage of clean white gauze around her wrist and paraded up and down the hall for everyone to see. I felt embarrassed, as if I had been unable to control her and had missed a crucial element or done something wrong in her treatment.

"She's just trying to sabotage the therapy," Kasdin told me. "She feels she's failed and that people have failed her. She's taking her rage out on you. She wants you to fail, too, to feel the same way she does—shitty. You have to point this out to her: that the only one who'll get hurt is her—not you. Even when she threatens to hurt herself, she wants to hurt Dr. Cameron for leaving her, or you in his place. Every suicidal impulse is really a homicidal one," he said. "It's anger directed at someone else. Her emotions overwhelm her. She can't stop to reflect on them, and she acts out."

"Is there anything else I could be doing with her?"

"No. She expects a lot from you—more than you can ever give her. Appeal to whatever healthy ego she has," he continued. "Let's try to send her out of here before she gets even worse."

Nancy was troubled by an illness that impaired her ability to relate to me appropriately. She wasn't purposefully trying to make things difficult for me and probably couldn't readily curtail this behavior, though other people might have been able to control such words and deeds consciously.

"We can't discharge you unless you see Dr. Cameron," I told her.

"I'll do what I want, and you can't stop me. I'm putting in a sign-out letter."

She submitted a letter but retracted it the following day and went out on a pass to see Dr. Cameron. Her pass was from ten o'clock to one o'clock. Yet at three, she hadn't yet returned to the ward. I phoned Cameron. "She never came," he told me. "She called to cancel."

At three-thirty, Nancy called the nursing station. "I'm at home. I'm highly suicidal and I'm not coming back to the ward." With that, she hung up the phone. I called her back. There was no answer. I spoke to Henry Nolan, who told me I had to call the police. An hour later, two policemen, both much taller than her, brought her back to the ward, leaving me stunned that she had gone this far.

She then put in another sign-out letter.

"Perfect," Henry Nolan said when he heard. "You should threaten to Two-PC her." To Two-PC someone means to complete a two-physician certificate in which two doctors write that the patient has an illness requiring treatment in a hospital, which the patient is refusing. The case is then presented in court. "If she doesn't agree to see Cameron she can't go home. She'll be shipped to a long-term facility. There, she'll at least be safe." A judge would decide whether she should be involuntarily hospitalized.

Two destinations were possible—an expensive private long-term hospital or the state mental hospital. She couldn't afford the first and the only alternative thus was the second—Rivershore State, known among patients as a "snake pit." Though recently euphemistically renamed Rivershore Mental Health Center, it was still called Rivershore State or just Rivershore for short.

"Would she really be committed against her will?" I asked Nolan.

"That's up to the judge. In the meantime, we'll hope that the mere threat of sending her to court will get her to pull herself together. If she does get committed it'll be to a state hospital, which should shake her up a bit." He smiled. "It'll be interesting to see what she does."

"Is a state hospitalization the best thing for her, though?" It sounded like a punitive threat: we would send her away if she didn't behave. It didn't fully or intuitively make sense—confining her because she was angry that therapists deserted her. Because she wouldn't leave the hospital, we would send her to one even longer. Moreover, she seemed verbal and intelligent, and somehow, I thought at the time, must be reachable and reasonable at some level.

"She's only regressing further since she's been here. She's become too attached."

"But a state hospital?"

"She has a treatable illness."

"But several years of treatment haven't helped much."

"She has to learn that this isn't a proper way to behave. Besides, nothing else has worked. She's failed the treatment. With patients like this, you have to decide if they're mad, or bad." The difference is whether they're mentally ill or merely being a nuisance and behaving badly. Nolan had decided in the end that she was "bad." I wasn't as sure and still thought she might not be able to control her behavior because of a psychiatric illness. "Anyway, frankly, I'm sick of hearing about her," he said, and with that, walked away.

"Your choices are either to keep the letter in or to take it back," I said to her when we met in my office. Her clothes were wrinkled and worn. Her hair hung down, unwashed for several days.

"I still don't see why I can't just leave here."

"You need treatment. You just tried to injure yourself again. If you don't accept going back to Dr. Cameron, we have to take you to court to have you transferred to a long-term hospital."

"Let some judge try to send me away."

"It could be to a large state hospital."

"That wouldn't be helping me now, would it?"

"You'd leave us no alternative."

"You can't make me do anything I don't want to do." She jumped up, shook her head, and stormed out of my office.

Nolan wanted her either out of a hospital altogether or in one for an extended stay of two years. The choice of options seemed oddly inconsistent. What Nolan didn't want for her was the middle road—a short-term hospitalization of about a month, which she was in now. We were either going to turn our backs on her suicidal behavior and ignore it, discharging her from the hospital, or take it very seriously and lock her away for two years as a result. It didn't make sense, except that either way, she'd be out of our hands. Nonetheless, the threat of sending her for a long-term hospitalization was the only leverage we had in getting her to see Cameron. Our approach wasn't based on biology or psychoanalytic theory, but seemed more a tactical strategy, a power play.

Yet that afternoon, she phoned Cameron on her own without telling me and promised to attend his sessions regularly. Cameron said okay, having known her well for several years. He phoned me and said that if we discharged her, he'd take her back into treatment and accept full responsibility for her. She had arrived at her own solution to our apparent impasse and had saved face.

She went to his office twice from the hospital over the next few days. Our two-pronged approach had worked. The threat of legally forced hospitalization provoked her to choose Cameron. I was surprised how seriously she had accepted my terms. They had prevented her from physically injuring herself and had changed her behavior. No drugs or hours of intensive psychotherapy had wrought as much change as a single sentence threatening long-term hospitalization. This maneuver wasn't what I had thought of as "psychiatric treatment," but it worked.

I met with her for the last time the following morning. "Who are you going to have to call you up at night now?" She laughed.

I smiled politely. "I hope things go well at home," I said. "Good luck."

She paused and then let out a long breath. "I know you tried to help me, and that I haven't always made it easy for you. . . . I'm sorry." Her comment surprised and gratified me. In the end, she had the insight to see that her behavior was difficult for me. And she could almost laugh at herself.

We shook hands, and she took her coat and left. Only now did I realize that the hospital had been a safe haven, protecting her and giving her ongoing contact with a psychiatrist until Cameron returned—though she could never acknowledge these needs at the time. She had gotten out of the hospital what she required. The events that had perplexed me as they had unfolded only now made sense. It was unfortunate that her psychiatrist's vacation had provoked all this turmoil.

This case, though I could just try to forget it, taught me a lot. Kasdin's and Nolan's initial expectations and plans had to be dropped. What worked with her in the end was neither a psychological nor a psychopharmacological approach. In short, the effectiveness of treatments couldn't be accurately predicted. They would have to be tried. That may sound obvious, but each supervisor had presented his approach to me as if it were clearly right, supported by theories and explanations, and guaranteed to succeed. However, solutions might be evident only after each approach has been attempted. Even then, neither might work. Moreover, the two different approaches—psychodynamic and biological—each sought to achieve the same outcome. I didn't understand how.

I also began to see what Kasdin had meant in saying that patients had to be treated differently from other people. I saw the need to be wary of my initial reactions. Only over time would patients' personalities become clear. An attractive, well-groomed woman who looked like she could almost be a friend could in fact be very disturbed and disturbing, frustrating me in new ways, tearing me between conflicting impulses I then had to reconcile. I had to focus on what patients said to me and how I felt inside. Appearance could provide valuable clues but could also mislead. Patients wouldn't always be as straightforward as they seemed, or even as my supervisors thought.

Nancy taught me the need for both concern and a certain detachment. Her behavior encouraged the staff and me to want to reject her. It is the reaction she stated that she wanted least, yet the one she provoked the most. I would often have to do the best I could for patients despite their efforts. Psychiatrists are often accused of being distant, ungiving, and unconcerned about those they treat, and I felt pressure to adopt this position, too. In the end I learned to be tough and firm with her, but I saw the need to remain compassionate and sensitive as well. This would be a difficult balance to achieve and maintain.

It was easy to blame her for failing the treatment, yet we didn't consider whether we, too, might have failed. None of our treatments worked, but no one questioned their effectiveness. The blame for her not getting better was implicitly placed on her, though this attribution seemed perhaps unfair. I began to think back to the witch doctor I had met in Papua New Guinea. Nancy was gone now, and the staff quickly busied themselves with other patients. But I began to wonder about how effective the field was, and how it dealt with its shortcomings.

A few weeks later, I was walking down a neighborhood sidewalk on a rainy evening. "Hello Doctor," I heard. A red raincoat fluttered by. Nancy Steele smiled broadly. Her white teeth sparkled, her hair swept lightly through the air. A dress swung around her body freely. She didn't stop but hurried onward. My eyes followed her for a moment in the lamplight until she disappeared into the night.

Roosters or Hens

Through the course of my training in psychiatry, I had to become more open to, and accepting of, my own psychological processes—both conscious and unconscious.

"Seventy percent of your choices are unconscious," Dr. Thomas Desmond told us in a noontime lecture a few days after Nancy went home. "Even what shirt or tie you buy or wear." Other residents and I looked around the table at what we were wearing. Our clothes seemed fairly standard: white or light blue Oxford dress shirts on the men, skirts and dresses on the women.

"Our aim," Dr. Desmond continued, "is to understand a person and his or her unconscious. This is one of your major jobs as a psychiatrist. To help you, I will be teaching you today about psychological tests."

"Remember that our image of the world is never 'reality,' " he continued. "Let me give you an example. I want you all to close your eyes." We looked at each other. Was he serious? "Go ahead," he urged. "Shut your eyes." I closed mine.

"Anne ..." I heard him say.

"Yes?"

"No, keep your eyes closed. Tell me, what color is the carpeting in this room?"

"The carpeting?"

"Yes. You've been in this room before."

"It's ah ... beige ... Oh no!" she exclaimed, I assumed, on opening her eyes. "It's gray!"

"Mike ..."

"Ah ... yes."

"What color are the walls?"

"White." He opened his eyes. "Yellow."

"Bob? What color are the chairs?"

Summoning up a mental picture of the furniture proved more difficult than I would have imagined. I hadn't really looked at the chairs but had taken them for granted.

"Orange," I said, that color faintly standing out more than any other. I opened my eyes. The chairs were rust. I wasn't too far off, but was still impressed by the weakness of our mental images of the external world.

"The brain is complex," Desmond continued. "You all have sat here several times but have never really observed what is around you. You looked but did not see. What we look at and what we see are different. As psychiatrists, you will constantly be assessing these differences between internal and external realities in your patients. And one way we do that is through psychological testing.

"The best way to tap people's experiences is to have them do a creative thing. In the first kind of test we use, we ask patients to tell stories about a series of pictures. Here's the first one. Sarah, tell me a story about what you see here."

"Me?" she asked.

"Yes." On the card, three chicks sat around a dining table with bibs tied around their necks as they held large spoons. In front of them was a big bowl of food. Behind them hovered the towering gray shadow of a parent bird. "Is this a rooster or a hen?" he asked.

"A hen," Sarah answered.

"What do you think, Mike?"

Mike looked around him nervously. "A rooster."

"Both," Anne said, sensing a trick question.

"No," Desmond said. "It has to be one or the other."

"Clearly a rooster," I said with exaggerated emphasis. Everyone laughed.

Desmond showed us some other images. "They're all scary and punitive," Mike said.

"Not necessarily," Desmond said slyly, peering at Mike. "That's all in the eye of the beholder.

"Next," Desmond continued, "we test patients with Rorschachs. Dr. Rorschach was a Swiss psychologist who made over two thousand ink blots, pouring dyes onto sheets of paper that he folded to produce patterns. He then performed experiments to pick the ten pictures that best elicited information about the unconscious. These images each uncover certain aspects of the person. Here they are." He picked up the top print.

"Mike, what do you see here?" On a card two splotches of black ink faced each other, with orange curls squiggling on top of each. "It's a simple picture."

"A pair of clowns talking to each other," Mike said. "They're happy and well adjusted," he added quickly, stabbing at what he thought a "normal" answer would be. The rest of us glanced at each other. None of us would have given quite that answer. Dr. Desmond jotted down notes about Mike's response on the blackboard to analyze it.

"Now card two," Desmond said. We all pulled back in our seats, afraid to be called on. What would we say? Would we be honest? This procedure seemed unfair, having us reveal our unconscious thoughts in front of the rest of the class. We all avoided eye contact with him. "What do you see here?" he asked Joe Tauber, a tall blond soft-spoken Californian who worked in a different ward of the hospital and was married to a lawyer. We all breathed sighs of relief that we hadn't been called on. To me the picture looked at first like a cartoon character, Snagglepuss. But my response seemed silly. I would have been ashamed to tell anyone, though now, in retrospect, I see it as no more or less valid than anyone else's.

Joe paused and blushed. "I see a penis and a labia," he said. The class was shocked. Normally reticent and reserved, he limited his discussions to work or polite but not overly personal social conversation. We were now talking about our own sexual thoughts more explicitly than we had ever done in an academic seminar through all our years of college and medical school. Dr. Desmond walked to the front of the room and rated Joe's response on the blackboard. I felt embarrassed for Joe. Tension mounted. We were all uncomfortable, nervous about saying something that might seem ridiculous or too exposing of ourselves. This technique seemed unfair of Desmond. When would he stop?

"What do you see here?" he asked Anne about the next card.

She examined it carefully. "Two rabbits?"

"Two rabbits? Where do you see *that*?" he asked, as if she were crazy. She pointed to the ears. "Hmm," he said, puzzled. "This card is *normally* described as showing two very feminine girls." Anne was a strong, assertive woman, but it didn't seem appropriate or fair to have her responses to this card revealed to everyone in the room, who now suspected that she might have "issues" or conflict around her femininity at some level. My heart beat faster. We felt threatened as he implied that we weren't as "together" or "healthy" as we tried to think of ourselves.

In principle, I liked his approach of trying to make us aware of psychological issues in ourselves, both in how we failed to perceive our environment accurately and how we as individuals responded differently to stimuli. It was one thing to think of psychological difficulties and the unconscious in relation to our patients or other people. But it was another matter to think of these phenomena in terms of ourselves.

Still, the topics Desmond explored didn't seem to relate much to the patients currently under our care. Presumably, though, these areas would be relevant to patients we would see later in our careers.

More astonishing at the time, however, was having our most intimate thoughts exposed in this way. Like most people, I had been schooled to keep my sexual thoughts to myself, especially in a classroom. But being a psychiatrist would apparently require me to break down these barriers. Nonetheless, I was surprised to see how personally threatening this exercise felt. I had taken my psychological defenses for granted. Not until they were threatened did I feel anxiety and realize that they were there. I had gotten through my training thus far in medical school and even internship without much emotional turmoil. Yet the wall that had protected my own private thoughts, fantasies, and whims was now being assaulted and cracked.

What Is T?

I began to see how residents occupied a peculiar role in the hospital hierarchy—in some ways akin to that of patients. The hospital shaped how we, too, behaved, dealt with stresses, and looked at ourselves.

After a few weeks on the ward, I received a memo about a "T-group" meeting every Wednesday at 1:00. I assumed it was a type of support group for residents, and looked forward to getting some psychological support and to meeting with other residents as a group. I enjoyed working with and getting to know others, and liked most of the other residents. But we were spread out on different wards and rarely got together to talk about our experiences. Moreover, I was interested in the process of education and in sociological issues of how groups shaped individuals' experiences, and I was eager to learn about group dynamics.

The meetings were to be held in a seminar room in the middle of one of the inpatient wards. When I arrived at the first session, most of the residents in my year were already present. The chairs in the room were arranged in an oval. At one end, an older gentleman in a navy blue suit stared at the floor, looking like he had been left behind accidentally from an earlier meeting. There were three seats empty—one on the man's left and two on his right. I sat down on the one farthest from him, next to Anne. Mike arrived next and was forced to sit down next to the man. A few residents had brought brown paper bag lunches and started bashfully eating. We were all present except for Sarah. I glanced at my watch—1:05.

"When does this start?" I whispered to Anne. Faculty usually started classes even if some residents weren't present yet, which was invariably the case, given our busy schedules.

"I thought one o'clock," she answered.

"So do we just start this thing ourselves or does he do it?" Mike asked, referring to the man at the head of the circle. Mike didn't point or indicate who he meant, but we all knew. I had heard that there was a group leader, a Dr. Leonard Nathan, and I assumed that this was he. Yet he sat stone-faced and said nothing. We continued to chat and mumble to our neighbors, occasionally exchanging puzzled looks. The door remained open.

Finally, Sarah arrived, about ten minutes late. She stopped just inside the doorway, sized up the situation, and walked to the far corner of the room where she started to lift up a chair that was against the wall.

"There's already a chair here for you," Anne said. The last seat was next to Dr. Nathan.

Sarah glanced around awkwardly and then sat down in it.

I looked to Dr. Nathan to start the meeting. But he kept gazing at the floor. His silence surprised me. We all looked at each other and shrugged. I glanced down at the armrests of my chair—durable, wooden, and of modern Scandinavian design, a model commonly found on the wards, though never studied by me as closely before. Its cushions, too, were rust colored.

Two or three minutes passed painfully in silence. Still no one spoke. I felt at a loss, virtually unable to talk, not knowing where to start.

"I have three hypotheses," Dr. Nathan finally said after ten more minutes, "about why the door remained open." We looked at one another. This wasn't what I expected him to say when he finally spoke. "First, you feel the institution doesn't have any boundaries. Second, you feel you don't have any boundaries. And third, you were all too afraid to close it."

I was confused. He hadn't said who he was or what the purpose of this group was.

"Frankly," Anne said, "I thought the door was open because we were waiting for Sarah." That seemed to be the actual answer, but was apparently too simple for us in our new roles as psychiatrists, supposed to be interpreting behavior on multiple levels. We sat completely quiet, all looking at the floor, embarrassed by our naïveté. Minutes dragged on. I heard my watch ticking on my wrist, then Joe's watch, clicking from across the room. I heard Mike breathing in and out in his seat next to me. I had never been in such an awkward and constrained social situation. Here we were, thirteen psychiatrists sitting in a room together saying absolutely nothing. I tried to avoid catching Dr. Nathan's eye. The situation was more awkward because through a decade of higher education, we had gotten used to sitting in a room with a senior instructor at the head of the class, but had been led to expect that he would teach, lead, and guide us. Yet here we all sat and nothing seemed to be going on.

"What's the experience of silence like for each of you?" Dr. Nathan asked after another five minutes.

Nobody spoke.

"It's anxiety-producing," Anne finally admitted.

"I think it's sort of nice," Mike said. "It's so rare to be in a room that's quiet around here."

We all laughed nervously. Still, no one wanted to take on the larger issues that hung in the background.

Was this the purpose—to have us be silent?

We again fell into a painful and uneasy quiet.

"I didn't know about coming in here," Anne said at last. "I was the first one here. I peeked in through the curtains on the door. No one was here yet. Only him," she said, her eyes glancing up slightly in Nathan's direction. He sat with his head cast down. "I waited outside the door until someone else showed up."

"I think everyone's just thinking their own private thoughts," Mike said.

"I was just at the dentist's and got novocaine," Sarah said, speaking out of the side of her mouth and breaking the silence. "So that's what I'm thinking about." That seemed oddly personal compared to the issues we usually discussed in class.

"Perhaps everyone is waiting for the anesthesia to wear off," Dr. Nathan countered immediately in a deep, prophetic-sounding voice.

How odd. He wasn't connecting with us emotionally or being very helpful or forthcoming.

"I didn't get that," Sarah said. We all looked up at Nathan to elaborate, but he wouldn't even lift his head up. More time passed.

I felt obliged to say something, to contribute to the group of which I felt a part. "I like the notion that the institution has no boundaries," I finally said after a long silence, "but I don't think it applies to why the door was left open."

"What's all this talk about boundaries?" Sarah asked. "That's too abstract and cerebral for me. I don't know what you're all talking about." I had a sense of the term metaphorically but was surprised she didn't understand.

"Well, what should we talk about?" Mike asked, getting me off the hook.

"Maybe we should set an agenda," Anne suggested. "We can make a list of things we want to discuss."

"What should we put on it?" Jessica, another resident, asked. This subject bored me.

"Maybe we should set some rules first," Anne suggested. This all seemed very formal.

"They didn't have rigid rules last year," Joe Tauber said.

"I heard that last year Dr. Nathan stared at the same spot on the carpet for six months without saying anything," Mike told us.

"This is ridiculous," Sarah said. "With all the stress we have in our work here, instead of providing us with people to help us or paying for our own individual psychotherapy, the administration throws us all in here together and says, 'Go help each other.' It's so typical of them!" She was right.

Dr. Nathan suddenly interrupted. "As potentially interesting as this conversation may be, it is avoiding the issue of setting rules." We exchanged glances of surprise. I had thought that Sarah had been appropriate, expressing the kind of feelings uttered in such a group. But apparently that was not what he expected us to be saying, either.

"Okay, well, how about everyone has to come?" Anne suggested.

"But what if you're tied up with an emergency?" Joe asked.

"A lot of times it can really wait, though," Anne said.

"Yeah," Joe said, "but what if a patient is dying or something?"

"That doesn't happen too often around here," Anne retorted.

"I've heard that some groups decide that you can't eat or come in late."

"How about you can't go to the bathroom, too?" Mike added satirically.

"We can spend a whole year here just like this," I joked, "talking about what we're going to discuss." Everyone laughed, and we drifted away from the topic of rules. I saw how I used humor to deal with difficult situations.

"Rules are being spoken of only after death and excrement," Dr. Nathan interrupted.

"Excrement?" Joe asked, puzzled.

"You all have been talking about going to the bathroom." His interpretation sounded far-fetched.

"We can always talk about the baseball season," Mike jested.

"Those who don't speak of setting rules may have them imposed upon them," Nathan announced loudly. Mike shrugged. Nathan seemed very abstract—not following the kinds of social interactions I was used to. We were being initiated into a very different world.

Sarah rolled her eyes. I felt peculiarly distanced from whatever he wanted us to do. Could we say what we wanted, or was this an exercise in which we had to be circumspect and appropriate to a classroom with a professor in front? If Nathan weren't here I would have said how weird and surreal it felt, but I felt constrained by this senior member of the faculty, who spoke regularly with our supervisors and the rest of the faculty.

"Frankly, I don't want any rules," Joe finally said. "I think we have enough rules and guidelines here as it is. I think we should do whatever we want."

"What are we here for anyway?" Mike asked, annoyed.

"I'm here because you all are," Sarah said, gesturing to all of us.

"I thought it might be interesting," I said.

No one else answered the question.

"I don't like this," Anne said. "We're doing all the talking. He's learning a lot about us and we're not learning anything about him."

"This is probably how patients feel in groups or with one of us," I volunteered. "We sit there as the authority figure in the room, and patients say what they're feeling while we don't say anything about ourselves." My brow sweat as I released my comment into the circle. I could have said something more personal, like, "I feel uncomfortable sitting here," but was still unsure what to utter to fill this void. No one responded. No one wanted to hear about how we could be learning about this process. Everyone was too angry at Nathan.

The meeting felt increasingly tense and forced. Something was expected of us, though we didn't know what.

"I don't know if I'm comfortable spilling my guts in front of this guy," Mike said. "How do we know we won't get knifed in the back?"

"I don't like this at all," Sarah said.

"Why?" Anne asked her.

"Because of this *thing*," she said, waving her hand. "Look at him! I think the problem is him. I mean you," she said looking at him, though he refused to tilt his head up from the floor. "What are we supposed to call you anyway? Do we call you, 'you'? Come to think of it, I don't think we were ever really introduced. I imagine you're Dr. Nathan because that's what it said on the memo we got, but you never introduced yourself or said why we were meeting here or what we were supposed to be doing."

"I've been addressed so far as 'thing,' 'it,' 'he,' 'him,' and 'you,' " he said.

"Well, are you a member of the group or not?" Anne asked. I was impressed that she was able to articulate an important source of my confusion and annoyance.

"The memorandum you received stated that I was a 'consultant to the group process.' "

"What does that mean?" I asked.

"The memorandum said I was a consultant to the group process," Anne repeated in a mocking tone, anticipating how psychoanalysts often respond—by repeating but not elaborating on statements made.

"I don't even remember getting a memo," Sarah said.

"Me neither," Mike added.

"I have it somewhere," I said, having saved it because of my interest in groups.

"Can you show it to us?" Anne asked. I agreed to.

"And what's a T-group anyway?" Sarah asked. None of us knew if T stood for "therapy" or meant tea, like a tea party. Was it supposed to be therapeutic, to help us cope with stress, or was it social, a chance for us to get together? I also wondered whether the purpose was to teach us about how groups worked, and if so, how. In any case, thus far it was producing more anxiety than it relieved.

"Well?" Sarah asked. "What does the T stand for?"

We all looked at Nathan, who said nothing. Suddenly, he rose from his chair, turned around, and exited the room. I looked at my watch: 2:00 exactly.

We continued to meet every week throughout the year, but the question of the group's purpose never got answered any more than at this first session. Dr. Nathan never said more than he did then, and the group continued to feel peculiar and unreal.

Nathan acted toward us not in a socially appropriate way, but as a therapist. The model he followed was that of a treating psychiatrist toward us. As a result, we were suddenly being put in the role of patients, our statements and actions interpreted psychodynamically and traced to psychological conflicts and drives. We weren't being informed about the rationale for his comments or approaches toward us. As in psychoanalysis, he refused to answer our questions about what he had said or done. He was encouraging us to examine and explore our own comments as indicative of underlying psychological themes. But he also adopted the detached distance of the psychoanalyst—disconnected, not direct or supportive or showing much concern. There was a lack of genuine human or emotional warmth from him, so we didn't feel comfortable discussing how we really felt. None of us ever got more upset or showed more emotion than we did in this first meeting, given Nathan's powerful but unpredictable and vague responses.

The problem was that we weren't here as patients trying to get better, but as residents, scheduled to be here as part of our curriculum. Still, this was the only thing resembling psychological support that the institution ever provided, even though the group never explicitly helped us to deal with the year.

School and training until now had been far more straightforward. It wasn't clear if he was instructing us, and if so, in what. The topics remained work related, and the institution was giving us a strong message that we should reflect on the experience of residency in a psychological way, in psychological terms. We were supposed to deal with our personal responses professionally, developing an appropriate vocabulary and tone for discussing them with colleagues that was different from how we would talk with close friends.

Yet because the rules and goals of these meetings weren't clear, we never felt more than partly engaged in them and never took them completely seriously. It was unclear how we were supposed to approach these meetings, and Nathan never said. Psychiatry was far murkier than internal medicine, in which our roles and actions and courses were well defined. I knew psychiatry would involve ambiguities, but the ways and extent to which this was the case were surprising me. Moreover, the institution acted as though psychiatry were very definite and *not* ambiguous. We had to realize these uncertainties on our own, not explicitly instructed or helped in coping with them, and grope and arrive at whatever resolution or reconciliation we could.

After Nathan exited the room at the end of that first session, we all remained seated silently for a moment, stunned. We didn't know what had hit us. Then, we all suddenly burst out laughing. We chuckled and guffawed for what seemed like several minutes. It was the first time we had ever laughed together as a group.

We finally stopped and sat quiet and still for a moment. We would now have to return to the wards to work and weren't eager to do so. Slowly, we gathered up our clipboards and books, empty cans of soda and bags from lunch, and held them in our laps, then rose together and left the room as a group.

Yellow Caps

The faculty, though teaching us the approaches in which they were expert, often ignored social and cultural issues in patients' lives. Frequently, patients confronted major social problems that the staff didn't address. As a result, occasionally, my sympathies for a patient ended up conflicting with my sympathies for the institution.

"You had a new patient admitted last night," Alice told me at rounds one morning a few weeks later. "And," she said, twitching her nostrils as she peered over the top of her nursing report book, "he itched all night. Co-patients complained about his hygiene. He smells and I think we should Kwell him." Kwell is a medicated shampoo that kills lice and crabs. It has neurological side effects, however, and like any medicine has to be prescribed only after seeing and evaluating the patient, rather than being blindly administered.

"I need to examine him first," I said.

"Let's just Kwell him anyway. I don't want any crabs or lice or fleas on *my* ward. He's a street person, a druggie."

"Let me just take a look at him."

"Well, hurry up!"

The staff clearly didn't like him already. After rounds I read over Ronald Bransky's chart and went to visit him.

He lay on the bed in Helen's old room, wearing a yellow ski cap and aviator sunglasses. A vinyl ski parka engulfed his body. A blanket was pulled up over him.

"Mr. Bransky?" He looked asleep, but on hearing my voice his eyelids fluttered and then opened. He looked at me standing over him and then reshut his eyes. "I need to examine you for a moment."

I bent over him, and my fingers picked through his scalp and body hair, looking for any bugs. He was dressed in jeans, a plaid lumber shirt, and boots. His hair was shaggy. He didn't seem particularly itchy, but I held my arms up in the air away from the rest of my body. I was working to help him and the staff, and straining to avoid getting any bugs on me if they were present. Yet he wouldn't even open his eyes. I was getting mad, putting myself at risk for getting lice. I really didn't want to be doing this, endangering myself. What for? I was sympathetic to the plight of street people, but also avoided them if I could on the outside, as they begged or harassed passersby. I didn't know any street people and, growing up in New York, had learned to keep to myself when walking down the street. Ever since I was mugged in a subway station, I kept my distance from strangers who approached me on the street. On subways, I would take the seat next to someone other than a street person even if the spot was farther away from me, or I'd sometimes even stand, rather than sit down next to him or her. Those who approached me on the sidewalk saying, "Hey, come here, I want to ask you something," rarely induced me to stray from my path. Certainly most homeless were probably harmless, but I usually didn't take any chances.

Yet here I was now having to take care of a street person. Bransky's hair was flecked with bits of fabric and dust. His clothing was ripped, brown, and crusted with spilled drink and food. He smelled—a dank, closed, dusty odor. He probably hadn't washed in several weeks.

The question was whether to Kwell him. I didn't see any insects, but I could have missed them and, after weighing the risks and benefits, decided to order Kwell, as a precaution for both him and others.

After I wrote the order and he showered, I completed the physical exam. His chart had said that he had bone cancer. My hand now lay over the left side of his chest, as required, to feel his heartbeat. Several ribs had been removed, and my fingers suddenly and unexpectedly sank into a soft mush of skin. His heart throbbed through the few remaining thin layers of doughy flesh, no longer protected from the outside by a grill-work of ribs. I had never felt a live human heart beating between my fingers, as vulnerably exposed. Most hearts can be felt only distantly and indirectly through the thick rib cage wall. I could have squeezed the pulsing organ.

I looked down at him as he lay there. He had dark brown

hair and eyes as I did, a similar large nose, and was Jewish, as was I. But he had cancer and lived on the street. I had neither of these problems.

Afterward I sat down and talked with him in my office.

"I can't go on like this anymore," he told me. "In the past thirty years, I've had fourteen or fifteen operations—I don't even remember how many anymore. They told me I'd only have a few years to live. Well, I've showed them, haven't I? I'm a survivor. But it's all finally gotten to me."

I asked him how he came to live on the street.

"My mother and sister refused to take me in anymore or help me out. They won't even accept my calls now when I phone them. So I have nowhere else to go. It's not easy, but I've managed to get by. My biggest problem is just getting treated like a human being, like everybody else. People think the homeless want to be homeless. Well, let me tell you something. No way do I want to be living on the street. I didn't ask for this. I didn't ask to be addicted to drugs. The surgeons put me on painkillers for my bone cancer, and I became addicted. You can't imagine what my life is like. A few weeks ago, somebody stole my cane when I was sleeping on a park bench. For a few days I couldn't get around. I was stuck on that bench. I couldn't leave it. I've also been mugged a few times—usually after getting my disability check. Last month three guys jumped me and took all my money. I tried hitting them with my cane, but I'm only one little guy. What can I do? It's very hard being out there all alone."

He described a life of hobbling from soup kitchen to shelter to welfare office, and from one doctor to another. He had been born and raised in Texas, but had left in his early twenties.

When we were done with our session, he slid off his chair to stand up, grabbed his cane with one hand, and shook my hand with his other. "Thank you for talking with me," he said. "A lot of docs don't give me the time of day."

I wrote orders for him and prescribed his usual dose of painkillers. Sandra, the social worker, managed to procure some money from the social work department to buy him a set of new clothes.

The next day, he approached me in the hall. "Dr. Klitzman, my arm hurts. Can I have some more pain medicine?" He had been to several drug detox and treatment programs, but had always ended up addicted again to painkillers and then methadone.

Still, I increased his dose slightly.

The next day, I was sitting in a small back room off the nursing station and overheard him at the doorway to the hall. "I want to see Dr. Klitzman," he told Alice.

"He's busy right now."

"But I need to see him."

I got up to speak with him. "Ronald, I can meet with you at three o'clock today."

"Can't I see you before that?"

"It's going to be hard."

"Can I have some more medicine in the meantime?"

"You got some this morning."

"I still ache."

Henry Nolan was watching from the nursing station. "That guy looks sedated," he said. "I wouldn't give him anymore." These medications were also addictive and could cause depression over time.

"It looks like you're on enough," I told Ronald.

"My surgeon always gives me a little extra."

"I think it's best not to increase the dose right now." He limped away sadly.

"How are things going?" I asked Ronald the next morning.

"I'm feeling better."

"Good. What have you been doing on the ward?"

"Nothing much. *Trying* to stay out of trouble."

"What do you mean?"

"I'll tell you, but please don't tell anyone else on the staff. I needed something, so I smoked a little pot in my room last night. Just half a joint. But please don't tell anyone. They'll get annoyed."

We talked longer, and then I left. When Henry Nolan met with me later to review my patients, I told him about Bransky's progress, without adding that he had smoked marijuana. Bransky had confided in me and asked me to keep a secret. I didn't want to betray him and side with the hospital against him. It felt unfair. Plus, if I did, he might not trust psychiatrists in the future. But I also felt uncomfortable allying with him over the rest of the staff. I thought about it further as Nolan spoke to me. Then, I told him that Bransky had used pot.

"That's against regulations," Nolan declared. "Throw him out."

"But he just got here and needs help. He wouldn't be here otherwise."

"If he smoked marijuana, he's out."

"But he may be depressed. Aren't we supposed to be trying to help him?"

"Policy is policy. He wouldn't have taken drugs if he really wanted to get better. The guy's simply a junkie—a druggie. Just hand him the address of the city shelter, and discharge him. Do it today. And make sure you document in the chart that you gave him the address."

"Can't we try to find him a place to go?" It was early fall, and getting cold outside.

"He can go to the shelter."

"But what if he doesn't make it there?" I was worried that he might end up sleeping on the street, and using more drugs.

"That's not our problem."

"If we throw him out, he might not come back again in the future if he needs help."

"If he doesn't come back, he doesn't come back. We have to be firm." The hospital's rules served, in part, to set an example to other patients. But kicking Bransky out didn't seem to be in his best interests. The institution could be harsh. Our ethical duty to help him conflicted with the policy of the institution. I suspected that if he weren't a street person, and unliked to begin with, he might have been allowed to stay.

Nolan was my boss and was more experienced, but didn't know Ronald as I did. Ronald was fighting cancer, on top of everything else. Couldn't we give the guy a break? Nolan thought not. In retrospect, I understand the need for rules. But at the time, the conflict between these issues wasn't even broached.

As a human being my feeling was to try to help him. But my professional role dictated that I kick him out. Professional requirements would sometimes oppose my personal inclinations. I would have to keep some patients I would have liked to discharge, and discharge some patients I would have liked to keep.

I met with Ronald to tell him the news. "I'm sorry, but using pot is against hospital rules. You're going to have to leave."

"Are you kidding me? I have surgical pain. I asked you for more medicine and you told me no. What was I supposed to do?"

"Those are the rules."

"Screw the rules. Aren't you supposed to help us patients?"

"Some rules can't be broken. You should have talked to me about it further. You're on more than your usual dose of opiates."

"What's wrong with needing drugs, anyway? You're just biased. You doctors just have middle-class values, that's all. Well let me tell you, a lot of great men have had drug and alcohol problems."

"Yeah. But a lot of not-so-great men, too."

He paused, and shifted his weight. "So now you're going to send me back out onto the street?" he asked, changing the subject. "That doesn't make much sense now, does it? When do I have to leave?"

"Today."

"Come on, it's cold out there. Can't I stay a little longer?"

"Dr. Nolan says you can't."

"You guys are incredible. If any of you faced the situation I did, you'd be in the same shape. You doctors just don't know. You're clueless. Don't they teach you anything in medical school? Unless you have the pain I have, you don't know what it's like. You think I want to be on drugs?" He shook his head and walked away. He packed up his single, worn bag with his one extra sweater and his few other belongings. An hour later he stood by the doorway, leaning his shrunken, asymmetric body unsteadily on his cane. "Thank you anyway," he said, shaking my hand. I handed him a piece of paper with the address of the shelter, even though he probably knew where it was.

"Do you need a token?"

He lifted his left shoulder up and thrust his hand into his pocket. He emerged with about seventy cents in change. "That's all the money I have."

I reached into my pocket, pulled out a token, and slipped it to him as he tottered precariously out the door. At least he could now make it all the way across town to the shelter. I had never before given something I owned to a patient. It was one of the only things he had gotten out of this hospitalization. Despite my initial wariness, I now somehow respected his fight and dream for dignity and self-preservation.

The following day was community meeting, where once a week doctors, nurses, other staff members, and patients all met, presumably to give patients the opportunity to feel we were all part of one community, and to avoid their feeling that the staff was somehow inaccessible. I announced that Ronald Bransky had been asked to leave because of using drugs on the unit.

"But he needs help just like we do," one patient said.

"Hear! hear!" an older man called out.

"I thought the hospital was for helping people," another patient said. "Not for kicking them out."

A few days later, Carol rushed up to me in the nursing station. "You'll never guess who I saw," she exclaimed. "Ronald Bransky. Sleeping in the train station. He had on the same clothes as when he left here. At least he was indoors and warm."

Outside, dried leaves had begun to fall from the trees and now scraped and eddied along the ground in the wind. I was relieved that Bransky at least had a roof over his head. I would have liked to have found out more about how he was doing, but couldn't call him or anyone else. It was impossible to know.

I was soon busy with other patients and their problems, and was surprised when a few weeks later a resident one year ahead of me, Lou Leftow, paged me. "Guess who I have?" he asked. I had no idea.

"Bransky."

Ronald had just been admitted to a surgical ward. Another of his bones had become tumorous and was removed. While recuperating, he had insisted that the tumor had also spread to his brain, though no evidence of this was found. Ronald believed the surgeons were lying. They requested that a psychiatrist evaluate him, which Lou had done. Lou now wanted to know if I'd take him back. I wanted to try, having sensed some of Ronald's vulnerability beneath his bravura, and concerned that another ward might too easily and unquestioningly dismiss him as a street person. I spoke to Nolan, who agreed to have Ronald readmitted if Lou Leftow would follow Ronald after eventual discharge.

"How are you doing?" I asked Ronald once he was back on our ward.

"I had an operation."

"How did it go?"

"They tell me okay. But I don't think so. There's cancer in my brain. I know it. There's something wrong with my thinking. Everyone's keeping the truth from me." He started to cry.

The surgeons had done a thorough evaluation.

I started to treat him with antidepressant and antipsychotic medications. At first, he dozed during the day and was frightened to leave his room. I visited him every day during the first week as was required for a new admission.

A few days later, he was standing against the wall in the corridor, grabbing at the air with his arm. "What are you doing, Ronald?"

"I'm reaching out for help." He continued swiping his fingers through the air with grave determination. I thought he was delusional and increased his antipsychotic medication.

A week later, he was walking up and down the ward more regularly. "My end is coming," he said. "I know it. It's just a matter of time." He still seemed depressed, and I increased his antidepressant. His depression and delusionality began to resolve.

"Can I talk with you?" he asked a week later.

"Okay. How about this afternoon?"

"Can you see me now?"

I paused, since I had several pressing tasks to complete. "Is it an emergency?"

He paused. "Sure," he said, "it's an emergency. I got pain. In my chest." He pointed toward his left breast. "Maybe it's my heart." Chest pain could be serious, and he was on drugs that could have cardiac side effects. I examined him, sent off blood tests, and performed an electrocardiogram to investigate the cause. But the tests were all negative.

"Why don't you try to lie down," I suggested afterward.

"Because that makes it feel worse. I don't feel right. Can't you give me more painkillers? I'm in pain."

"We'll leave the regimen as it is."

"Then I want to leave."

"How come?"

"Because you're not trying to help me." I suspected he was angry I wasn't giving him what he wanted.

"I am. Treatments take time. You need to be treated. Do you really want to go home now?"

"I have no home," he corrected me. "But I want to leave here, I can tell you that. I'll stay only on one condition: I get more pain meds and better food."

"No conditions."

He sneered. "I'm just another patient to you, while you're all learning."

"I think you should stay and get better."

"Maybe I'll stay a little longer. Maybe. But I'm only going to give you two more days. Do you hear that? Two more days." He spoke as if he were in a position to give orders and make threats. He was clearly getting better, returning to his old self. Yet he also wanted me to engage with him more. I would try, if possible.

The next day he waited for me by the door of the nursing station as I was leaving.

"Dr. Klitzman, I want to talk with you."

"Can it wait until tomorrow?" I had already met with him that day. Kasdin had advised residents to draw limits with patients and meet with them only three times a week, after the first week of a hospitalization.

"I'm hearing voices. . . . You know, in my head."

"When people aren't there?"

"No. Just when they're talking to me." He was confused and partly trying to feign psychosis.

I had to figure out exactly how much time to spend with him—in large part a subjective decision. "I'll meet with you tomorrow," I said with determination.

Ronald didn't leave as he had threatened and over the next few weeks improved further. He became less agitated and began to teach me about his life on the street and his drug use, explaining the street names of various drugs, and how people bought, sold, and used these substances.

Sandra submitted applications to housing facilities on his behalf. The waiting lists at these city-run agencies stretched from three months to a year. In the meantime, the hospital became a home for him. He was fed and protected. He began to chat with the nurses each day, joking with them. He also volunteered to be the patient representative on the ward, helping orient new patients to the floor, tottering around the halls giving them tours, showing them where the bathrooms and the laundry rooms were, introducing newcomers to other patients, and asking if they had any questions—always while wearing his yellow ski cap. One afternoon, I overheard him making numerous calls on the pay phone, arranging for a friend of his to be admitted to another, nearby hospital for help, phoning that hospital's admissions office and making all the necessary administrative arrangements.

Many substance abusers whom I had met in the hospital devoted themselves exclusively to seeking drugs. Ronald, however, now tried to extend himself to others in small ways. Drug abusers were generally hard to identify with. Some staff clearly thought he was "just another addict." But Bransky's pain had more obvious sources. He had medical problems, and had been utterly rejected by his family. He was more than someone just trying to get drugs.

Every Friday, the staff held walk rounds. We traveled from room to room, speaking with each patient briefly.

"How are you doing, Ronald?" I asked when our entourage entered his room.

"Fine, thanks."

Nolan interrupted. "Why are you still here?"

"I'm not ready to leave yet."

"But we can't keep you here forever." Medicaid might not reimburse the hospital for the period while he was awaiting a housing program.

"But I don't want to go."

"I think you're ready. Talk to Dr. Klitzman about it." Nolan turned and we all began to leave his room.

"Wait, team," Ronald called out. We halted. I wondered if he would try to plead his case. "Can I join you all on walk rounds?" No patient had ever requested to join us before. He was asking, in effect, to be made an honorary member of the staff. Everybody burst out laughing—including Ronald. He knew we wouldn't let him, but it was the biggest laugh a patient had ever managed to elicit from the staff.

Still, his humor was a sign that he was better. Depressed patients rarely joke or laugh. Sadly and ironically, his jest indicated that he was ready to return to the street.

Nolan set Ronald's discharge date for the following Monday, right after Thanksgiving.

That Saturday, while I was on call, Ronald and some other patients organized a Thanksgiving party in the hospital gym.

"Dr. Klitzman, are you coming to the party tonight?" he asked when I passed him in the hall.

"Maybe." I would be the only doctor there, which would make me feel out of place.

"I'm going to be there," he said, poking his thumb into his chest. "It's sort of my going-away party, too. You should join us. You get to see what we patients are like when you doctors aren't around. That's important for you young doctors to know about. I want to see you there." He pointed at me with his index finger and winked. I was surprised at the extent to which he liked me and was attached to me beneath his gruff exterior.

That evening, the hospital wards were quiet. I stood by the elevators, about to press the down button to return to my sequestered on-call room.

Instead I pushed the up button, to go to the gym.

Patients had decorated the large room. Strips of yellow, orange, and brown crepe paper looped down from the ceiling, and maple leaves, turkeys, and Pilgrims painted by patients decorated the walls, affixed with Scotch tape. A mirrored ball hung in the middle of the room. The gym was darkened. Disco music shook the floor. In the center of the dance floor Ronald in his yellow cap was rock-and-rolling with Carol. His two legs were of unequal length, and he tottered unevenly as he danced. Because of the limited motion of his body, he rocked backward and forward, his weight balanced primarily on his stronger and longer leg. His arms, one of which was shortened as a result of surgery, swung back and forth in the air. His face was solemn but energetic. He probably hadn't danced in years.

Several other patients discoed as well. One lightly pranced, another cavorted sloppily but with enthusiasm. Jimmy Lentz, who was still in the hospital but had been doing better and was about to be discharged, danced as well. He came over to me and pointed out two watercolor paintings on the wall he had made—one of a turkey, and another of a roller coaster, the track rising up and down flat against the surface, with buildings and small people behind the metal grid. His mother was dancing, too, and probably hadn't enjoyed herself this much since her son had been hospitalized several months earlier. She smiled and swayed her arms about her with smooth rhythm. She probably hadn't been out dancing in years. The nurses asked several patients to join them and many patients walked onto the dance floor with the staff, though not with each other. I hovered near the doorway, watching, my clipboard still in my hand. The patients were having fun, unlike during the week, when doctors were continually hovering about, scrutinizing them. Tonight they were not being watched, observed, and treated. Here, for once, they were free, moving their bodies as they pleased, not acting like patients but like dancers at a club. For the first time since I had begun to work in the hospital, they were not identifiable as patients. On the ward, even when sitting on chairs, some stared off into space or seemed zombielike—in part because of medications. But now they looked like anybody else.

If it hadn't been for Ronald, I wouldn't have been there.

A short-haired woman approached me, smiling. "Hi. I'm Diana from OT." She was wearing a red jumpsuit with a white stick-on name tag that said "diana" in lowercase letters, written with a red magic marker, with a circle dotting the i. "Do you want to put down your clipboard and join us?"

"I have to leave in a few moments," I said. "No, thank you."

Carol sent one of the patients over to me. The patient offered me her arm to escort me onto the dance floor. "May I?" she asked.

Again, I politely declined.

Carol herself eventually sauntered over to me. "The party is bringing out lots of sexual energies and tensions between the patients," she said.

"I can see."

"Would you like to dance?"

I would have liked to participate. I generally liked dancing but felt constrained in my white coat. Somehow dancing with patients went against the sense I had been given of how a psychiatrist was supposed to behave. If I were with friends, I would have danced. But I felt very much that my position here was different. "No, thank you," I answered.

"Why not?"

"Because I'm the only doctor here."

"That doesn't matter." But I wondered whether my relationships with patients would change if I looked ridiculous boogying on the floor. In my long white coat, I felt the force of social roles keeping me apart from patients and felt obliged to preserve a professional distance between us, in part to make it easier to be clear and effective with Ronald and other patients when necessary. I was their psychiatrist, not a dance partner. I didn't want to blur my role as a therapist by socializing with patients. I felt bad not taking part, and not being as spontaneous as I would have been if at a party of friends. I didn't enjoy this position. My job required me to adjust and restrict my behavior, which disheartened me. I was surprised at how strongly this division had already been ingrained in me.

But, most important, the evening belonged to the patients and was their chance to be away from doctors. Few had spotted me in the corner, and I thought it best for them not to see me, reminding them of the fact that they were in a mental institution. If they wanted momentarily to forget it, I would let them.

I stayed a few moments longer and then left.

That night on my ten o'clock walk rounds, the patients were all asleep, which was extremely unusual. Ordinarily several were up, troubled, but tonight they were all exhausted. I had never seen the hospital as calm.

On Monday, Ronald was discharged. He packed his small sack, and shook my hand. As he left, a tear rolled down his cheek.

Lou Leftow followed Ronald as an outpatient. I occasionally spotted Ronald teetering on the sidewalks around the hospital, working his way through the building's revolving doors with his cane. "Dr. Klitzman," I would hear. There would be Ronald in his yellow cap. "I had another operation," he told me a few weeks after his discharge. "But this time I'm doing better."

Lou Leftow also kept me updated. With each welfare check, Ronald now paid to have his ski parka, his hat, and his few other articles of clothing dry-cleaned. He stayed at different shelters, so didn't pay any rent or utilities.

Ronald never kept appointments with Lou Leftow. He just came by whenever he could. Other patients were required to have scheduled appointments. No other patient had such a special, ad hoc relationship with the hospital.

Ronald started staying at a small shelter affiliated with a local church. The director of this shelter, Gerald Turner, called me up one day. Ronald had given him my name as one of "his doctors." Turner wanted to know how to reach me if he ever needed to get help for his "client." "Ronald can be a pain in the ass sometimes." Turner laughed. "But you have to admit he's a character."

"That he is."

Guests on Checks

The fall continued to pass quickly, as countless patients were admitted and discharged. Before I knew it, the weather grew even chillier, and winter arrived.

On Christmas Eve I was on call. It seemed everyone else in the city was out celebrating with friends and family except for the patients and me. Almost all the patients remained locked on the wards.

I was busy with various tasks, though there were no new admissions as the evening progressed. Not many families chose Christmas Eve as the time to bring a loved one to the emergency room to be admitted. An insulated tranquillity pervaded the building, as if we were together on a ship during a long voyage, isolated and unable to leave, but sailing along, secure thus far, and hopefully free of any oncoming storms.

"I can't believe it's Christmas Eve," I heard one patient say to another in the lounge. "Look at us, just sitting here."

"What do you want to do?" another patient asked. "Sing Christmas carols?"

As I was walking by the patient cafeteria on the twelfth floor, having finally completed my errands, I passed a patient, Sally McIver, in the hall. "Merry Christmas, Dr. Klitzman," she said in a frail voice.

"Merry Christmas, Miss McIver."

"Thank you." She crinkled the edges of her lips upward slightly, a faint, barely perceptible smile. It was the first time I had ever seen her smile. "Would you like some cake left over from our holiday party?" she asked.

"Yeah, have some cake," another patient added.

Alice had frequently told residents, "Never eat food from the patient dining room. It's for the patients only." A small

97

kitchen attached to the dining room usually stored leftovers and snacks. But now the patients themselves were offering me food. I was starved, not having had a chance to eat dinner yet, though it was around 11:00 P.M., and having been working nonstop.

"And have some punch," Sally said, pouring some from a plastic pitcher into a paper cup. I wasn't supposed to be accepting food from them, but it was Christmas.

"Thank you," I said, grateful for their gifts.

"You're welcome. I hope your Christmas Eve is okay here."

I returned to the on-call room and found myself humming as I sat down with nothing to do for the moment. "Have yourself a merry little Christmas, a merry little Christmastime . . ." I hoped it would stay quiet and that I wouldn't be awakened that night.

Yet like everything else in the hospital, Christmas was filled with the unexpected.

My beeper suddenly started squeaking shrilly.

A patient was being admitted downstairs, and I went to meet her. Denise Neston was a thin woman with long blond hair. Earlier in the day her boyfriend had said he wanted to break up with her. She thought of jumping from her roof but instead left a message on her answering machine that she was about to kill herself, and then hailed a taxi and came to the hospital.

"Have you called your boyfriend back to tell him you're okay?" I asked her.

"No way. I bet he and his friends are sitting around Christmas Eve dinner right now worried about me and talking about how I sabotaged their holiday." She smiled.

"It would be important to tell them. I'm sure he's concerned about you."

"Tough shit." She crossed her arms.

"I think it would be good for you to call."

"I'm going to wait a little while longer," she said, "and let them all worry about me."

This, I realized, was textbook sadism. Christmas brought out the best and the worst in patients. They were a hard group to categorize as a whole.

I spoke to one of the nurses on the floor, who said, "I'll put her on checks," and went to the nursing station blackboard and in a box that said "Guests on Checks" wrote "Neston." Every twenty minutes a staff member would go by and make sure she was okay. The nurse also agreed to talk with her about the situation with her boyfriend. I went to write up an admission note and finish other tasks that had arisen.

I was walking by the twelfth floor nursing station when the doorbell rang.

"Bransky!" I heard Carol exclaim when she opened the door.

I looked down the hall. Ronald was leaning on his cane, wearing his yellow cap. His hair, hanging below the band of his hat, was clean and neatly cut. "What are you doing here?"

"I came to wish everyone a Merry Christmas. I was in the neighborhood and thought I'd stop by."

"What were you doing around here?"

"Well," he said, looking down at the ground. "I really didn't have anywhere else to go."

Most patients are relieved to leave the hospital. I had never heard of any returning to visit socially. But Christmas was a time to visit close friends and families. Ronald, living on the street, was visiting us.

"Merry Christmas, Ronald," Carol said, smiling. "But how did you get in here?"

"They all know me downstairs. How's Donna doing?" he asked, changing the subject. "How's Jimmy Lentz?"

"He finally went home."

"Did he manage to go back to high school like he wanted?"

"No, he's going to a day program."

"Oh well. That's too bad. But at least he got home. How's Dr. Klitzman?"

Carol looked up at me, standing halfway down the hall. "Dr. Klitzman!" Bransky yelled. I started toward him. He reached out to give me a big hug. Though I was glad to see him, it didn't seem appropriate to hug him, and I reached to intercept his hand to shake it. He lifted his other hand up into the air and patted me on the arm.

"Hi, Ronald. You got a haircut."

"And I got my beard trimmed, too!" he said proudly.

"It looks good."

"You think so?" he beamed. "Thanks. I did it for the holidays."

"How have you been doing?"

"Okay. Except," he lowered his voice and moved closer to me, "for the one time when I almost seized."

"You what?"

"I had taken a Valium or two . . . and a few other things . . . Sinequan and . . . that's about it."

"You have to be careful with street drugs. Your body's more sensitive than it used to be." He looked thinner. "It reacts more strongly to smaller amounts, Mr. Bransky . . ."

"Ronald," he corrected me quickly, smiling. He had caught a change in my tone from friend to professional.

I spoke with him for a few minutes but had other duties awaiting me. "I have to run," I finally said. I felt bad but didn't have a choice. "Good luck," I said, shaking his hand on his shorter arm. Carol and Ronald remained standing in the hallway conversing for a few moments. There was nowhere else on the ward they could go. He was neither a patient with a room nor a staff member with an office. Carol offered him some desserts that patients' families had donated to the staff. He loaded his hands and coat pockets with cookies and candy, then left. I didn't know when I'd next see him.

Two weeks later, in the first week of January, changeover occurred, when residents switched wards, severing ties with patients and staff on one floor, only to start new ones elsewhere. For weeks, every time Dr. Kasdin saw us, he asked, "How are your patients dealing with your leaving?" I had assigned them to Joe Tauber, the resident who was replacing me on the floor. The patients accepted it. A few said they'd miss me. Many had been through decades of young residents rotating through their lives.

I didn't know the fate of many of the patients I had seen and was leaving behind. Unless patients happened to cross my path again, there would be no way to find out what became of them or how they fared. We were continually overloaded with concerns about new patients whom we would see only briefly, as they passed quickly through our purview. The fact that we would know these people for only short periods of time encouraged us to focus only on particular aspects of patients' cases, rather than entering their lives more fully. Residency continually taught us to distance ourselves somewhat from our patients, to be less involved than we might otherwise be in the care of any one patient, and not to see our interactions with them as ongoing, thus justifying less of an emotional investment. It felt unfair to them. I would miss many of them and the staff as well. A few days later, Kasdin said, "It's the end of your rotation." I repeated the phrase to myself. I didn't think of it as a rotation, as something I was just passing through. It was the longest job I had ever had in one place: even as an intern I had stayed on wards for only one month at a time. As a result, my education before had been more external to me, more easily contained. Now, work had become a part of me, the ward a home. Here, I had gotten to know the patients over weeks and months, and had developed a rapport with the nurses. I would leave them all now, probably never work with them again, and would go on to get to know others. This system also served to keep residents and nurses separate. We trainees were just revolving through. The nurses stayed behind. It made us different.

Anne, Mike, Sarah, and I went out to dinner the night before leaving the ward. After eating, we strolled back to Anne's apartment, put on music, and danced around. She had a goofy Snoopy hat with floppy ears and sunglasses attached. We each tried on the hat and jumped, swinging our arms up and down to make the ears flap. We had come to know each other fairly well. We had all started out together and had seen each other's beginner's mistakes.

"I'm on tomorrow," Mike finally said with hesitation, meaning he was on call. Quietly, we all went home.

On the last day, the staff scheduled a goodbye party for us. They served us fruit punch and cookies.

The staff gave each of us a gift. Mine was in a small box wrapped in yellow and green printed paper, tied with thick white yarn.

"Should I open it now?" I asked Carol.

"Yes."

It was a glass mushroom paperweight—shiny, clear, and filled with air bubbles reflecting and refracting the light into glints of color like a prism. It was the first gift I had ever received in a professional setting.

A card was attached. "Congratulations," it read, "on surviving the 12th floor."

"Is that a phallic symbol?" Kasdin immediately asked me, slinking over.

"What do *you* think?" I retorted.

He didn't answer, but quickly scurried away.

The other residents had also been given glass paperweights in different shapes—a strawberry, an apple, and a pear. The nurses and other staff had been very kind to give us presents.

Kasdin came up to me at the end of the party. "I want to sit down with each of you for a few minutes before you go."

"Tell me about the unit," he said when I met him after the party.

"What specifically?"

"How were the nurses?"

"They were good."

"How was Alice? ... How was Carol? ... How was Henry?" I told him there were occasional problems with the staff but that they generally tried hard to do their job. I felt awkward reporting on everyone else, as he wanted both formed opinions and fleeting, subjective impressions. Everyone apparently talked about everyone else on the ward. I'm sure he asked them about us. This intense reporting felt excessive. Everything I said to anyone was liable to be repeated to someone else. The subjective and personal were blurred with the professional and scientific. This community felt very enmeshed and intrusive. Yet he was asking me what I thought of others and was accepting and respecting my opinions. I was now considered one of the authorities on the floor, offering criticism of the nurses and other staff members who only a few months ago had been the experts, while residents were all novices.

Kasdin also gave us our evaluations—nine-page forms with more than sixty questions that he had answered about each of us.

Yet though he knew a lot about us, we knew almost nothing about him. I had worked with Dr. Kasdin and Dr. Nolan for several months, yet didn't know where they lived, if they were married or had children, had hobbies or outside interests, or anything else about their lives. I had had jobs during summers where I had gotten at least some sense about my boss's life. But here, no one seemed to find it odd that nothing was known about them. In their relations with the staff they followed a psychoanalytic model. Yet these men weren't conducting psychoanalysis with anyone here.

Later that day, I bumped into Joe, who was finishing on the fifteenth floor where I would be starting Monday. "All ready for the changeover?" I asked.

"Are you?"

"Our floor's been talking about it for weeks."

"Not on fifteen," he said. "It was brought up once a week ago. Someone said, 'We should talk about the changeover.' 'Okay,' everyone agreed, but no one had anything to say about it. Then today, the nurses just freaked out about it. Time passes slowly up there. You're on your own and get little help or attention from the attendings"—that is, faculty members. "The unit chief's never around. Some say it's the Land of the Dinosaurs up there. It's another world—completely different from what I hear about twelve."

PART II

House Wine

I had gotten used to one ward and would now have to learn about and adjust to another. I had seen how various issues were important on the twelfth floor but didn't know if they would be on other wards as well. Wards differed only by the staff—particularly the unit chief and associate unit chief, and their respective areas of expertise, personalities, and styles.

But it soon became apparent that, as a result, each ward constituted a different social environment—a different culture—each framing what I did and learned, and how I grew and developed as a psychiatrist, and each shaping the experiences of patients as well. As it turned out, the twelfth and fifteenth floors could not have been more different.

On my first day there, Pam, one of the nurses, came up to me and squeezed my arm. She was short and had black hair with dyed red streaks in it. She was wearing tight black jeans, a black blouse, and black sneakers. "You have a new admission," she told me. "She's in the lounge with her daughter. Name is Blanca Díaz. She's a winner."

"What do you mean?"

"You'll see." She walked off, giggling to herself.

I walked down the hall to the lounge. There in the middle of the room stood an elderly woman wearing a simple, light blue day dress and a pair of light blue bedroom slippers with faded gold stitching.

"Hello, I'm Dr. Klitzman," I said, approaching her. She smiled and nodded. I reached out to shake her hand. She raised her hand and shook mine. "And you're her daughter?" I asked, turning to a younger woman slumped in a chair, looking exhausted.

107

"Yes. Bonita López."

"Why don't you come to my office, Mrs. Díaz?" Mrs. Díaz smiled and nodded but didn't move. "I'd like to talk to you in my office." She looked confusedly at her daughter.

"Mrs. Díaz?"

"She doesn't speak English, Doctor."

"She doesn't speak English?"

"Not really, Doctor. No. I just brought her here from Honduras to be seen here in the hospital." Unfortunately, I don't speak Spanish.

"Okay. Why don't you both come to my office?"

In my office Bonita said, "My mother's not been herself. For the past two years she's been getting more and more confused. She had been living by herself. But I don't think she can anymore. She wanders out in the middle of the night. My sister and I are afraid and don't trust her by herself anymore. My doctor suggested we bring her here to America to have her seen. Our whole town pooled money together so she could come. I'm hoping that maybe you can do something that will make her better."

Mrs. Díaz rose from her chair. Her gray hair was pinned up. She patted my arm and wandered over to the window behind my chair, her hands clasped behind her back as she surveyed the streets below.

Mrs. Díaz shuffled back over to my desk and sat down. She leaned over toward my blotter and pulled a tissue out of a small flat box of Kleenex issued by the hospital. She removed another tissue, then another. She soon removed all ten remaining in the box. She smiled at me, then refolded each, flattened them neatly, and inserted them back into the box. She nodded again as if looking for a small sign of approval from me. I nodded back. She still seemed aware of her environment and tried to engage with it as best she could.

"Can you help us, Doctor?"

"We'll see what we can do."

Some causes of dementia are treatable. "Dementia is not normal even among the elderly," Nolan had once told us. Mrs. Díaz could have a medical problem—cancer, infection, neurological disease—potentially "reversible causes" to be ruled out. I ordered a barrage of blood tests, X rays, and scans, hoping to find a cause that we could correct.

* * *

The next day, Pam read the morning report. "Blanca Díaz appeared to be settling in, though she wandered around into other patients' rooms and took other patients' combs, hairbrushes, and cassette tapes."

"Does she have a tape player?"

"No. She swiped an Elton John tape with a colorful cover. I think she just liked it."

The blood results began to come back, all within normal limits.

At community meeting that afternoon, there was no patient agenda, and Roy, the floor's fourth-year resident and thus the assistant unit chief, asked if there were any complaints. No one said anything. I scanned the circle of patients and staff. Mrs. Díaz caught my eye, smiled, and waved to me, no doubt not understanding what was happening, but perfectly content to be a part of the gathering.

"How's everyone feel about the treatment here?" Roy asked.

"Fine," one woman said.

"We're all sedated," another patient added.

I wanted to speak with Mrs. Diaz and procured a translator— Gina, the secretary in the outpatient department. I asked Mrs. Díaz some questions. She had problems with addition and subtraction but seemed to appreciate my attention.

"Tell her she's not allowed to take things from other patients' rooms," I told Gina. Mrs. Díaz on hearing the translation smiled and nodded. She reached out and patted me on the hand.

"Does she understand?"

Mrs. Díaz again smiled at me and nodded. I still wasn't sure.

The next day Pam read through morning report. "Mrs. Díaz gets more confused at night and continues to wander into other patients' rooms." Pam looked up from her book. "It's getting to be the social event of the evening around here, retrieving things from her room—sweaters, shampoo, books. She seems more organized during the day but becomes disoriented at night"—a phenomenon termed "sundowning," and often seen with elderly demented patients.

"I think it's time to start an antipsychotic," I said. We usually watched patients who were off medication at first to see exactly what was wrong without the confounding effects of drugs.

"How about Navane?" Cynthia Nelson, the occupational therapist, or OT, said. "That's the house wine up here." Navane was an antipsychotic medication or so-called major tranquilizer. This medication was popular, as it produced only a moderate amount of the two kinds of side effects commonly seen in this family of drugs. Some drugs produced a lot of sedation and possible drop in blood pressure when standing up. Other drugs produced a lot of muscle stiffness. Navane could result in both sets of side effects, but to lesser degrees.

"I think a little vitamin H would be better in this particular case," Roy said. He was referring to Haldol, used in elderly psychotic patients to "organize" their thinking and in geriatric patients on many medical wards to help calm agitation or confusion. The medicine caused much less sedation and blood pressure decrease than Navane and other drugs, though it could yield more stiffness. Added sedation and a drop in blood pressure, however, were particularly unwanted in elderly people who may already have some cardiac or cognitive impairment which wouldn't be exacerbated by stiffness. In general, sedation bothered some patients more than others. Navane could be used more widely in younger patients for psychosis. But the point is that these medications could be tailored to individual patients, and selected in order to produce the least undesirable set of side effects for a particular person. Unfortunately, we could predictably adjust these medications' side effects far better than their relative benefits.

I started Mrs. Díaz on a low dose of Haldol.

"Do you know where you are?" I had Gina ask her in Spanish two days later.

Mrs. Díaz answered and Gina translated. "This is the House of God, the Gateway to Heaven."

"Do you know who I am?"

"An Angel of God."

"How have you been doing?"

She looked worried. "There is evil in this world."

I nodded in agreement, but ordered her dose of Haldol to be increased.

Mrs. Díaz began to wander less and soon understood she was in a hospital, though she was still not aware of the date. She became calmer but remained forgetful.

The tests continued to come back negative. I ordered others, but as is usually the case, there was no clear reversible cause of her dementia. As a result it was concluded that she had Alzheimer's dementia. As a diagnosis, I coded in her chart, "NDDAT"—nondiagnosable dementia of the Alzheimer's type. There was no treatment for the illness. Haldol helped one symptom and organized her so she wouldn't wander as before, but we couldn't reverse the dementia or treat its underlying cause.

I asked the unit chief, Dr. Randolph Johnson, if there was anything else I could be doing for her. He shook his head. I also asked Roy. "No," he said, "they came here to the Mecca and got an answer." Mrs. Díaz wasn't going to get any better.

I hadn't entered her life very much compared to my treatment of patients on the twelfth floor. The case seemed much more straightforward than cases there. Faculty were also much less involved. I was, indeed, more on my own.

I phoned Bonita, had her come in, and told her that we wouldn't be able to make her mother any better than she was now. I was disappointed and felt bad that after all their effort and expense, we couldn't offer more. "I'm sorry," I said.

"Thank you, Doctor," Bonita said, patting my hand twice, and then resting her hand on the table between us. "At least you tried. And we did, too."

Medicine and psychiatry provide order and the possibility of hope, even if no treatment. I relieved some of the helplessness Mrs. Díaz's daughter and family must have felt. They had gotten the answer that nothing else could be done—definitive, even if not good news, and better than no answer at all. How odd that we would manage a patient for a few weeks, but in the end do very little to change his or her situation. Clearly, we served other functions than treating or curing. This conclusion was surprising, given how much effort and expectation we invested in remedying every case. No one commented that in some regard our work with Mrs. Díaz had been for naught. Our efforts with her were over, and we would simply go on to the next case, busying ourselves with the problems it presented, and all but forgetting patients who had recently departed.

Bonita said she would take her mother back home and continue to look after her there. In the United States, Mrs. Díaz undoubtedly would have been shipped to a nursing home where she would eventually die. But in her native land, few such institutions existed, and Bonita and her sisters would take their mother in and care for her. In that respect Mrs. Díaz was fortunate and would probably have a higher quality of life.

Though she had a language barrier and dementia, she was still clearly a person, a human being with strong emotions. Though her brain had cognitive impairments, she liked me and I liked her. She couldn't add or subtract, but she could still love and feel wanted. Though from a poorer country, she would be surrounded by loved ones more than if she lived here. Despite our country's technological sophistication, in some ways we were very limited.

Bonita and Mrs. Díaz finally departed. "If you ever come to Honduras, let us know," Bonita said, handing me a piece of paper with their address. I told her I would.

My own family was in town that night and took me out to dinner.

"So how are all the crazies doing?" my younger sister Lisa asked. She was now a sophomore in college. Her question annoyed me, crudely labeling the varied individuals I cared for in many ways. I found myself being protective of them. She was implicitly criticizing them. Friends and family frequently posed similiar questions. It reflected a certain distance people try to create between the so-called mentally disturbed in mental institutions, and the rest of us, supposedly normal.

"I had a dream last night," my sister went on. "Are you going to tell me what it means?"

"If you want, I will try. What was the dream?"

She relayed an anxiety dream she had had before going that morning to an interview for a summer job. "Well, what do you think?" she asked.

"What are your thoughts about what it means?" It was important to understand her associations to it and to see how aware she was of what I suspected its underlying themes to be before I presented my impressions. I wanted to tell her my interpretation in a way that would make most sense to her, be most palatable, and tap into whatever sense of it she had, into her own understanding of herself, so that the comment would be most helpful or interesting, and least foreign to her. People can be resistant to issues raised in their own dreams, defending against unconscious conflicts. Our unconscious puts into our dreams many of the themes with which we are having the most trouble dealing.

"Oh God!" she moaned. "That's such a typical psychiatrist's thing to do. Ask a psychiatrist a question and he just asks you one back. What use are you? Why are you so interested in psychiatry anyway?"

It was very hard to describe the profession and what went on inside a psychiatric hospital to someone who hadn't been or worked in one, even to a member of my own family who saw my ordeals and travails.

Two weeks after I started on the ward Dr. Johnson's birthday arrived.

I was invited, along with the rest of the staff, to a birthday party for him.

The event was held in his apartment, a penthouse in a tall apartment building not far from the hospital, furnished with conservative Americana, Currier & Ives prints, and English antiques.

"Hey Bob Big Boy!" I heard when I entered the party. Pam sidled up to me. She was wearing black leather pants and vest, and a black T-shirt. Her black hair was even more moussed up and blown-dry than usual. "Let's party. Are you going to dance with me?"

"Maybe." I walked into the next room, where Cynthia Nelson, the occupational therapist, had arrived earlier to line up the dining table and several bridge tables end to end to form one long surface. She had unrolled a sheet of white paper twelve feet long and a yard wide, and had dumped boxes of crayons along the edges. "We're making a big mural," she called out to me. "Everybody has to do some. Then we're going to display it." Several nurses had drawn a picture of the hospital building, looking small and homey with a few curtained windows and a peaked roof, as if in a fairy tale. On the outside stood big bushy apple trees and yellow daffodils with long green leaves sprouting gently out of the ground all around. The nurses also drew smiling self-portraits. These drawings, with their innocence, could never have been done on Steve Kasdin's ward, where even the littlest gestures were interpreted. Yet the fifteenth floor seemed to function just as well as his. Perhaps all his added psychoanalytic interpretations and overlay weren't, in the end, necessary.

Part of the mural was a mock nursing station blackboard. But instead of—"Sharps Alert," "Matches Alert," and "Guests on Checks"—the categories in the nursing station—someone had written "Husband Alert" followed by a colon and Pam's name. Someone had written "Boots Alert" and put in Anne's name. "Black Loafers Alert" and put in my name. I wrote "Mousse Alert" and wrote in Pam.

Henrietta Baker, the head nurse, rolled out a cake. She was tall and thin, with graying, curly black hair, and was in her fifties. She was considerate but somewhat formal and reserved.

"Just don't ask me how old I am," Dr. Johnson said as he stood before a dense patch of birthday candles. He was an elderly, dignified-looking man—of medium height, bald, and with silver spectacles. He was an exception in the hospital in that he had expertise in neither psychoanalysis nor psychopharmacology, having trained decades earlier when a faculty member could get by without specializing in either.

He spread out his fingers, arms behind him, and leaned forward—a baseball umpire's gesture for "safe." Then he blew out all of the flames. Everyone applauded.

"Thank you, Henrietta," he said, going over to her and kissing her on the cheek.

No residents had spoken to him all night, but I decided to go wish him happy birthday. When I approached his group, he quickly turned away. I was surprised. He went around speaking at length to all of the nurses, greeting and kissing them, especially the older ones who had been there as long as he had—for two or three decades. Throughout the course of the evening he didn't talk to any residents for more than a quick moment, and rapidly left them as he had me.

It suddenly occurred to me that the other residents and I were transients here. Everybody else had known each other and worked together for years. Although the ward was a crucial place in my training and education, residents were just passing through—like the patients. What was valued here was length of stay, time of association. In that regard, this ward evoked those in mental institutions in the 1950s and 1960s before deinstitutionalization. Time passed slowly. The fewer changes, the better. I stayed for a while longer at the party and then slipped out.

Home

Increasingly, I saw that though psychiatry viewed itself as a science, much of what happened to patients resulted not from psychotherapy or drug treatments, but from complicated social and administrative problems unfolding and getting worked on. I was learning, for example, the importance of knowing and negotiating about different social settings.

When one of the other residents on the floor, Todd Spitzer, went on vacation, he assigned me to cover his patient Maxine Bailey. He hastily introduced us the day before he left. "This is Dr. Klitzman, who'll be your doctor while I'm away," Todd informed her.

"I'm leaving to get my own apartment soon, you know," she told me as the three of us stood together in the hallway. She was a small, thin black woman with straightened hair.

"I'm not sure you'll be ready," Todd said, shaking his head, clearly indicating that he thought she wasn't. "But you can work that out with Dr. Klitzman."

The following Monday when we met she announced, "I'm getting my own apartment. And I don't like this medication."

"Why not?"

"The side effects."

"What side effects are you experiencing?"

"It's making my head swell."

"Where?"

"Here." She pointed to her temple. Head swelling is not a side effect of the medication. But if she said her head was swollen maybe something was wrong. My finger pressed against her scalp to check. Her hair was greasy, but her head wasn't swollen.

"It doesn't feel swollen."

"But it is. I know it is." She seemed delusional.

I continued the drug. That afternoon, the team met and felt that she had benefited as much as she would in the hospital from the medication, and that it was time to figure out her discharge plans. "She wants her own apartment," Audrey Cahill, the social worker, said. Audrey had short black hair and long polished nails.

"She can't possibly handle her own place," Cynthia replied. "She has to be transferred to a residential facility." These institutions, for psychiatric patients on public assistance who usually had been homeless, were generally not very pleasant.

"Why can't she have her own place?" Audrey asked.

"She's too disorganized. She can't shop for herself or keep the place clean or balance a checkbook. In art therapy, she tried knitting a scarf for herself but had trouble with the different colored yarns. She needs to be in a residential facility."

"But she refuses it. If she wants her own apartment, who are we to say she can't have it?"

"You're her physician," Cynthia said, turning to me. "What do you think?"

"I've had her for only one day. But she still seems somewhat delusional to me."

"See?" Cynthia said proudly, grinning at Audrey.

"Are there any other options?" I asked, not wanting to coerce the patient.

"No," Cynthia interrupted. She wasn't being very flexible.

"Doesn't she have some family?" I asked.

"Two sisters."

"Will they take her in?"

"They both said no," Audrey reported. "They've tried before and think she's too difficult to live with. Both have families of their own, and live in small apartments without any extra room."

"So she has to be told she needs a residence," Cynthia said.

"I'm warning you," Audrey said, "she won't go for it." I wondered how this debate would eventually be resolved.

"Bob, why don't you tell her?" Cynthia suddenly suggested.

"But I barely know her."

"But it'll sound best coming from a doctor."

Everyone agreed with this solution.

"The team," I said to Maxine later that day, "has decided that you need to go to a residence." I didn't like telling her that she couldn't try living outside of an institution, especially as we had just met. But my medical degree apparently gave me the authority to determine important domestic, nonmedical aspects of her life.

"No. I'm getting my own apartment."

"The team feels you can't handle that."

"Yes I can. And if not, I'll stay with my sister Roberta."

"Has she agreed to that?"

"Yes."

"How do you know?"

"I asked her."

"She told us you couldn't stay there."

"She's my sister. It's okay with her."

A few hours later, she went up to OT and eloped. I called her two sisters to tell them.

That night, two huge policemen in blue uniforms hauled Maxine back to the ward in handcuffs. She had showed up at her sister Roberta's, who had promptly called the cops, saying that an escapee from a mental institution was in her home. Roberta demanded the police transport Maxine back. When the officers arrived, Maxine refused to go and sat on the sofa, adamant that she would not move. The police handcuffed her, yanked her up off the couch, and dragged her out.

"Why don't you want to go to a residence?" I asked her the next day.

"I've lived in a residency before. It was dirty, and I didn't like it. I want my own apartment."

"But we don't think you'll be able to manage in your own apartment."

"Well." She shook her large head back and forth. "Then I'll stay at my sister Valerie's."

"But she can't have you there either."

"Oh yes she can."

"Have you asked her?"

"Yes."

"And what did she say?"

"That I can stay there."

"But you said that about Roberta—that she was willing to have you stay there."

"Yeah."

"But when you showed up there, she called the police and had you returned here in handcuffs."

"Well, I never said I'd stay there."

"You did."

"No, you must be confused." I must be confused? "So what, anyway?" she continued.

"Now you're saying Valerie will let you stay with her. But that doesn't sound realistic."

"It is."

"Where would you sleep?"

"In the living room."

"Does anyone else sleep there?"

"Her three daughters."

"How long would that work out for? You need somewhere you can stay for a year or two."

"I can do it there."

"Does that make sense to you?"

"Yes. She's my sister. And I'm only going to stay there until I find an apartment." We had gone full circle. What a pain. She had her own logic, and it was impossible to reason with her. A little bell went off in my head. This was psychotic-like resistance—a different entity from what I was used to in my day-to-day interactions. Medical school and classes on psychological theory hadn't trained me for this.

"Next case," Dr. Johnson announced at team the next day.

"Maxine Bailey," I said.

Cynthia and Audrey immediately started arguing.

"Bob, what do you think?" Cynthia interrupted to ask.

In principle, I agreed with Audrey, and couldn't blame Maxine for not wanting to live in an institution. Philosophically, I believe in individual liberty and freedom. But Cynthia—the expert on social and occupational functioning—thought Maxine couldn't handle it. Also, Maxine was still mildly delusional, about this issue for example. To prevent her from doing what she wanted felt punitive and restrictive. Maxine might be able to make it on her own. But as a psychiatrist, my professional recommendation had to be that she not take the risk of failure and of subsequent exacerbation of her illness. I would have to put aside my personal sympathies for her plight. Officially, I had to remain opposed to what she wanted, and do what the profession considered to be in her best interests by avoiding future increases in symptoms and subsequent hospitalizations. Yet I appreciated Maxine's frustration with that approach. I didn't like being in charge of this decision and casting the swing vote, but felt obliged to do what was right professionally.

"I think she's still psychotic," I said.

"Why don't the three of you form a subcommittee and decide?" Dr. Johnson suggested. We agreed. Cynthia, Audrey's social work student named Rebecca, and I would meet later to make a final decision.

The official subcommittee gathered in my office the next day. It was an otherwise lazy afternoon. A committee can make for strange alliances. Cynthia and I were teamed up as allies. Still, with just the three of us, the atmosphere was more relaxed.

"Don't you have any qualms about sharing the patient's delusions?" I asked Rebecca.

"It's what she wants. And we should always try to give patients what they want."

"Can Maxine really not take care of herself?" I asked Cynthia.

"I don't think so."

"Maybe she needs to try and fail," Rebecca said.

"We can do ADL"—activities of daily living—"testing," Cynthia suggested with a sigh. "And we can also apply for residencies. The testing process may force her to acknowledge that there are things she can't do, and it may be therapeutic for her." We agreed.

The next day at morning rounds, I announced the subcommittee's decision. Audrey became indignant. "It's going to take time for her to do ADL testing, and in the meantime, she can be looking for an apartment. I think we should let her look for one now."

Johnson roused. "Let's move on. You all can discuss it again in the next team meeting or in another subcommittee meeting."

On Friday, the debate still raged. "This is controversial," I said. Everyone laughed. "And come Monday morning, Todd Spitzer will return, and I will no longer be involved." Everyone laughed again. My efforts had gotten nowhere. I had tried to be sensitive to all of the issues involved but had to recognize that I wouldn't always be able to advance or alter what happened to patients.

"There's an old Scottish proverb," Dr. Johnson said: "Most things in life don't matter very much. And many things don't matter at all."

Much of clinical care was social and political, and involved negotiations. Medications in psychiatry were often only one part of what was needed, though studies in psychobiology and psychopharmacology received almost all of the available research funding, and led to almost all faculty promotions.

On Monday, Todd returned. Changes of psychiatrists weren't optimal but allowed for vacations. He followed the course I had taken. Maxine started ADL testing, got frustrated, and eloped again. She tried to get what she wanted in spite of our rules and meetings. But this time her sister Valerie, upset about the police having trucked Maxine away in handcuffs from Roberta's, let Maxine stay and made room for her. Psychiatric patients sometimes had a way of finding solutions that were acceptable to them despite us. Maxine didn't get her own apartment, but she didn't have to go to a residence either.

Comrades

More and more, the importance of larger systems issues in psychiatry became apparent and began to interest me. Though senior psychiatrists focused on interventions applied to patients one-on-one to influence the mind or the brain, a broader social perspective seemed to make sense of problems that Nancy Steele, Maxine, and others faced in ways that individual psychodynamics or psychopharmacology, by themselves, did not.

Yet I began to wonder about how the social contexts in which we worked—both the wards of this hospital and our larger culture—affected our treatment of psychiatric patients. How specific to our culture were our views of and approaches to mental illness?

Residents were budgeted time for vacations, and my own arrived a few weeks later.

My sister Robin—Lisa's twin—had been teaching English in

mainland China for three years. I had never been there and decided to visit. Two years earlier, during my last year of medical school, I had met her in Japan during Christmas. On our last day there, I had looked up a friend's cousin who turned out to know several Japanese psychiatrists interested in combining Western psychiatry and psychoanalysis with Eastern philosophy and culture. Unfortunately, I didn't have time to meet them. I decided now to take advantage of my trip to China by visiting psychiatrists while there, to glimpse how psychiatry in China differed from what I was doing each day.

For years, the communist government had claimed that there was no mental illness in China. Communism had made everyone happy, they claimed. How could there be, for example, any depression? Such problems, the Chinese claimed, were strictly the result of capitalism, and hence avoidable.

I toured around with my sister and then arranged to visit a small outlying hospital, where I was introduced to a psychiatrist, Dr. Hwang Chi. He was a short balding man with a smiling round face and black plastic glasses. He had been imprisoned for several years during the Cultural Revolution and his entire library confiscated and burned because, having been to medical school, he was educated and thus considered to be an intellectual and a danger to society. How much more fortunate were doctors in the West, including myself, by comparison.

He led me upstairs. The hospital was spotless. Bronze pots of blooming yellow chrysanthemums were placed on each landing of the stairway and on low wooden tables in a reception room and a conference room into which he escorted me. Almost the entire staff of the hospital showed up to meet me. The nurses were arrayed in white uniforms and hats with stiff fronts rising up from their heads. I was introduced in Chinese as "Ka-li-tzi-man-Gu-ga," or "older brother Klitzman."

The head psychiatrist told me about his hospital. Some patients received traditional Chinese medicine, others Western medication, and some a combination of the two. The doctor was proud of his institution.

He asked if the staff could ask me questions, to which I agreed. The first question was from the head psychiatrist himself. I didn't know what he would ask, whether about the latest biological research in the United States, or psychoanalytic theory, or the problems of Western medicine. He cleared his throat. "Do patients in the States wear uniforms as they do in China?" he asked.

I was surprised. "No," I answered. A man in a dark suit sitting in the corner recorded my answer, I assumed for reporting later.

"What do you see as the benefits of wearing them here? Do you think it is better for patients to wear them or not to wear them?"

"I don't know. But I'd be concerned that it would make them feel more like patients."

"Do nurses wear uniforms?" the head nurse asked.

"No. Not usually." The staff, on hearing my answer translated, was amazed.

"What do they wear then?" a young nurse asked meekly, confused.

"Whatever they want." They giggled when they heard my answer translated.

"Can the ladies wear pants?" one nurse asked bashfully.

"Sure."

"How about the psychiatrists?" Dr. Hwang asked. "Do they wear uniforms?"

In China, they wore long white coats and ties. "At some hospitals the doctors wear long white coats and shirts and ties. But at other hospitals they don't wear coats and at some they don't wear ties." All of these, I realized, were symbols of our authority. "At institutions where neither patients nor doctors wear uniforms, the two groups are thought to seem more equal. Patients might also feel more at ease with their psychiatrist as a result," I added. It occured to me that this was again mere ideology and that we didn't really have data or studies to support our policies and customs one way or the other.

"What is your open-door policy?"

"If patients are elopement risks, the door is locked for them. Patients follow a step-by-step system, going to occupational therapy, and recreational therapy first with staff members, and then by themselves. Patients may be motivated, seeing gains they would accrue by becoming healthy." As I said it I wondered if the system actually helped patients improve.

"What is your occupational therapy?"

I described individual patients creating art projects and making shopping lists, balancing checkbooks, looking for apartments, and assembling résumés. My hosts were shocked.

"Here," I was told, "we have patients work in factories, reminding them of the importance of being a worker. We help our comrades return to the workplace." In China, the patients helped make products then sold by the state as any other product and not identified as having been made by psychiatric patients. OT in the West encouraged creative self-expression, individual identity, and financial skills. It was hard to know if either system worked as therapy, but they both seemed to reflect the culture's prevailing values.

"Who does the psychotherapy?" the psychiatric chief asked.

"Mostly the doctors." In China, it was mostly the nurses, I was told.

"What is the ratio of doctors to patients?" someone else wanted to know.

"At better hospitals, one psychiatrist for five to eight patients." In China, there were several times the number of patients per doctor.

"How about nurses?"

"About the same at any one shift. The ratios are probably not as high at large state-run institutions with many chronic patients."

"Is the staff the same there?"

"No. There are some differences."

"Like what?"

"More are foreign-trained."

"Do they receive the same salary?"

"Yes."

"Are there Chinese doctors there?"

"Yes."

"Do residents get paid?" a resident asked.

"Yes."

"How much do psychiatrists get paid?"

I told them. They were all shocked.

"Do they own cars?"

"Some do. Some don't." More astonishment. So much for interest in the role of cultural factors in conceptions of psychiatry and the mind. The possible differences between patients, treatments, or theories of mental illness were much less interesting or important to my listeners than the basic human differences in the workings of the institution and particularly, despite communism, in the finances involved. But I did see the importance of social issues in psychiatry. Despite the fact that our hospitals couldn't be more different in numerous ways—the Chinese lacked Freudian theory and many of our psychiatric medications—we faced similar basic logistical and economic issues and problems in psychiatric treatment. Despite the very different cultures and the use of newer and more sophisticated medications in the United States, the staff's concerns were similar to those in our country.

Also, though, for the first time I saw that I knew quite a bit about the field and was perceived as an expert. I was able to represent the profession effectively in ways that interested this group.

Afterward I asked to see patients and was taken on a tour through several wards. The patients all wore uniforms: red corduroy coats for the women, brown corduroy coats for the men. Each jacket was numbered with Arabic numerals in white stitching—an identification number that had been assigned to the patient. The wards were segregated by gender. The building had no dining hall, but instead long shelves ran along the narrow corridor, used as dining tables by the patients. Stools squeezed side to side. White painted numbers, chipping away, labeled each place and each stool with a patient's assigned number.

My last stop was once a missionary church, now part of the hospital compound. The Spanish Baroque edifice boasted curved stone cornices and a portico of Doric columns—now woefully out of place amidst the prefab buildings sprawling over the suburban neighborhood outside the hospital's gates. A hand-painted sign above the ornate carved wooden doors of the cathedral read in Chinese: "Occupational Therapy." By the carved doors stood stacked crates of small milk bottles into which patients had poured bright pink liquid perfume that another group of patients had mixed. A third group of patients, Dr. Hwang told me, had capped the bottles. Inside the church, Baroque balustrades and stone garlands adorned balconies encircling the huge hall and decorated spiral staircases leading up to the gallery. Light poured in through paned windows several stories high. Throughout the room stood large round folding tables, at each of which a huge pile of small cardboard boxes towered in front of five to eight patients who were staring off into space. The church was now a factory. The boxes—for holding staples—arrived as cardboard sheets, which one table of patients was supposed to cut and fold. At the second station, halfway down the nave of the church, the patients were to pick up one lid at a time and snip semicircular holes at each end to enable the top to be lifted off the bottom of the box easily. At the next group of tables, near the transepts, patients were to pick up the top of a box, try to find a bottom, and push them together. In the choir, at another table, the completed boxes were to be stacked and tied.

The patients looked chronic—suffering from severe and unremitting mental illness. Even these tasks were too much for many of them. Nurses seated at each table worked busily. But the patients stared at the empty gulf separating them from the mountains of boxes before them. Others focused vaguely on a lid before them or in their hands. They seemed unable to rouse themselves to search for the complementary box half. I couldn't imagine these patients returning to the workplace. I wondered further how many assumptions in psychiatry were accepted because they sounded good or fit our values but were, in fact, incorrect.

I exited the church and walked back into the sunshine. Off to the side was a male patients' ward. The patients had just had lunch and had now been allowed out and paced in the courtyard behind a metal fence. They saw me and crowded to the end of the yard, sticking their arms through the black iron bars to reach me or to try to shake my hand. Some looked preoccupied, confused, or depressed, reminding me of patients back home. But here, despite the similarities, the patients were uniformed and permitted outside only when locked behind a fence. Still, I wondered how much freedom we actually gave patients back in the West, and whether, though clearly more than here, it was in some ways less than we thought or wanted to believe.

To Walk in the Valley

When I returned from China it was late winter. The streets were covered with snow. Fierce winds howled at night. The trees were bare, the days short.

On my first morning back at work, Lou Leftow paged me. "When did you last see Bransky?" he asked me.

"Christmas Eve," I said, remembering his visit fondly.

"He died last week."

"He *died*?" I was shocked. It didn't sound real.

"What happened?" I asked.

"He came to the ER two weeks ago. I heard he looked a little worse this time," Lou told me. "But he said he wasn't suicidal or homicidal, so he wasn't admitted. The resident just assumed Ronald was chronic," meaning his problems, presumed to be persistent, could more readily be ignored, with resources channeled to other, needier patients.

"He had been taking a lot of drugs, maybe because he was more depressed or anxious. Perhaps his tolerance for them had sunk too far, leading to an accidental overdose. But no one will ever know for certain what happened, whether his death was an accident or a suicide."

Though psychiatry was more stressful than medical internship in many ways, in one regard it had thus far been calmer: it hadn't involved death and dying. During my internship, many patients were expected to die. It was merely a question of time, and we worked to postpone the inevitable. Psychiatry, I thought, would be cleaner, unshadowed by the finitude of death. Decisions in the end were not as literally life-and-death as they had been in medicine. The work, therefore, in at least one regard, had been lighter, less onerous.

Ronald's death left me even more stunned since he had

126

seemed a paragon of resilience and survival against the odds. Some patients are suicidal, and death hangs over their treatment as a risk. But I hadn't thought of death as an imminent possibility in Bransky's case.

"There's going to be a memorial service," Lou continued. "Gerald Turner is putting it together. I'm going to attend. Do you want to go?" I had never been to a patient's funeral or memorial service before—let alone a street person's. But Ronald had affected me as few other patients had. As a medical student and intern, I had kept more of a professional distance, rarely entering deeply into patients' personal lives and struggles or seeing their problems from their point of view, focusing instead on the biological disease processes in their bodies.

But with Bransky and other psychiatric patients, being aware of and responsible for their emotional lives as well, I experienced and knew them more fully as people. My hand still remembered the soft doughy flesh around Bransky's heart, how my hand had sunk in and cupped his small heart. He seemed more vulnerable and unprotected than many other patients, despite his tough exterior, bravura, and threats, and the battles I had had with him over drugs. He felt like more than merely a patient. He had tested and pushed the limits of the definition of that term in my mind. I had seen his humor, his pride, and his disappointments. I had gotten to know him. Compared to patients' deaths I had seen as a medical intern, Ronald's felt more like that of a friend or family member—even though I was not very acquainted with death in my personal life.

Two weeks after Lou had called me, I went to Bransky's service.

The church was located on a narrow side street. The massive Gothic building was dark and foreboding. It also housed the shelter where Ronald had spent many nights.

The foyer was cavernous and somber. In one corner stood a stairwell. A cardboard sign read "Shelter," and an arrow pointed down toward the basement.

I went down the shadowy steps to see it. A long low-ceilinged passage led to a small but clean white room. Narrow cots were lined up. Three black men lay on the bunks with their shirts off. The odor of stale clothes and perspiration permeated the room. I nodded hello to the three men. Here was another side of Ronald's life. He was not merely someone hustling for more drugs, but was struggling to get by, and to survive, seeking warmth and shelter.

"Are you here for Bransky's service?" one of the men asked me.

"Yes," I answered. "I was one of his doctors."

"I only hope they don't put him in potter's field." The man sighed. He looked down at the edge of the bed and fell silent.

"The service is about to start," I said, gesturing toward the door. But the three men shook their heads, not wanting to go. Perhaps it would have been too disturbing.

I said goodbye, wandered back into the lobby, and entered the small chapel where the service was to be conducted. In the front of the sanctuary was a shelf on which stood a black marble urn and a vase of yellow flowers.

I sat down on a hard wooden pew. I couldn't fully believe that Ronald was gone. It seemed like I had just seen him. His memory remained firmly in my mind. Yet he had left nothing physical behind. He had no real possessions, other than those that fit in the little bag he toted, barely able to transport because of his deformities. He had no children, no home, no mementos of his life. He wasn't bolstered by any family or friends or "support system" other than Turner, Leftow, and, I now realized, myself. We were the closest thing he had to a network, a family, as he roamed the streets between us.

I mused about the urn straight ahead. As a homeless person, he would be utterly forgotten, his death unnoticed. The jar might have been empty, and always stood in the chapel for decoration. Or, I imagined now, it might contain Ronald's remains. Where *would* his remains go? Would he be buried, placed in a marked grave, given the lasting home he had lacked during his lifetime? Or would he be cremated? Would his ashes be collected in an expensive urn, or scattered, and if so, where?

The chapel was brightly lit with fluorescent bulbs. I glanced around at the other people present. The only one I recognized was Lou, who had brought his wife.

The group quieted as a bearded man stood up before us in a blue parka and a yellow ski cap just like Ronald's. He looked like a larger version of Ronald, only healthier and with lighter hair. "I'm Gerald Turner," the man said. I had spoken with him on the phone, but had never met him. He removed a folded piece of paper from the rear pocket of his jeans and opened it. "Ronald Bransky was a special guy," he read. "He didn't die. He lives on . . . here . . . with us, each time we walk down the streets which were his. Ronald Bransky wasn't just another faceless homeless person." Turner's voice rose with urgency and passion. "He walked around and referred to himself as 'Me: little guy.' Always in that yellow hat of his." He laughed. "At methadone clinics, he had to wait on line at dirty windows for his small cup of salvation. He finally said: Enough. He didn't die of an OD or of his addiction. The problem was partly us. Us in here and us out there—our neglect of homeless people, our willingness to tolerate their problems and ignore them. Finally in the last month of his life, for the first time in ten years, he had a home, his own home. One room. An SRO"—or single room occupancy hotel. "But it was his and he decorated the walls, and was proud of it." Gerald stopped. He looked away from the page and tried to hold back his tears, as he slowly uttered, "God bless him."

Turner sat down and was replaced by a young woman dressed in a white cardigan sweater and a pink skirt. The top button of her white blouse was fastened. She was a divinity student and carried a small book, from which tiny pieces of paper stuck out between the pages. "The Lord is my shepherd, I shall not want," she started. She read the psalm. "Yea, though I walk through the valley of the shadow of death, I will fear no evil . . ."

For once, those lines took on a special meaning. Here, they referred to the deceased, not merely to our grief, as solace to us. It was Ronald's pain, more than ours, that she was describing.

I couldn't fully concentrate, sitting there. Other tasks, waiting to be performed on other patients, kept rising in my mind—forms to complete, blood samples to draw, and laboratory results to check. I didn't want any other patients to die as Ronald had. He had reminded me of the fact that death hung over us all.

The memorial service continued. A few other prayers were said. Then we slowly and silently filed out. The group broke up into small clusters and, almost as an afterthought, we paused along the fringes of the large foyer. The service had brought us together. If the funeral had been someone else's, there would have been somewhere to go: a cemetery, or the home of a relative or a friend. But now, there was nowhere. We hovered at the edges of the room before dispersing. I stood next to Lou. Gerald joined us. "I have another patient for you," Gerald said to Lou. "To replace Ronald."

Lou hesitated. "Call me," he finally said. I suspected that

Lou felt devoted to Ronald as a person, more than to home-lessness in general as a social cause. But Gerald was responsible for an entire shelter of people, many of whose needs were as great as Ronald's. Lou was compassionate and concerned about social issues. But as a trainee like myself, he had only a limited amount of free time.

Gerald stared down at the slate floor, rebuffed.

"Ronald was really something," I said to him quickly to change the topic.

"Yes sir." He suddenly looked up, momentarily forgetting Lou's hesitancy. "You know he was always replacing that yellow hat of his. It would get lost or stolen in the streets. He was always buying a new one with the little money he had."

Some people in the hallway started to drift away.

"Wait," Gerald suddenly called out. "I don't think we all know each other. Let's go around and introduce ourselves." We collected back together and formed a big circle.

Lou went first. "I'm Dr. Lou Leftow," he said. "I was Ronald's outpatient psychiatrist. I just want to say that I learned more from Ronald than from any other patient."

I was next in line. "I'm a psychiatrist, too. Ronald taught me a huge amount about how much I can and can't do as a physician." It is easier to list symptoms, make diagnoses, and prescribe medications than to understand and change the peculiar social worlds in which some patients live. The larger issues in Ronald's life—the ceaseless spread of his cancer, his homelessness, and his family's rejection—stood gaping before us, unresolved. I saw the limitations of my role. All my efforts seemed meager compared to the enormity of what patients often needed.

The other members of the circle spoke, too. Most lived in the neighborhood, and they or their spouses were volunteers at the shelter.

One man said, "I was Ronald's friend." He was gaunt and disheveled. His eyes focused on the empty space immediately before him. "I used to be on methadone, too," he continued. "Now I'm off it. But I'm having a hard time. I don't want to have to go back on it." He started to cry. "But it's so hard. I don't know if I'll make it." One of the shelter volunteers put her arm around his shoulder and hugged him.

The clergy student broke down in tears. "You all make it worthwhile doing this each day," she said, pulling a Kleenex out from a small package of them in her purse. She dabbed her tears from beneath her glasses. "Only this man could have brought us together." She was the last one to speak. We stood together there, joined in a circle for a few more moments. Then we nodded to each other and drifted out.

A few days later I saw Lou again. "Gerald Turner just called me," he said. "Bransky's sister in Texas won't claim the body. It's still in the morgue after three weeks. Only a blood relative can have rights to a corpse. Turner wants to get it to have Bransky cremated, but can't." Lou paused. "By the way, my wife and I are thinking of volunteering in the shelter. Are you interested?"

My schedule was packed, and I was soon to start my next rotation. But I still felt a strong connection to Ronald. Other people in shelters needed help, too. "Yes," I said to Lou, "that's a good idea."

Over the next few weeks, I thought about it further. When I saw people sleeping on stoops or in subway stations I looked at them differently. But after being on call all night or completing my long hours of regular duties, I would collapse at home, exhausted. My training didn't permit any flexibility or lessening in its demands. I didn't have much spare time in which to volunteer.

I, too, was committed more to Ronald as an individual than to homelessness in the abstract, though it was an important issue. And I knew I'd treat my future homeless patients differently as a result of knowing Ronald, seeing them more as individual human beings, concerning myself more with their care during and after their hospitalization. I would be more aware of the abyss into which we often again sent them and of the limited effects of our efforts. We spent time adjusting medications for patients who might not continue them once they left the hospital to live on sidewalk benches or cardboard boxes on the street, alone.

None of us ever went to the shelter. Lou and his wife never mentioned it again. Neither did I. But on the subway, I no longer avoided street people, and whenever a staff member said that a patient was "just a druggie," I thought of Ronald.

The Man in My Head

Just as I would feel confident about the work, as if I had the hang of psychiatry, new problems and challenges presented themselves. Seemingly familiar issues became configured in unprecedented ways. Over time, the stakes also got higher. I was learning a lot through this first year, and had expected that residency would begin to get easier. But in many ways it got harder, since compared to medical conditions I had encountered as an intern, mental illness remained far less predictable.

Enrico Gómez was assigned to me one morning, brought to the hospital after he tried to jump off a moving subway onto the tracks. He was a twenty-year-old Latino, short with straight black hair. "I just wanted to get out of the subway car," he told me. He had been filled with an ominous foreboding that something bad was about to happen to him if he stayed on board. He insisted he wasn't trying to kill himself, "just escape." I conducted a mental status exam, part of which consists of asking patients the meaning of standard proverbs, the most commonly used of which is "What do people mean when they say, 'People who live in glass houses shouldn't throw stones'?"

"It'll break the glass," Enrico replied. His response was concrete, not abstract, suggesting a thought disorder.

A standard part of the exam is also to ask patients about similarities between objects.

"What do an apple and an orange have in common?" I asked him.

"They're both stuff you can't depend on," he replied.

"What do cats and mice have in common?"

"I don't like mice."

His answers sounded bizarre.

I decided to start him on a neuroleptic. "Try Navane," Dr. Johnson suggested.

Over the next week on the ward he began to improve, becoming more appropriate in some ways, though not entirely.

From the day he arrived there was a question of where he would go when he was eventually discharged. As insurance companies were cutting back the length of their hospital coverage, we had been instructed to think about discharge plans from the beginning of patients' admissions. On some wards, a patient's discharge date was determined on the first day of a hospitalization, scheduled to use up the full amount of time the insurance company would pay for, which was usually needed to enable the patient to improve as much as possible.

Enrico's parents were divorced. His father, Rafael Gómez, wanted to be in charge of Enrico's care after the hospitalization. But Mr. Gómez didn't have room in his house for Enrico. Mr. Gómez wanted the patient to live in a residential facility in Cedarville, west of the city, near Mr. Gómez's own home. Enrico's mother wanted the patient to live with her in Hightown, to the south. Enrico, when I met with him alone, told me he'd prefer to be with his mother.

In the meantime, Enrico needed to be on medicine in the hospital to help him as much as possible. The full effect of the drug could take a month to be achieved. Gradually I increased his dose, and he slowly settled into the ward. He was very calm, though like many schizophrenics he remained exquisitely sensitive to stress and conflicts around him. He was not very talkative—even when he had been well. I tried to engage him as best I could. When I found out he liked shooting pool, I played with him a few times in RT. He was a good player and I was not. He won and felt proud and more trusting of me as a result.

Two weeks after his admission, his cousin Ernestine, to whom he had been close, died.

"I'm sorry to hear that your cousin died," I told him.

"She didn't die."

"She didn't?"

"No."

"But that's what your family said."

"She's still here. Her spirit is still here. I feel her inside me." His voice had a serious tone. He was still psychotic.

"I wouldn't let him go to the funeral," Roy said. "Let him visit the grave afterward." I also further increased Enrico's medication.

Gradually, he started to sound more organized, and I began again to consider discharge options.

His father asked to meet with the patient and me together about Enrico's future.

"Enrico should do what he wants," Mr. Gómez said.

"Good," I said, thinking that we would now be able to reach agreement about where he would go when he left.

"And what he wants," Mr. Gómez continued, "is what's best for him. Right, Enrico?"

"Yes."

"And what's best for you is to live near me, not with your mother." I was astounded. "And Enrico is smart enough to realize this, aren't you, Enrico?"

He hesitated. "Ye-es."

"And so it's a very simple matter. Enrico knows he cannot go home with his mother. Isn't that right, Enrico? He knows he must go to live with me."

"Yes," Enrico said, his head cast down.

"But I don't think Enrico has decided," I said.

"There is nothing else for him to decide."

"I think it's best not to make a decision now," I said.

"You are siding with his mother," Mr. Gómez accused me.

"No, I'm not. I'm just interested in arranging what's best for Enrico."

"We have already decided what's best for him."

"You've decided. But I'm not sure Enrico has."

"Of course he has!" his father shouted, banging his fist on my desk. "Haven't you, Enrico?"

"Yes," he said very quietly.

"Look, Enrico," I interjected, "it's your decision. You don't have to do what your father wants."

"But he knows what's best for him," Mr. Gómez said. I looked at the clock on my desk and realized I was late for another meeting.

"Why don't we stop there for today. I think we should continue to talk about this," I said. His father got up to leave.

"Enrico, can I speak with you for a moment first?" I asked. Enrico stayed behind.

"You know you don't have to do what your father wants."

"I know," he said. He looked uncomfortable, and quickly jumped up and joined his father in the hall.

* * *

The next day, I was paged while sitting in a class.

It was Henrietta, the head nurse. "Bob, you'd better come to the ward." She sounded shaky and pressured. "Enrico just fainted."

"Is he okay?" I was in the middle of a class. If he was okay now, I could perhaps wait until the end of the class to see him.

"You'd better come up here now." I couldn't imagine why he'd have fainted or why it was such an emergency. Something didn't seem right.

When I arrived on the floor a few minutes later, Pam was running down the hall. The patients' doors were all shut. I hurried down the hall after Pam in the direction of Enrico's room, and gaped at the doorway. Enrico's bed was surrounded by a throng of doctors and nurses with an EKG machine whirring, green metal tanks of oxygen, like ammunition, behind. This was the code team, called in emergencies whenever a patient is "coding"—that is, thought to be undergoing a cardiopulmonary arrest, in which his heart or lungs have stopped or might stop.

"What happened?" I asked Roy.

"Enrico just tried to drown himself."

"He what?"

"He called his mother on the phone and said he was going to join his dead cousin." He then hung up, went back to his room, covered the bathtub drain with a piece of cardboard, and turned on the tap. He lay down in the tub, held his nose, and lowered his head below the surface. "Luckily, his mother called back. Francine Blair," another patient, "answered the phone and ran to tell the nurses. Enrico just had put his face under the water so it looks like he'll make it. The amazing thing is that Dr. Johnson and I had just talked to him on walk rounds half an hour before, and he had seemed okay."

Enrico was now breathing on his own. The code team started packing up to leave.

"What happened, Enrico?" I asked.

"I wanted to join Ernestine," he whispered.

"Were you trying to kill yourself?"

"No, man," he said as if I were crazy for even asking. "A voice in my head told me to do it."

"What do you mean?"

"The man in my head."

"Huh?"

"The person who tells me what to do." It sounded psychotic. The man in his head was himself.

I increased Enrico's Navane and put him on MO. A community meeting was called, and I informed all of the other patients of what happened, reassuring them that Enrico would be all right. I felt distracted, troubled, almost slightly faint myself, yet thankful he was still alive, without serious consequences. Also, Roy and Dr. Johnson had seen him just half an hour before and had spoken to him at length. I wasn't solely responsible. Still, Dr. Johnson said nothing to me that day.

At home that night, Roy called.

"I wonder if I could have somehow prevented this," I told him.

"Don't be so damn narcissistic."

"How do you mean?"

"We psychiatrists think that whenever a patient tries to hurt him- or herself that we caused it or could have prevented it if only we had somehow acted differently. That's just ridiculous. Patients do what they do with their lives, and we can't always stop them. You did everything you could for him. It just reminds us how unpredictable things are with crazy people. We were lucky."

"Johnson didn't even say anything to me about it."

"That doesn't surprise me. I feel totally unsupported by him on the floor, as well." I appreciated Roy's support as a fellow resident.

Mike also phoned. "I hear you had a brush with death today. How are you doing?"

Sarah called. "I'm tired of being responsible for what crazy people do with their lives," she said. "I hate it. I'm tired of Dr. Johnson."

"I'm tired of Dr. Johnson, too."

"I want to quit."

Joe Tauber, my fellow resident, had had a patient successfully complete a suicide six months earlier, and also called. "The only thing that keeps me going is playing with my eighteen-month-old daughter at home," he said. "That's what saved me. Why don't you come over sometime this week and play with her? It's great."

I thanked him and agreed to.

Enrico hadn't been able to communicate the depth of his reactions. I still felt responsible, but I also felt shut out by him, with no control over what happened. We were both at the mercy of his psychosis. The experience showed yet again patients' fragility. Despite my best attempts, disastrous events could occur. There was no way to know for sure. The possibility of catastrophe underlay daily activities on the ward. Enrico's case was traumatic for me. I started to have trouble sleeping, and my confidence was shaken. Something kept me going: other patients to see each day, meetings and decisions to make. But part of my feeling of innocence and ease in the hospital seemed permanently lost.

The next day, Enrico denied any thoughts of wanting to hurt himself or join his deceased cousin. Dr. Johnson came up to me that afternoon. "All I can say is, 'Those things happen.' Let's DC," that is, discontinue, "the MO."

"DC the MO? But his attempt was totally unpredictable. He might try again."

"What are you going to do, keep him on MO the rest of his life?"

"Let me talk to Roy about it."

"All right, if that's what you want to do," he said hesitantly, shaking his head.

Johnson's suggestion astounded Roy, as well.

"Enrico just tried to kill himself and came very close. Now Johnson wants to DC the MO? I don't think that's right. I agree with you. We should keep the MO, at least for now."

"Who has more experience around here," Johnson asked at morning report the next day. "Me or you all?"

"I'm just concerned about him," Roy said.

I increased Enrico's medication further. He was on so-called megadoses: more than I had ever given any patient before, but he still complained of a person's voice whispering in his head.

"He's just soaking up the drugs," Roy said.

I ordered blood tests to be drawn to check that Enrico was taking the medication and that it wasn't having any adverse effects. But when the blood drawer came around in the morning, Enrico refused. I had to draw the specimen myself.

"I don't want to give my blood to anyone," he told me.

"It's for us to make sure the medication isn't having any bad effects on you."

"I think you just want to keep the blood for yourself, Dr. Klitzman."

"How about ECT?" Dr. Johnson suggested the next day. Though most effective for major depression accompanied by delusions, ECT had been reported to be useful also in the treatment of some cases of refractory or nonresponsive schizophrenia. Ironically, it had once been used widely for schizophrenia, until other medications—the neuroleptics—had been found to be more effective in most cases. Yet Enrico wasn't responding fully to these drugs. I sat down with him and gave him a pamphlet written for patients, "ECT and You."

"It's Dr. Klitzman who needs ECT," he said. "Not me." He held the white stapled pamphlet up in the air and ripped it in two, laughing. He let the torn pieces drop onto the floor.

I spoke with his father as well, who was subdued after Enrico's attempt, but agreed that something else should be done and supported ECT. He spoke to Enrico, who then agreed. A few days later, Enrico signed the consent form.

I had his father sign the form as well, officially documenting his support.

I announced in rounds the next morning that they had both consented to ECT. Dr. Johnson walked up to me afterward and put his arm over my shoulder. "Nice going, Bob," he said, nodding and smiling. It was the only time he had ever touched me and one of the only times he ever complimented my work.

The next morning, Johnson said to me, "Let's DC the MO as soon as we can. Roy is going on vacation soon. I'd like to get Enrico off MO while Roy's away."

Enrico went to ECT. We planned twenty treatments, three a week, to take seven weeks altogether. We would have to wait until the end of that period to evaluate his response and know what approach to take next.

The Great Door Debate

Part of the difficulty of becoming a psychiatrist was learning to deal with a wide range of staff views and interpretations that were based on neither biology nor psychoanalytic theory, but on philosophical and highly subjective opinions. Patients presented complex decisions and dilemmas that led to intricate negotiations.

"I have an admission for you down here in the ER," Judy Van Meter, a third-year resident, told me one morning a few days later. "You may want to come down and see her."

I headed downstairs to the ER. The patient, Susan Parr, was just waking up. She opened her eyes, looked around her at the brightly lit hospital room, and said, "Fuck!" Then she reclosed her eyes.

Her mother, Lucille Parr, had tried phoning her at home incessantly the day before. Lucille, not getting an answer, went to the apartment, and called the police, who knocked down her daughter's front door, found Susan unconscious, and brought her to the ER, where she was now resuscitated.

Susan was still frail and shaken when she came up to the ward. An IV coiled into her arm.

"How many times have you tried to hurt yourself?" I asked her.

"Twenty-five. I've been in ICUs," intensive care units, "a whole bunch of times." It was amazing she had always survived.

"How many psychiatric hospitalizations have you had?"

"About the same . . . twenty-five." That was by far the highest I had ever heard.

"Where were they?" I asked, still not sure whether to believe her completely or not. She reeled off four or five other hospitals in the region in addition to ours where she had been three to five times each. She was short and gaunt with thin curly black hair and a voice that trembled as she spoke.

I ordered her chart, but it didn't arrive all day. I decided to trek down to the medical records department myself, rather than wait longer. The clerk handed me four fat charts, each three or four inches thick. That was more than I had ever seen for a patient. On the cover of the last volume was glued a large red and white sticker. "WARNING!" it said in bold red letters, "THIS PATIENT IS NOT *EVER* TO BE READMITTED TO THIS HOSPITAL." I had never seen such a declaration on a patient's chart, and was surprised that the hospital felt it had the right to keep out a patient who needed help, in effect selecting patients it wanted to exclude. Her chart said that each time she had been here, she had difficulty leaving, refusing to accept plans the staff made and refusing to attend outpatient appointments they set up for her. One time she cut her wrists while on a pass to ensure that the staff would keep her longer. The administration had decided at a certain point that it was better not to admit her at all.

At morning report the next day, I presented her history. When I listed her series of suicide attempts and hospitalizations, Roy, at the far end of the circle, held up an index card and panned it across the room, letting everyone see. "Transfer to Rivershore State," he had written in block letters.

"Send her straight there," he said, "as soon as you can." The staff seemed eager to get rid of her.

"The staff thinks it best to have you transferred to the state hospital," I said to her. "Would you be willing to go?"

She rocked gently back and forth in her chair. "Okay," she said in her frail voice. "I've been there before."

I had never heard of a patient being transferred there willingly. I didn't even know if Rivershore would accept a voluntary admission, but I called them anyway.

"First send me paperwork on her," Dr. Bhimani, the psychiatrist in their admissions office, said.

"How long will it take?"

"I can't say. Maybe a couple of weeks."

I checked Susan's blood to make sure that she was recovering adequately from her OD. For the moment, I continued the three medications she was on.

The next day at staff meeting, Henrietta said, "Let's talk about the door."

"What about the door?" Roy asked.

"Why don't we have it open?" Pam asked.

"I think we should still have it locked for Enrico."

"But he's starting ECT."

"Yes, but he's been very impulsive in the past. I don't think it's worth risking. Plus we have Susan Parr on the ward."

"She's not still suicidal, is she?" Henrietta asked.

"She says no, but we're still just getting to know her."

"I think she's fine," Pam said. "She wouldn't do anything here on the ward. She's the kind that would first inform the staff how she's feeling. I can tell."

"You never know. Besides, she's had attempts here before."

"I don't see what the rush to open the door is," Roy said.

"This isn't a jail!" Pam said.

"It seems to be," I joked, trying to ease the tension. People turned to me, angry. My attempt at levity hadn't gone over big.

"I want to quit," Pam declared, "and go work in a hospital that has *real* unlocked units. When we lock the door, it seems like a prison. These patients are supposed to be here voluntarily, not involuntarily."

"We shouldn't confuse locked and unlocked with voluntary and involuntary," Roy said.

"It makes for a better environment overall for both patients and staff," Henrietta argued.

"The staff seems more affected by having an open door than the patients are," I commented. People again looked at me, not wanting their discussion interpreted.

"It's important to the patients, too," Pam said. "To all of us." But the patients hadn't talked about the door at all.

Henry Nolan had once told residents that the open-door policy started in Britain during World War II because of air raids. To have people locked up was thought to be unsafe if there was a bombing. It was found secondarily to have therapeutic advantages. "Although like many therapeutic interventions," Nolan had said, "it probably doesn't matter: one-third of patients are helped, one-third stay the same, and one-third get worse."

At the moment, it was Roy's decision whether to unlock the door, and he kept it closed. Dr. Johnson wasn't even at the meeting.

"I can't believe the nursing staff," Roy complained later. "We barely avoided a suicide attempt, and we've had elopements and have a new, suicidal patient. The nursing staff is working in a psychiatric hospital, but they just won't accept it. They want it to be otherwise. By the way, what you said in the meeting—that the door mattered more to the staff than to the patients—was true but inflammatory."

Later that day, in T-group, I talked about what had happened.

"You're the anti-leader," Dr. Nathan said disapprovingly, "because you interpreted group process to all and also because Johnson himself apparently is philosophically in favor of having the door open. That puts you in a very vulnerable position." I thought I had been pointing out what was accurate and important.

"Aren't we in the business of trying to seek the truth?" I said.

"Not necessarily on an inpatient ward. You have to be careful." In short, following the political hierarchy was more important than helping others to understand the psychological and social issues that arose. Conformity was more important here than the truth.

"I don't see how it makes Bob the anti-leader, though," Jessica, another resident, said.

"You," he said to her, "are the group skeptic."

"The skeptic? Why am I the skeptic?"

That night I was on call and was working through most of the night. Several patients were admitted. I went to sleep for half an hour, only to be awakened when an elderly woman fell out of bed and had to be evaluated. By then it was morning and another day had to start. I dragged myself to morning rounds and more meetings, and saw other patients.

Finally, at the end of the day I staggered home, after being in the hospital for thirty-six hours, working the entire time, except for my half-hour nap. When I straggled out of the building it was twilight. I shuffled home and opened my mailbox, filled with bills, junk mail, and an alumni magazine. Upstairs, I dumped the pile on my desk and plopped into an old easy chair I had bought at the Salvation Army. Outside, dusk settled over the city. To sit inside there all night would be stifling. I had been too tired even to make plans to have dinner with friends. Screw this. I got up, shucked my white coat, unknotted my tie, pulled on a light jacket, and breezed out, the door slamming behind me. A public bus heading downtown was stopping on my block, admitting the last of a line of passengers. The front door still gaped open. Inside, a line of small yellow lights ran the length of the bus. From outside it seemed a lantern in the twilight. I quickly jumped on board, entering the cool dark green interior of tinted windows. The bus lurched forward, pulling away from the street and the hospital neighborhood. The bus, like a boat full of light, plowed through the evening darkness. Buildings and streets floated past. I had nowhere in particular to go but had just wanted to get away. I had never done that before—gone somewhere just for the sake of going. An older resident I had once asked for advice about residency had offered only one suggestion. "Make sure," he said, "that you go out every night after being on call. Even if it's just to a movie and you can't stay awake. At least you've spent some time out of the hospital. Otherwise you'll die."

Downtown, a long avenue was lined with a record store, a bookstore, clothing shops, and outdoor cafés. I exited the bus and bought a few CDs—a new Michael Jackson album and a Mozart piano concerto. Music had become one of my few refuges during residency—quickly and easily reminding me of something purer or more exciting—soothing or reinvigorating me, depending on my mood. With my new purchases in hand, I meandered down the street, browsing until drowsiness overcame me. A bus then swept me back home. My short trip had been a needed, if momentary, escape. The world still existed and glittered outside the ward.

Residency was embroiling me in conflicts not only with patients and their families but with nurses and other staff. Within the hierarchy of the hospital, residents were accorded less respect than many other staff members. My medical degree did not give me the kind of authority that I had as an intern in other medical specialties. Here, the nursing and social work and occupational therapy staff, who had known some of the patients for decades, challenged my decisions and actions. Because of how little was known about the mind and the brain, everyone's opinions about a patient's behavior were heard, leading to frequent disagreements and debates.

A week later, Roy went on vacation. He had chosen me to be the acting assistant unit chief in his absence. Arguments about the door continued. Nurses asked me more about it and about what I thought of putting various patients on MO. With Roy away, they got nervous and asked me questions more frequently. I had to run meetings as well as handle their doubts and anxieties.

"Can I divide doses of this medicine?" they would ask about particular patients. If problems arose during the day, as they inevitably did, I had to answer them, handling two jobs at once.

"If anything comes up," Dr. Johnson said, "we can talk about it during our usual supervision time, okay? Unless it's an emergency or something. Then, you can call me before." He walked away. He was implicitly saying, "Don't bother me."

The only thing Johnson did ask during this time was that I take Enrico off MO, which I eventually agreed to after Enrico started receiving ECT.

In the end, Enrico received all twenty ECT treatments and began to improve, becoming more organized. He started to deny hearing voices and stopped uttering delusions. He and his father agreed he would live with his mother, at least temporarily, when he left.

Susan Parr felt restless and couldn't "sit still," a possible side effect—known as akathisia—from one of her medications. I tried lowering the dose to simplify her regimen. "I'm being attacked by my thoughts," she cried a few days later. Since she seemed more anxious and possibly psychotic, I put her on a similar medication that had fewer side effects.

Monday morning a note sat in my box on the ward. "Dear Dr. Klitzman. I feel much better. The best in a long time. That restless feeling is gone. Thank you. Sincerely—Susan Parr." The next day, she put in my box a poem she had written entitled "Flowers Seen from the Ward," surrounded by crayoned drawings of daffodils. "In pots outside my window, yellow flowers bloom," the poem read, "I hope that I can, too—some day."

The social worker, Audrey, met at least once with each patient's family.

"I don't think we need to meet with Parr's family," Audrey said. "We're just shipping her to a state hospital."

"But we meet with every other patient's family at least once. I think we should meet with her mother anyway," I said. "Susan's a patient just like any other, even if our plan is to transfer her."

We arranged a meeting.

"I just don't understand what's wrong with my daughter," Susan's mother said when we met with her. "I have tried so hard with her. I don't see why she just can't get her own apartment like everyone else." She started to cry, opened a large brown leather purse on her lap, and dug for a Kleenex. "There are some nice new apartments in my neighborhood. She used to have her own apartment a number of years ago—I don't see why she just doesn't get one now. I'm sure it would help her feel better."

"But she has an illness that makes it hard for her to do that," I said.

"Well I think that if she really wanted to, she could."

"But a symptom of her illness is that she has trouble organizing herself."

"Is that really true? Or are you doctors just telling me that?"

"It's true."

"What's my daughter's illness, anyway?"

"Have doctors discussed it with you in the past?"

"In the beginning they did. But in the past few years when she's been in the hospital, nobody's talked to me at all." Her voice shook slightly. Her eyes, round and moist, looked directly at me pleading, "Please, Doctor, tell me what's going on with her."

"It's not exactly clear, but it may be schizoaffective disorder, which is related to schizophrenia." We had been told to be careful when telling patients' families this diagnosis, since in the past it was blamed on patients' parents.

"Oh yes," she said, interrupting momentarily, "that's what they've said in the past. But I still just don't understand her anymore." I gave her some information about her daughter's illness and recommended that she speak to her daughter and call Rivershore hospital once Susan went there, since her doctor there hadn't yet been determined.

"Thank you," she said, drying her tears.

"It was a good idea to meet with her," Audrey later conceded.

Rivershore said they'd send an ambulette to pick up Susan but didn't know when. It could be as early as 6:30 some morning. Every few days, she left in my box other poems and paintings she had made of frail flowers in pale washes of blue or pink watercolor. Slender green leaves and single blossoms reached up into blank white pages of stiff cardstock.

A week and a half after my meeting with Audrey and Mrs. Parr, I arrived on the ward to find that the ambulance had come at 6:40 that morning, an hour before I entered the building. Susan was gone.

In only one week, my PGY-II year would be over, and my rotation on the floor would end. Parr's chart remained to be dictated, but other tasks and responsibilities—finishing up on the ward and getting ready for the new year—soon crammed my time. In the meantime, I walked down to medical records and dropped off the notes and poems she had written to me for inclusion in her chart.

* * *

Liver rounds—a monthly hour of beer and pizza for residents and faculty—were held a few days before the changeover. As we stood around with drinks, I asked Greg Halper, who had been the assistant unit chief on the twelfth floor, "How did you find the three year?"

"It's very tough. It's worse than the two year. By the end of it, I felt chewed up and spit out. Being on call in the emergency room can be a killer: you see folks there for half an hour or forty minutes, only now you're by yourself without any other staff around watching them. Then, after you've sent most of these patients back out into the world, if anything happens to them, you can be nailed. One medical intern at a hospital downtown had an ER patient die and was sued for criminal charges before a grand jury."

Roy walked up to me. "Getting ready for the three year?" he asked.

"I think it'll be exciting but hard."

"That's probably right. I thought it was better than the two year. Except for the nights on call, it can actually be quite pleasant."

"Any survival tips?"

He tilted his head to the side and screwed up his eyes, thinking. "Make sure you eat dinner," he said. "You'll be stuck in the ER seeing several patients at once, with more waiting. But make sure you sneak out to grab a bite—for your own sanity as much as anything else. You'll learn a lot this coming year," he said. "For the first time you begin to feel like a Real Psychiatrist. But the ER is the most stressful thing I've ever done in my life. The thing to remember is that it never lasts more than twenty-four hours. I had to keep telling myself that whenever I was on. 'Twenty-four hours and it will all be over.' A lot of us entered therapy ourselves. It's a good time to begin. As a three your time is more flexible since you schedule some of it yourself, so getting out during the day to see your shrink is easier. Plus, your own therapy is helpful for dealing with some of the cases you'll treat." I had hoped and assumed that residency would get easier over time, but I now got the sense that it might not.

I gulped down my beer, tossed out the bottle, and walked home with a sinking feeling in my gut.

Strings

I had gotten used to working on inpatient wards but would now have to learn a whole new set of skills and approaches with outpatients. It was one thing to help patients already on a ward. The ultimate goal was clear: to discharge them, hopefully by making them better, though not necessarily. But with outpatients, the tasks were much different: determining whether they had a mental illness or not and, if so, figuring out whether they should or shouldn't be psychiatrically treated and hospitalized. These decisions had enormous impact on people's lives, from stigmatizing to lifesaving. I would also be more on my own than ever before and thus have more responsibility. Outpatients wouldn't be watched around the clock as they were in the hospital. By comparison, inpatient work was much more secure.

My first morning in the outpatient department, or OPD, Gina, the OPD secretary, paged me. "Your ten o'clock eval is here," she said. Downstairs, she handed me the appointment slip with the patient's name in block letters, printed neatly in pencil.

"Gary McClintock," I called out.

"Yes." He was sitting in the waiting area, huddled in a chair against the wall, wearing a plaid lumberjack shirt, work boots, and jeans. His black hair was parted on the side. He gathered his green army-navy jacket in his hand and closed a glossy, embossed-cover Stephen King novel he was reading. Compared to inpatients, he didn't look "sick." He could easily be someone on a subway or a bus.

I introduced myself. "My office is over here."

"Okay," he said springing up to walk along with me.

147

"What brings you here today?" I asked when we were seated in my office.

"My OCD."

"Your OCD?"

"Yes." He had obsessive-compulsive disorder and told me his history. "I've had it for years. I'm forty-five now. It started in my twenties. I've had every kind of treatment available. I need something else."

"What treatment have you had?"

"First ECT, but it did nothing but make me confused for a while. Then I had a cingulotomy. Then—"

"A cingulotomy?"

"Yes," he said matter-of-factly. "They removed a portion of my brain." He tapped his finger on the side of his head. "They went in over here." He pointed with two fingers toward the upper corner of his eye socket, under his eyebrow and beside his nose. Initially, lobotomies had been performed by piercing that spot with an actual ice pick. Psychosurgeons had removed a portion of his brain in an effort to cure him. A hollow chill tingled from the base of my neck down my spine, and a coldness clutched my bones. I had never before met or even heard about a patient who had received psychosurgery, though textbooks describe it. In a cingulotomy, part of the thalamus, a portion of the brain, is snipped away. Cingulotomies were rarer than lobotomies, which clipped off prefrontal lobes, thought to be the seat of planning for the future and, perhaps as a result, anxiety and psychosis.

"How was it for you?"

"It helped for about thirty days. Then my OCD returned." He was missing part of his brain. Little was known about the full functioning of subportions of the brain. What if too much live tissue or other memories and capacities had been cut out? What if the bit of plucked-out brain was later found to be involved in other functions as well? Recent theories about neuronal processes have suggested that many intellectual functions depend on the integration of the brain as a whole. What if the tests used in the past had failed to detect more subtle deficits? Psychiatry seemed to me to be about guiding people to interact differently, not about intervening this irreversibly, permanently excising parts of their brains, making them biologically different people. Psychosurgery has been heavily discredited, at least in many of its uses, and employed with much less frequency than in the past. Yet according to textbooks, cingulotomies are still occasionally performed for severe OCD that doesn't respond to any other treatment. Gary had subsequently been hospitalized several times, and had received individual psychotherapy, group psychotherapy, psychoanalysis, extensive behavioral treatments, and various medications, including clomipramine—much heralded recently, though it hadn't worked on him either. In his place, I might have been more wary of psychiatric treatments as a result, but he was eager to try something else, something new.

After meeting with him I spoke to Dr. Shelly Tarr, an attending in the outpatient department.

"How about clomipramine, *with* behavioral treatment and group all at the same time?" she suggested.

None of these had worked individually, but she felt they could be a solution together. I was skeptical but went along. If that failed, no doubt some other addition would be made, perhaps a second or even a third medication added simultaneously. Perhaps over time the illness might naturally abate by itself, with credit given to whatever the treatment was at the moment.

I told Gary of the plan. "Maybe that'll help," he said. "It's something." He struggled to grin and looked searchingly at me to share his hope. Clearly, much of what I offered was the possibility of improvement. The placebo effect, though derided by some, has been shown in a number of studies to alleviate a variety of woes in about one-third of patients. The glimmer of hope is worth a lot, allowing patients and psychiatrists to believe that treatment is effective, that helplessness can somehow be relieved.

As Gary looked at me in my office, I smiled back at him. His lips then widened until he beamed, glad that something else would be tried.

Evaluations in the outpatient department had a leisurely pace, scheduled in advance and allowing me ample time to meet with the patient more than once and discuss the case with an attending physician. But the emergency room, where my on-call nights would now be spent, differed dramatically from all of my previous work. I would be the only psychiatrist on duty in the ER, the only one to act or make decisions about patients. Quick decisions would be called for, often based on little information. Even on inpatient wards, when on call, other staff were around who knew the patients and watched them at night.

In the past, the patients I had seen on the wards had been judged by more experienced psychiatrists to need hospitalization. Someone had decided that each patient had slipped above a certain level of dangerousness to himself or others. I hadn't thought much about what separated those who needed to be in the hospital from the rest of us. Yet now I was to begin making these decisions myself, assuming the role of gatekeeper.

I started working in the ER late one afternoon. The ER was open to the street through big glass doors. Just inside stood a registration desk, where a secretary checked patients' insurance information, and a triage desk where a nurse assigned patients to appropriate specialists in the ER, prioritizing the cases.

Anyone could walk in off the street and see a psychiatrist. Patients who came here were often the most in need of treatment, and most vulnerable to stresses outside. I would be the first one to evaluate the patient fully. Any person with any problem could enter the glass doors from the street and be my next case.

"You psych?" a nurse asked me after I arrived in the ER, having been paged for the first time to see a patient. I introduced myself.

"I'm triage. My name's Karen. The sheet's in your box." She gestured toward a stack of slots with black labels on them, reading, "Med," "Surg," "OB," "Ophtho," and "Psych."

Inside the slot was a triplicate ER registration form. "Doris Perkins. Thirty-eight years old." Chief complaint: "I'm nuts."

"You'll be having some fun," Karen chortled.

"What do you mean?"

"You'll see. She was brought in here by the police. I put her in cubicle ten. Medicine is using the psych room at the moment."

That's all I knew about my new patient.

I knocked on the EKG machine parked by the entry to the cubicle. There was no door—only a torn curtain. "Doris Perkins?"

"Yes?"

She was seated in the corner of the room, at the far end of a stretcher, a tall thin woman with bouffant blond hair, wearing a waist-length fur jacket. And nothing else. No shirt. No pants. No skirt. No dress. No underwear. From her shoulder, on a gold chain, hung a designer pocketbook, its soft leather hide embossed with a diamond pattern.

"I'm Dr. Klitzman," I said, reaching out to shake her hand, almost automatically, as I had been taught.

"Nice to meet you." She smiled politely—unconcerned about her appearance, as if unaware of it.

"Let me see if there's something else I can get for you to wear." I found a pair of hospital pajamas on a cart outside and returned. "Here," I said, offering them to her, "put these on." She opened them over her lap to cover herself partially.

"You're wearing only a fur coat," I observed, unsure if I was asking her or telling her.

"I thought it might be cold out and I didn't want anyone to steal it."

"I see. What happened to your other clothes?"

"They were contaminated."

"Contaminated?"

"Irradiated. I'm afraid to wear them."

In retrospect, I'm surprised I didn't crack up. But she elicited my concern, sadness, and protectiveness.

"How long have you felt that?"

"Since yesterday."

"And what made you come here today?"

"I was going uptown."

"Oh."

She wasn't suicidal or homicidal—the two criteria for admission discussed the most. But another criterion, far less frequently invoked, was inability to care for oneself, which seemed to be the case here. She seemed delusional and was placing herself in enough potential danger to warrant admission.

"Do you have any insurance information with you?"

"Yes," she said, reaching into her purse and handing two white cards to me between two fingertips. Her other fingers spread away in the air, far from the pieces of paper. "But be careful," she whispered, leaning closer to me. "I'm warning you: they're hot." She accented this last word. She apparently thought they were irradiated, too.

"Okay," I said, lowering my voice as well, going along with her. I followed her example, and held them with only two fingertips. "Thank you."

I didn't know anything about her past, and she wasn't able to tell me much.

I spoke to the policeman who brought her. He reported that she had been staying for several days in a penthouse suite at the most expensive hotel in town, ordering champagne, caviar, and lavish meals through room service and telephoning around the world, tracking down old friends and family members, some of whom she hadn't spoken to in years. She had run up a bill of several thousand dollars and didn't have the money. The hotel finally called the police.

"Is there anyone who knows you whom I can speak to?" I asked her.

"No one here. I'm from out of town."

"Anyone?"

"My sister in Florida." She gave me the number.

I left and phoned to relay the story. "Not again!" her sister exclaimed in exasperation. "She did this three years ago, too, but recently she's been doing better on her lithium." Lithium is a naturally occurring salt successfully used in the treatment of mania.

"What happened with your lithium?" I asked Doris back in the cubicle.

"I ran out."

I admitted her to the hospital. She signed the form readily. I had her put on the pajamas, over which she slipped the fur coat, and I brought her up to the fifteenth floor. There, I introduced her to Carol Walters, the nurse on duty, who had Doris sit in the lounge. Alone, in the middle of the lounge at 2:00 A.M., wearing her pajamas and fur coat, Doris looked woefully out of place, defenseless, and confused. My contact with her was now officially over. I would probably never see her again and might never find out how she fared. I felt worried about her. She was exposed and unaware of how she appeared or came across. I had momentarily been a guide, helping her in ways she couldn't help herself, defending her from situations in which she might end up. I said goodbye, and wished her luck.

I would actually get to see Doris one more time. A month later, I spotted her leaving the building one evening. I did a double take, almost not recognizing her except for her fur coat. Everything else had changed. She was now wearing a blouse and a skirt and high heels. She stopped, looked at me, trying to remember my face, then glanced at my name tag and grinned.

* * *

When I left her on the ward that first night, I was very concerned about her but had no way of continuing to help her, having done all I could.

I walked slowly downstairs, unlocked the door from the inside, and stepped out into the fresh air. It was now dark out, but I was free. The evening air was scented with soft fragrances from a boxwood hedge along the street and a flowering tree, through whose branches a light breeze played.

The sky opened up above me. Through the leaves, tiny stars glittered. At the end of the hospital driveway, almost at the curb of the street, I started home, when suddenly my beeper squawked again.

The number flashed was that of the emergency room.

Disheartened, I turned around to return to the hospital. Up in the sky, the stars now looked fewer and fainter.

"You have another patient down here," the triage nurse told me on the phone, as if reminding me, and surprised I wasn't there already.

I headed back to the ER.

On the ER sheet for my new patient, under "Name," were the words "Banana Bush."

"Banana Bush?" I asked, walking into the small psychiatry interview room. A short Hispanic woman sat with her legs crossed, smoking a cigarette.

"Yes?"

I introduced myself.

"I'm related to the president, you know," my new patient told me. "I married one of his sons." She was wearing a pair of sunglasses with one of the lenses missing. The empty frame encircled her left eye. She wore a tattered and dirty red sweater and a pair of blue jeans, ripped, sooty, and stained. The seam unraveled along both legs.

"Me and Barbara are real close," she continued. "Like this." She crossed her middle and index fingers and held them up in the air. Her fingernails were long, yellowed, and clotted with dirt along the edges. Her other hand held the lit cigarette. Flecks and bits of cotton and fabric and threads nested in her matted, unwashed hair. "Sometimes I stay at the White House."

"Is that right?"

"Yes." She took a drag on a cigarette, then turned her head and exhaled the bluish smoke between us. On her registration form, under "Address," the triage nurse had written "Undomiciled." She was a street person.

"Have you ever seen a psychiatrist before?"

"Plenty."

"Have you ever been in a psychiatric hospital?"

"They don't always tell you what it is."

"How many times?"

"I lost count."

"What would you guess?"

"Four times at Rivershore State . . . Twice here . . . Three times at . . ." She rattled off the names of four or five other hospitals where she had been several times each.

"When was the last time?"

"About three months ago."

"What brings you here now?"

"I want psychoanalysis." Psychoanalysis was usually indicated for "high-functioning neurotics."

She looked psychotic. "Are you hearing any voices when no one is speaking?"

"Yes."

"What's the voice?"

"The president. He speaks to me. We're related. I married one of his sons."

"What does the president say?"

She took a drag on her cigarette and blew out another thin stream of smoke, then tapped the ashes twice into the ashtray.

"I can't always make it out."

"Is there anyone I can speak to who knows you?"

"The president."

"Anyone else?"

"My caseworker. At the shelter."

I phoned the caseworker. "I have a patient here named Banana Bush."

"Oh, you have Banana there? Great. How's she doing?"

I glanced back at her sitting in the psych room, making paper fans out of the pile of admission forms and fluttering them back and forth in the air. "Well, it's kind of hard to say. I'm wondering if you can tell me about her, and about how she's been doing lately."

"She thinks she's the president's daughter-in-law."

"So I gather."

"It's a delusion she has. She tells everyone about it, and actually tried phoning the White House once when she was broke. She sees a psychiatrist, but often stops her meds and gets crazier."

"Have you noticed any change recently?"

"She's slowly getting worse."

"Over how long a time?"

"I'd say the past few months."

"What kind of change?"

"She gets into fights here at the shelter. Nothing too serious. A lot of our clients fight periodically. If you could do something to help her it would be great."

"Is her ability to take care of herself being affected?"

"It's beginning to, yes."

I wasn't sure if I should admit her. She could benefit from hospitalization and was clearly sick and getting worse. She was also asking to be admitted by coming here. Yet we had been instructed that that was not enough. There was an implicit prejudice against admitting patients at night unless it was an emergency. It was a point of honor. Dr. Sidney Ostrow, a senior attending in the outpatient department, had told us during a brief orientation to the ER, "If a patient can be admitted electively during business hours rather than as an emergency at night, then do it." Residents sometimes admitted patients anyway, since once a patient was in the ER, admitting them took less time than sending them out, having to make further calls to ensure that outpatient treatment was in place. But the wards hated it when we admitted patients at night, as they were less staffed, and we were admonished to "be a wall" down in the ER. Other residents told stories of patients they had managed to keep out, easily justified by the low resources generally available. There was particular pressure not to admit chronic patients, such as the homeless, who, though ill, might not be much sicker than their usual baseline state. I still remembered that Bransky hadn't been respected or treated well during his first hospitalization, and was eventually kicked out. Indicatively, he hadn't been readmitted from the ER shortly before his death. To keep patients out was seen as being strong, to admit them was a sign of weakness.

Banana did have an outpatient psychiatrist and had an appointment scheduled in a few days. There were also only two beds left for the weekend. If Banana took one there'd be only one left for any sicker or more desperate patients who came in.

Unable to reach Banana's psychiatrist, as it was night, I left a message. The decision was up to me. I would have to make a choice as to who would be helped, doing my own triage.

I decided to let her go, in large part because of institutional pressures that, I was seeing, sometimes ended up prevailing over concerns for the individual.

I told her that she wouldn't be admitted. She slid down off the ER stretcher. I had heard that the registration desk could give patients bus fare if necessary, and asked them to give it to her. I shook her grainy, rough-skinned hand, and she left.

Of my first two ER patients, I had thus admitted one and discharged one. I could help some, but not all. The issues were very different but also seemed manageable. So far, so good.

I was completing the paperwork, including a note outlining my findings and reasons for not admitting Banana, when a short man with a gray crew cut tapped me on the shoulder.

"You wanted a chart on Bush?" He read off the name. "Banana Bush. Number 5703481?"

"Yes."

"Here it is. Sign for it over here." According to her chart, she had been seen in the ER six times over the past month and a half, though she hadn't told me. Each time a different resident had assessed her.

I read over their respective notes. Everyone had come to the same conclusion as I had—not to admit her. But the notes indicated that she was slowly getting worse and that she seemed to want to be admitted. I felt glad about arriving at the same conclusion. I hoped that if she ever got much worse she'd be able to find her way back to the hospital.

A week later I saw her on the low balustrade by the steps to the hospital's side entrance. She was crouched down playing with a handmade wooden yo-yo. It ran up and down a thin, rough white string over the edge of the hospital steps, as crowds of doctors and nurses strode by during lunchtime. She watched the yo-yo roll up and down. None of the staff noticed her at all. In the past, I might have rushed by and not seen her either.

Vows

My world was being increasingly divided into that of psychiatrists and nonpsychiatrists. My role and experiences as a resident were difficult to explain to others, going against popular, commonsense views about the mind and mental illness. Most of the lay public, as psychiatrists called them, believed that doctors only did what was clearly of immediate good for patients, and that helping patients as much as possible at all times was the goal. It was hard to express how the situations I encountered were often much more complicated than that. The difference between the public image of psychiatry and the reality continued to astound me.

As I proceeded deeper and deeper into psychiatry, I felt increasingly separated from those outside the profession. Many psychiatrists dated, married, and socialized almost exclusively with other psychiatrists. During the summer, flocks of psychiatrists all go to the town of Wellfleet, Massachusetts, for the month of August and constantly see each other on the beaches, around the swimming lakes, and walking in town. No other profession vacations together as widely and predictably. It is a clan that clings to itself. A wide gulf quickly separates psychiatrists from others, partly as a result of the kinds of experiences I was having in residency. The process of dealing with the furthest, most disturbing reaches of the mind alters and warps one's ability to socialize as one has in the past. Nonpsychiatrists become wary of members of the profession, segregating us even further. Psychiatry is not well understood by those outside the field.

This gap was soon made clear to me one weekend when I attended a wedding in Vermont of some friends from college. It was nice to get away for two days. At the reception, I was introduced to an intelligent-looking couple—an architect and a lawyer.

"Bob here is a psychiatrist," a mutual friend said.

The couple stepped back. "A psychiatrist?" the architect asked. He sported a goatee and wire rim glasses and held a scotch and soda in his hand. "Doodoodoodoo— Doodoodoodoo," he sang, imitating the musical theme from Rod Serling's *The Twilight Zone*, twiddling his fingers in the air between us as if performing magic. "I'd better be careful what I say, huh? Are you going to psychoanalyze me while we talk?" This last was a common question. I now understood why Dr. Farb, the psychiatric hospital's director, once said that he never tells strangers he meets, such as people sitting next to him on an airplane, that he's a psychiatrist. When a stranger asks him what he does, he says he's an internist. In contrast, a successful film director I know of always tells strangers who ask that he's a psychiatrist. "You wouldn't believe the stories people then tell you," he says. "It's amazing."

"Say, how does that work by the way?" the architect asked. "To become a psychiatrist do you have to get psychoanalyzed yourself?" He seemed intrigued by the notion of being able to explore one's inner life.

"That's if you want to become a card-carrying psychoanalyst," I said. "But you don't have to be psychoanalyzed"—that is, by lying on a couch three to five times a week—"if you just want to become a general psychiatrist," in which case psychotherapy is not required. Even well-educated people weren't clear about these distinctions. Perhaps the field didn't make them clear.

"Do people treat you differently because you're a shrink?"

"I hope not."

"So do drugs really work? Do they change the mind?"

"Many times, yes," I said. "Though often, more than drugs alone are needed."

"Don't you get tired listening to crazy people all day?"

What would I say? "Sometimes, yes."

They asked me more questions. The low level of general knowledge about psychiatry and mental health surprised me. Once I had joined this specialty, it was hard to remember how little I, too, knew about it beforehand. Moreover, only in meeting nonpsychiatrists did I now see how much I had, in fact, become a member of the profession.

Wire Glass

Psychiatry was often stressful because of the impossibility of knowing patients' outcomes. The unpredictability of mental illness kept raising its ugly head. Some patients did better than anticipated. But others did far worse.

A few days after returning from the wedding out of town, Lou Leftow, who was now the chief resident—chosen from his class to stay on for an extra year and have administrative duties, helping to run the residency program—paged me during the middle of a class and asked me to report immediately to his office.

"Do you remember Susan Parr?" he asked after I sat down across from him.

I had transferred her to Rivershore State several weeks before. Why was he bringing her up now? "Yes," I said, hesitatingly.

"She suicided over the weekend."

"She what?"

"She hanged herself."

"At Rivershore?"

"That's right."

I didn't understand. It didn't fit. How did she kill herself while in a hospital, especially one supposedly most suited to caring for severely ill patients like her? She had been fairly stable at our hospital only a few weeks before. Somehow, her twenty-sixth suicide attempt had succeeded. She was no more. I suddenly thought of her limp hair, her frail voice, her thin, quivering smile, her drawings and her poems. I respected her attempt to express herself creatively through poetry and art, in the face of a disease she could not control. Even though she had been under other psychiatrists' care at a different hospital, her death was still unnerving—too much for me on the heels of Enrico's attempt.

"They're having an M and M next week," Lou continued, "and asked me if you would go." My heart beat faster. An M and M is a morbidity and mortality conference, where technically either a patient's illness or death—but, in fact, in my experience always death—is discussed and analyzed by a room of physicians. The patient's doctors present the case, implicitly defending their decisions before official scrutiny. Was I somehow culpable? "You'd just be there as an observer," he continued. "You don't have to say anything."

"I haven't had a chance yet to dictate her chart," I said, "because of the changeover."

"That's okay."

"Should I mention what happened in my summary of her hospitalization?"

"I wouldn't. Just write a separate note about it in her chart since it occurred post-discharge."

I returned to my class. "Is everything okay?" Anne asked. I told them all what had happened. The group fell silent for a moment.

"That's too bad," Sarah finally said.

The professor quickly resumed his discussion, but I sat in a state of shock and grief.

The instructor called on me to answer a question at one point. I was surprised. Couldn't he tell I was preoccupied after the news? He assumed that nothing would prevent me from paying full attention to his lecture. What mattered most to him was his class. But I kept thinking of Susan Parr, the tragedy of our hospital's passing her on to a larger, impersonal institution that had been unable to save her from herself.

Death is never easy, particularly that of patients. The fact that she was gone carried with it a hard certainty, permanence, and irrevocability unlike any aspect of my care of other patients I was then treating. I felt a gap, a loss. I had tried to help her. Despite my better judgment, I felt somehow guilty and wondered whether I had done everything I could for her. I sensed yet again how suicide was seen as a flaw in the therapy, as potentially preventable through hospitalization and maximal observation until treatment took effect.

It was clear that the stakes in clinical psychiatry were far higher than I had thought or had been led to believe. Nothing in this profession would now be the same for me.

One week later, I hailed a taxi to Rivershore State in the rain.

I had never been there, though several patients I knew had been sent there, often against their will. The taxi took a highway to the outer edge of the city. In the distance, across a river, a conglomeration of buildings slowly emerged out of the mist. Steep walls, pierced only by rows of tiny black windows and topped by towers, rose up rigidly against the dirty gray sky. Dark trees hugged the shore and climbed up at the base of the building as if trying to soften the imposing brick facade. Somewhere in that fortress, Susan had ended her life.

I had occasionally driven by the buildings on the highway, but had never known what they were or thought to inquire, and no one ever mentioned them. They looked like an abandoned prison.

The cab exited the highway on a ramp with only one destination—the hospital. We followed a line of dirty sanitation trucks under the belly of the highway. The cab sloshed through muddy pools, past patches of weeds and piles of stones and debris fallen off the overpass. Dripping graffiti streaked the walls. The air smelled rotten and stale. We filed slowly over a concrete Depression-era bridge the gritty color of cornmeal, and entered the hospital grounds. Rows of neatly clipped trees lined the road and looked stunted in their growth. The wide lawns were empty and silent.

Once inside, I followed the directions I had been given, making the second right, the third left, and the third right, passing the "B Well Clinic," en route. Patients shuffled by stiffly in the halls, slowly and without energy. The M and M was held in the cafetorium—the patient cafeteria with an elevated platform in front allowing the space to serve also as an auditorium.

Dr. Lee, the hospital's chief psychiatrist, presented Susan's case. "Ms. Parr was clearly a suffering person," he concluded. "But why did it happen now?"

"She was afraid of the insight she was getting," one doctor suggested. I was dubious of that as an explanation, of how much insight patients get in state mental hospitals.

Along the side of the room were tiny windows made of small panes of glass embedded with metal chicken wire mesh. A few windows were hinged, enabling them to tilt open—but only slightly—to let air in through a narrow crack. Through the trees outside, a boat calmly passed in the distant river, seeming strangely out of place in this closed institution—almost an optical illusion. I looked around me at the hospital, with its cinder-block walls, wondering if she had succeeded this time because of where she was: here in this institution, where the severely mentally ill were housed when they were beyond the help of outpatient psychiatrists or more pleasant, shorter-term hospitals. In some ways our own hospital had just dumped her here. She might have felt rejected, unwanted.

"It was luck when it happened," Dr. Lee said. "But she also had apparently recently spoken to her mother on the phone, which she hadn't done for a while. Had anyone here spoken to her family during her hospitalization?" The audience hung their heads, sad and embarrassed. None of them had. He had found something that they had done wrong. He was suggesting that if only that were done, if only her mother had been spoken to, Susan might have lived. Yet, as Nolan once told me, "In every hospitalization, of the four hundred things done, we probably do forty wrong. They usually don't matter, and we usually don't think about them—unless the patient dies."

Still, it felt like Dr. Lee was blaming the staff. I didn't want to say that I *had* spoken to her mother previously, and make them feel or look worse at that moment, rubbing it in that there was something they hadn't done. More important, I sensed that it probably wouldn't have made a difference.

I sat on the dais, in numb shock. A patient of mine killing herself—even a former patient no longer under my care—shattered the soft and comfortable cocoon of this profession, the sense that the work was often pleasant, and that I could talk to and act toward patients as I felt appropriate. I now saw that disaster lurked much closer than I had thought. Bransky's problems had been beyond my control and also my purview. Enrico had ultimately lived. In the end, nothing had happened to him, and, consequently, it was easier to dismiss the burden of responsibility, the sense that perhaps—just perhaps—a death might have occurred. But the potential dangers and risks were far more visible and real now. I would have to be more careful and couldn't just act spontaneously, blithely proceeding, but would have to be more vigilantly on guard against disaster. This may sound extreme, but in fact, recent studies have shown that the most stressful experience in a psychiatrist's entire career is having a patient commit suicide. Indeed, some psychiatric disorders are more fatal than medical disorders. According to some studies, roughly twenty-five percent of patients with major depression eventually kill themselves, as do ten percent of schizophrenics and ten percent of patients with borderline personality disorders.

In some ways I was lucky because in no case did a patient under my care successfully suicide. And with neither Bransky nor Enrico nor Susan had I actually done anything wrong. Yet I was still left unsettled, especially by the cumulative effect. I felt guilty that I had sent her here, even though everyone had seemed to support that. Maybe I was angry with her that she had done this and had risked soiling my reputation, though that seemed selfish. But mostly I felt vaguely threatened and somehow hollowed out, removed and speechless. I had always been a bit of a perfectionist, trying to do the best I could in my work. But here something had gone wrong. I thought back to nurses on our ward saying that Susan wouldn't kill herself while hospitalized, yet here she had.

The M and M proceeded. The meeting felt like a funeral or a memorial service, in which we talked about the deceased and tried to make sense of his or her life and death, to find some explanation, some meaning.

I felt somehow partly responsible and that to be more cautious, I would no longer be able to trust the straightforward ease of some parts of my job. Since psychiatry relied heavily on our own impressions and subjective judgments, bad outcomes were more difficult to attribute to external factors. In medicine, for example, failures were ascribed to patients' high sodiums or low potassiums. When disaster occurred in psychiatry, I had nothing to blame but the subjective impressions that had led to my decisions—not objective factors. I was left questioning myself more.

After the M and M I exited the cafetorium and retraced my steps through the hospital's mazelike corridors, getting lost several times. In the foyer, I telephoned for a cab and waited. A large mural stretched behind me, filled with ladders and houses all askew. Static bubbled on overhead speakers. I felt confined just standing there, and stepped outside into the cold damp air to wait for my taxi. The grounds were still deserted. No patients were outside. As I crossed the driveway, a huge flock of pigeons flapped noisily into the air from the asphalt where they had been resting undisturbed. They scattered dirt and dust about them.

A black cab finally pulled up and we drove off, soon merging with traffic on the highway. The buildings of Rivershore soon stood behind me in the distance, silent monuments, their inhabitants out of sight. Out of mind.

When I returned to the hospital I was paged about an emergency I had to attend to. I had to walk an older patient to the ER, then to the business office to arrange for her admission. As a result, I was delayed for my next appointment, a new evaluation. I mentioned to Shelly Tarr, the attending, that I had a new patient waiting. "Just make sure he's not suicidal or homicidal," she told me, "and then reschedule him."

"Edgar Weintraub?" I called out, back in the OPD.

"Yes. That's me," he said.

He was a thin man with pale skin and freckles and long blond hair, dropping down from the sides of his head and pulled back into a pony tail. He wore tight blue jeans, cowboy boots, and a tight-fitting leather jacket. I had seen him when walking my admission back and forth and remembered him scanning me.

"I'm sorry about the delay, but I had to take care of an emergency." He frowned. In his eyes it probably hadn't looked like an emergency: no flashing lights, crash carts, or blaring beepers. An elderly woman and I had merely tottered back and forth in front of him. "My office is around the corner." We sat down inside. "Unfortunately, we're going to be able to meet only briefly today, but we'll set up another appointment."

"Do I get charged for this one?" I didn't know and assumed not, but had never had to deal with fees for an evaluation before. If he were in a crisis, it might take up the full time—I'd just be late for my next appointment—and he might need to be charged.

"Let's talk for a few minutes first, then we'll discuss that. What brings you here today?"

"I'm fed up. I get bummed out a lot."

"Are you feeling depressed?"

"Depressed? Yeah, you can say that."

"How long has it been going on for?"

"About six months. Since my girlfriend left me last winter." His sleep and appetite were decreased.

"Any feelings that life isn't worth living?"

"Sometimes."

"What do you think?"

"That I'd like to end it sometimes."

"Do you have a plan?"

"I've thought of taking an overdose. I have enough pills in the bathroom cabinet."

"Any thoughts like that now?"

"Right this second? No."

I spoke to him further and decided we could stop and meet again next week.

"So do I have to pay for this?" he asked.

We had met for about twenty-five minutes in all.

"I don't know. I don't think so, but I can check downstairs."

"I'm self-pay," meaning, I assumed, that he didn't have insurance, "and I don't really want to pay."

"They'll tell us downstairs."

"I don't know about coming back here."

"Why?"

"Because all you did was ask me short questions. You didn't really talk to me much. I didn't like it."

"I just wanted to speak with you for a few minutes. Next week we'll have more time."

"If I come. This wasn't helpful."

"Look, I don't really know you, but you say you're feeling depressed, and I think it would be important to come to try to see if there's something we could do that might help you."

He pulled back in his chair. "You *don't* know me."

"I realize that, but it seems that psychiatric treatment might help you, and I think that not to pursue it might not be a good idea." He made another appointment, got up, and left.

The next day, Dr. Ostrow paged me.

"What are you doing right this minute?" he asked abruptly.

"I'm just starting with a patient."

"Come down to my office as soon as you're done," he barked. Click. He hung up.

I had no idea why he wanted to see me.

"You met with a patient yesterday—Weintraub?"

"Yes."

"What happened?"

"What happened?"

"Yes. What happened?"

"I had an emergency right before. I told him we could meet only briefly and scheduled another appointment."

"That's not what he said."

"Huh?"

"He says you made interpretations to him about himself without even knowing him."

"What? No, what happened was—"

"Don't get defensive," he snapped, cutting me off quickly, leaning forward, and spreading out his hands in front of him to block me from continuing.

"I wasn't getting defensive, I—"

"There you go again. I'm going to reassign this patient to someone else. You're off the case. But I don't like this. I don't like it at all. I don't want it happening again, understand?"

"Yes, but that's not—"

"There you go again being defensive. Now I have to go. I don't have time for this kind of thing." He leaped up, thrust open the door, and ushered me out.

"But . . ."

He glared and pointed his finger at my lips telling me to shut up. It wasn't worth pursuing. I staggered out of his office, utterly stunned, bewildered, and mortified. Only later would I fill with rage. He had criticized me and then wouldn't even give me a chance to respond. My heart raced. After walking around in a daze for a while, I bumped into Roy in the hallway and relayed the story.

"That's the same exact thing he did to me once," Roy said.

"Really?"

"Yes. He called me in and bawled me out about something that hadn't even really happened and then jumped on me and said, 'Don't get defensive' when I started to answer his attacks, which were all incorrect. He does that to people, I've heard," Roy said. "It's just him."

Roy was a talented psychiatrist who would later do very well in the hospital, receiving several large research grants that were difficult to obtain, and getting promoted quickly.

Still, I never saw the patient again. He was assigned to Anne, who continued to see him in long-term therapy. She later told me that he had felt slighted and cheated—which were major issues for him, ways he saw the world that interfered with his life, on which Anne was working with him in therapy. In retrospect, what he most minded was the possibility of having to pay for the session. Self-pay was rare, and sliding scale fees were available. But residents were given very little information about how payments in evaluations worked.

Yet most surprising was Dr. Ostrow's presumption that when

a patient complained, the resident was wrong. He pounced to keep people in line, but since a real offense might not even have occurred, his policy served to maintain his own power. He routinely interviewed job applicants to the hospital early in the morning, before many would ordinarily be up—sometimes before dawn. He got to work then, anyway. But he'd note when the applicant arrived and how he looked. Ostrow did little to create anything resembling understanding or humaneness. Only later did I realize that his interrupting, "Don't get defensive," was simply a clever tactic, proclaiming, "I am right, you are wrong. Don't even bother to try to defend yourself."

"It's like the Marines here," Judy Van Meter had told me before I began. I now knew what she meant. The situations we faced were almost always gray rather than black and white, and filled with ambiguity. Scientific grounding was often weak, and successes were somewhat subjective. In this environment, inappropriately harsh criticism squelched any questioning or dissent, stymied discussion, and reinforced the hierarchy in the institution. We were learning to be on guard at all times with everything we said and did. We couldn't just be ourselves. The tactics showed no empathy toward us, which could in turn affect how we dealt with those under us in the hierarchy—our patients. It was a shame for all involved, for trainees, and for our patients.

That night, I went out to dinner with Mike and ordered a beer as soon as we sat down. I had never in my life felt as strongly that I needed a drink. I sure wanted one now.

Talisman

In the ER, I was more personally vulnerable than in any other setting. Here at the entry point to the hospital, as a resident, I would be most exposed and most threatened—both physically and psychologically. Whatever patients walked in from the street and the wild night, the resident here confronted—unbuffered, and unsupported by a staff of nurses, other doctors, or mental health aides.

A few days after Susan's M and M, I was again on call in the ER. Patients came and went all night without stop. No sooner did I finish one case when the next one arrived. I also had to see patients on medical wards who had psychiatric emergencies. No time was left even to get dinner.

Susan's death hovered over me throughout the evening, shaking me up more than I would have expected: I was awed and terrified by how much of patients' lives was beyond my control. Bad outcomes, even deaths, could occur. I was up against the raw harshness of mental illness, but had to keep going—another patient always waiting to be seen. I was driven by a schedule made weeks in advance, the ambition to do my best, and the belief that residency couldn't get any worse.

At 2:00 A.M. I was finishing with my last patient, who was on a medical ward. I was eager to return home, when triage paged me. "You got another one down here," she told me. "And he's violent."

"Put a security guard on him until I get there," I said. I headed downstairs a few minutes later, and as soon as I walked through the automatic double doors to the ER heard a man screaming. As I neared the psych room, the voice rose.

"I'm not staying!" he was yelling. "It's political. It's all political! They're putting me away for political reasons!"

A young man was standing in the doorway, his hands raised, pushing against the two sides of the blue metal door frame. John Tefferello was twenty-eight, with greasy long light brown hair tied back in a pony tail. The buttons of his plaid shirt were unfastened down to his stomach, exposing a hairy chest. He wore blue jeans, a wide leather belt with a big metal buckle, and work boots. "There ain't nothing wrong with me," he shouted. An indifferent security guard was leaning against the wall diagonally across the hall, at a safe distance.

I walked up to the patient, introduced myself, and held out my hand to shake. His arm didn't move.

"Can we sit down?" I asked, gesturing to the empty room behind him which he was barring.

"I'm getting the hell out of here."

"Why don't you sit down and tell me about it?"

"Fuck you, man. I'm bolting."

"I'd like to find out what's going on first."

"No way."

"I think it's best if you step into the room and sit down."

"Fuck off, buddy."

Suddenly, a cold, slimy glob smacked my face and rolled down my cheek. I was shocked. My finger reached up and touched the goop clinging to my skin, which had landed fractions of an inch from my eye. He had spat in my face. Good God!

The security guard called a colleague to join him and the two uniformed men in police hats were soon standing between John and myself.

"Come on, pal," one of them said to the patient, "step in the room here like the doctor asked you to."

A short elderly man had been pacing halfway down the hall, cowering underneath an old brown raincoat, and grinding a worn hat between his fist and his palm. He nervously stepped toward us now. "John, do here as the doctor says." The man was apparently the patient's father.

Under the combined pressure, John yielded, stepped back, and collapsed into a chair.

"Watch him," I told the two security guards, while dabbing the gooey saliva with my fingertips, which were soon coated with the frothy fluid. I started to raise my arm up to wipe the mess with my sleeve. "I'll be back in a minute." I went into the bathroom, bolted the door, and looked in the mirror. Below my left eye a wad of fluid had splat. I wiped it off with rough brown paper towels from the shiny stainless steel box on the wall, moistened a second towel with tap water and pink liquid soap from the plastic dispenser, and cleaned the area. Should I wash my eye out? What if he had some infectious disease—TB, syphilis, or AIDS? Luckily, it hadn't gotten directly into my eye.

My heart pounded. I felt assaulted, barely wanting to be there at this hour and being brutally repaid for my labors. It made it even harder to care about patients. But here I was with a job to do. Professionalism required separating myself from my work. I would have to take a different tack. Slowly, my neck cooled in my collar. I exhaled, shut my eyes for a minute—soothed by the blackness—then reopened them, and glanced in the mirror one last time.

John was now seated in the back of the room. His father hunched over in a chair near his side. One security guard leaned his rear end against the fake wooden armrest of a chair, the other guard stood at the door, his hands on his hips.

"Can I speak with you for a moment?" I asked his father. He nodded and we exited the room.

"I'm so sorry, Doctor, about what happened," he said to me in a thick Italian accent. "I'm sure he didn't mean it. But this is what he does at home, too."

"What's been going on?"

"He's been acting strange." John had been released from a psychiatric hospital five months before. At first he attended his outpatient appointments and took his medications, but then he complained that he didn't like or need the drugs. He stopped taking them and then stopped keeping his appointments. He had started mumbling to himself and stayed indoors most of the day, talking about the FBI coming after him. The few times he went out, he yelled at strangers on the street about government plots against him. His father only managed to get him to the ER by promising to take him out shopping and then telling him that he was going to the hospital himself, and merely wanted John to accompany him.

Back in the room I finally spoke to John, keeping my distance now. "What's been going on?"

"Nothing."

"How have things been at home?" He didn't answer. "Have you been taking your medications?"

"Fuck the medications."

"I think you need to come back into the hospital."

"No fucking way."

"You can either sign yourself in voluntarily or be sent against your will."

He eventually agreed to sign in. But there were no longer any beds available at the hospital. I would have to transfer him elsewhere. I made numerous calls without success. Two additional patients had now arrived and were sitting in the waiting room. I wondered how I'd ever get through this and despaired, overwhelmed.

Finally, after several more phone calls, I found John a bed at Rivershore State.

"How do I arrange for an ambulance down here?" I asked the triage nurse.

"Dispatch." I looked at her quizzically. "Down the hall. Second door on the left."

I followed her instructions and came to a thick wooden door, on which a basket of heavy-duty metal, open at the top, was screwed, presumably for dropping off memos or letters. I knocked. A muffled voice said, "Come in," and I entered a darkened, windowless room, much cooler and more air-conditioned than the rest of the ER.

A chubby woman sat in a padded swivel chair, her short black hair pulled back and held with a rubber band. She wore a loose rugby shirt of wide pink, yellow, and green horizontal stripes, and sneakers and jeans. In front of her on a Formica ledge lay an unwrapped half-eaten meal from McDonald's—Big Mac, fries that now looked cold, and a medium soda. It was 2:30 in the morning. A large machine with dials faced her—a combination of shortwave transmitter and switchboard.

Beside her burger stood a microphone on a nine-inch-high base. Huge street maps of the city and the surrounding counties sprawled across the walls, covering the cinder blocks. The only light in the room emanated from a dented gray metal desk lamp.

The air conditioner whirred and purred in the dim background. The coolness and relative tranquillity felt removed from the pressures and hubbub of the emergency room on the other side of the wall. It could be day or night in here. They were the same.

"Can I help you?" she asked.

"I'm from psychiatry. I need to send a patient to Rivershore State by ambulance." She reached up behind her along the wall to a five-foot-tall rack of slanted brown plastic boxes, each open at one side and storing a packet of blank forms. "Here," she said, slipping out pages from the different piles, "fill out these transfer forms. I have a driver who'll be back in about three hours. That's the best I can do. Can it wait?"

"I suppose."

"Okay." The patient probably wouldn't leave the ER until the next working day.

The various sets of forms—fronts and backs—were often redundant and took another hour to fill out. I Xeroxed all of the papers and confirmed the ambulance with the dispatch office. Then I had to see the two other patients, and finally was able to head home. A drizzle fell, wetting my clothes. Over my head I pulled my thin white coat, but it barely protected me.

Until now, during my nights on call—as a medical student, as an intern, and as a second-year resident—I always had to sleep in the hospital. For the first time, I could take calls from home, even sleeping in my own bed if there were no emergencies to handle. But I would have to be ready to rush back to the hospital at any hour of the night at a moment's notice. A week earlier, I had bought a television set for the first time in my life. I anticipated that during these periods of unknown length between visits to the ER, the uncertainty would hang over me and impede my doing any kind of reading or work. Watching TV seemed the right antidote, the only activity of which I'd be capable.

It was now 4:00 A.M. I had been in the hospital since 8:30 the previous morning, and had been looking forward to getting home. My answering machine was blinking and I played back the messages.

The taped first message started to roll. Through the crackling static of a bad connection, and odd noises, a gruff voice spoke. "Fuck you, asshole," a man yelled. Loud but indistinct voices mumbled in the background. "I'm going to get you . . . asshole . . . I'm going to kill you!"

I was horrified, and could hardly breathe. The little safe haven of my apartment had been invaded. It felt like a bad dream. The telephone could have been John Tefferello, or several patients in the ER during the day and night, or a random crank caller. The speaker didn't mention my name, yet I was frightened and helpless at the same time, without recourse. I could contact the police, but didn't have any information to give them—no name, no suspect. It wasn't realistic to list all the ER patients that day. It could have been a patient from the past, if it was one at all.

I decided to keep an extra close lookout on the street for any recent patients or other threatening people. I couldn't do anything about the threat now and decided to go to sleep. Dangerousness was impossible to predict with precision.

I carried the beeper into the kitchen with me to pour myself a glass of milk before going to sleep, and then put the beeper down on the tiled bathroom floor while brushing my teeth. I couldn't miss any pages. Finally, I lay down in bed, not knowing if I'd have to rush back to the ER in a few minutes or could sleep several hours until the morning. I set the beeper next to my alarm clock, and slept only lightly, having the sensation that I didn't go fast to sleep, though in fact having dreams.

Birds chirping outside awoke me. It was morning. No one else had called during the night.

A week later, Anne, Mike, Sarah, and I went out to dinner together. We had started our residencies together and still felt closer to each other than to the others in our group.

"So, I finally admitted Banana Bush last night," Sarah said as soon as we sat down. "She came in again. I read everyone's notes, and she was clearly going downhill." Mike, Joe, others, and I had all evaluated her. "I didn't want to be the softy—the one to admit her. But I did."

"She sounds endearing," Anne said over her shrimp salad, not having met her.

"You should have seen the patient I evaluated in the ER last night!" Mike said. "I got dragged out of bed at four-thirty in the morning to see the guy. I must have looked like hell, all unshaven, because he turned to me and said, 'You're the psychiatrist? You look worse than I do.' "

Two nights later it was again my turn in the ER.

"You have a patient in the psych room," the triage nurse paged me to say.

I picked up the patient's registration sheet and headed to cubicle ten.

The patient had rearranged all of the furniture in the room, moving one of the orange vinyl chairs from the left wall to the middle. The stretcher now abutted the door. The trash can, rising on a hollow black metal base, was now rolled on its side in the corner. He had torn up the pile of admission packets, ripping each one in half sideways, systematically proceeding through the foot-high stack, one set of forms at a time. They were scattered, matting the floor.

"Mr. Rothstein?"

"Yes."

"You've moved around all the furniture in the room!" I said, partly in astonishment, partly questioning his rationale.

"I didn't like the way it was. It bothered me."

"I see." I spoke with him further. It seemed he was very disturbed and would benefit from being admitted. There were no beds or cots left in the hospital, so I would have to transfer him. I dialed his local hospital. The telephone rang countless times. Someone must be there, though. Finally, after fifteen minutes: an answer.

"You want the ER?"

"Yes, please."

The operator transferred my call. The phone again rang incessantly. A gruff voice finally answered.

"I'll give you psych," she said, putting me on hold yet again. The line clicked faintly every second, as if searching, waiting.

"I'm sorry, we have no beds," a psychiatrist finally said when she answered.

"No beds? But he's from your catchment area." The county was divided into catchment areas around each hospital.

"I'm sorry, but we're full."

"We don't have any beds either. What am I suppose to do with the patient?"

"That's not my problem. He's in *your* ER." She hung up on me.

The call had taken me forty minutes and left me back where I'd started. I dialed another hospital and held the receiver as the phone rang for about fifteen minutes. An operator finally answered, paged the resident, and put me on hold for another ten minutes.

"Okay," the resident eventually said after picking up the phone and hearing about the case. "I'll take the patient. But I'm doing you a favor. What's your name, again?" I told her. "If we ever meet, you'll have to buy me a drink."

"Sure," I said. "It's a deal."

"Have the patient transferred. Fill out *all* of the paperwork, or I'll be annoyed."

"We're going to transfer you," I told the patient.

"You are not, Doctor," he said, standing up before me to his full height. "Because I am from the FBI, and Dr. Klitzman, you are now in deep trouble. I am here posing as a patient. We recently had a complaint about you that you transferred a patient illegally without his consent."

I was stunned. Had all this been a plant, having him look crazy to fool me?

I sat down on the orange plastic chair that he had moved into the center of the room. Had all of his redecorating also been a ploy to make me think he was disturbed? Had I previously done something incorrect? Nothing came to mind.

"Do you have any identification?" I finally thought to ask, having watched my share of television detective shows.

"Yes, I do," he said confidently, unperturbed.

"Oh shit!" I thought to myself, feeling defeated and stung. My career threatened to take a gigantic step backward.

He reached into his pocket and pulled out a piece of paper. It was small and pale blue. I leaned forward and squinted. It looked like a ticket from a movie theater.

"Can I see it please?"

"Yes."

He handed me the ripped stub. "Admit One," it said.

"This is your identification?"

"Yes."

I stood back up. "On the basis of what you've said, you need to be admitted to a hospital."

"Oh no I don't!"

He eventually refused to sign in, and I had to transfer him against his will.

It could be impossible solely on the basis of one interview to distinguish a real psychiatric patient from a fake one posing. It wasn't always easy to tell if someone was really crazy.

The ER exposed me to the vagaries and erraticism of the street and made me appreciate the inpatient wards where patients had all been screened and were being watched. The unpredictability of the ER filled me with dread. Mental illness was often impossible to gauge or evaluate with certainty. Just when I was getting the hang of it, new twists and problems would appear.

Thursday's 9:30 meeting started with a buzz. "Did you hear what happened last night?" Anne said under her breath as we were on line to get danish. "Joe Tauber was on. You won't believe it."

Just then, Dr. Farb started the meeting. "Sounds pretty agitated in here," he said.

"We're all talking about what occurred with Dr. Tauber last night," someone said.

Joe walked in and sat down. Everyone around the room turned to look at him.

"Good morning, Dr. Tauber," Dr. Farb said. "Do you want to tell us what happened overnight?"

"This man kept calling, claiming he was . . ." He mentioned the name of a world-famous celebrity, a multimillionaire closely tied to the worlds of politics, finance, and high society, someone's who's been on the cover of *Time*, *Newsweek*, *People*, and *The National Enquirer*. His name was a household word. "Anyway, he kept calling claiming it was he and that I should admit his niece to the hospital, and he mentioned a patient's name. I had seen this patient in the ER and didn't think she needed to be admitted. The caller started screaming at me, saying he would stop donating money to the hospital unless I admitted her. Then the hospital nighttime administrator called me. It seems this caller was bothering her, too. Finally, when the guy phoned again, I just hung up on him. I figured he was just a crank."

"He wasn't," Dr. Farb said from the front of the meeting. Gasps sounded around the room. Then silence.

"You mean," Joe started, clearing his throat, "that was . . ."

"That's right."

Joe blushed.

"So is the hospital screwed?" Anne asked.

"We've been on the phone all morning calming things down," Farb answered.

"But there's no way I could have known."

"What you should say," Farb told us, "whenever anyone calls saying he's someone and wanting to talk to you about a patient, is that you have no way of telling if that is really he on the phone."

"But what could I have done?"

"Said that—that you have no way of knowing who he is over the phone; it's a problem I'm sure someone like him is aware of—and that if he wants to come to the ER you'd be happy to talk to him."

"He wouldn't have done that."

"The other thing you could have done was to call me."

"At three in the morning?"

"You can reach me anytime at home." Yet residents never called the director of the hospital, let alone at home and at night. We tried to keep our dealings with him to a minimum. He was busy, important, and removed. None of us knew much about him or were even certain, for instance, what part of town he lived in, who his wife was, or whether he had any children. We all wanted to make a good impression on him, not come across as needy, pushy, weak, or uncertain. It was important to seem confident and in control.

* * *

A week later while on call, I admitted Lori Cardell from the ER. She had been depressed, had started drinking and using drugs, and had tried to overdose.

"Oh, and by the way," she said as I was completing the packet of necessary paperwork. "I don't want my family to know I'm here."

"Why not?"

"They'd hate me if they found out that I was using drugs and tried to kill myself. I couldn't ever face them again."

"I'd imagine though that they'd be concerned and want to help."

"No. You don't know them. Take my word for it: all hell would break loose."

My job was only to admit her to the ward. But I was concerned and said, "It's important you talk to your therapist about telling your family, once you're on the ward."

Every night, anyone calling the hospital to speak to a doctor is referred to the doctor on call in the ER. Later that evening a woman phoned and was given my name. "This is Edith Cardell," she said. "I understand my daughter went over to your emergency room a few hours ago. I haven't heard anything, what's wrong with her? Is she still there?"

What would I say? I didn't think the patient's stance of not wanting her family to know was good in the long run. But Lori was just settling into the hospital. "I'm sorry," I told the caller. "But I can't give out any information about a patient over the phone."

"What? Now you listen here—she's my daughter and I want to know where she is."

"I can't tell you."

"Why not?"

"If you want to come down to the ER, I'd be happy to talk with you."

"The hospital is way across town. I'm not going all the way over there—not at this hour. This makes no sense. Your hospital has my daughter, and I demand to get in contact with her!"

"I'll tell you what. Give me your name and number and let me call you back."

I explained the bind to the second-year resident on the ward. He was Lori's treating physician in the hospital for the rest of the night. "See if you can convince her to change her mind," I said.

I was back in the emergency room with another patient

when he called me back. "Cardell still doesn't want her family to know."

"Are you sure?"

"I just spent half an hour talking to her about it. She's adamant, and she has her rights."

"Tell her the bind we're in."

"I did. But it's a no-go. She wants her mother to worry. But our hands are tied. If that's what the patient wants, we have to respect her wishes. We don't have a choice." The patient was already on the ward at this point and under his care. There was nothing I could do.

My beeper emitted piercing squeals and I jumped. It was Mrs. Cardell. She hadn't waited for me to return her call.

"Well?" she asked. "Are you going to tell me where my daughter is?"

"I can't."

"This is crazy. Young man, if you don't tell me, I'm going to call the police. And television stations. And every major newspaper in town. I'm going to tell them that you, Dr. Klitzman, are holding my daughter and refusing to let her go or tell me where she is!"

"I'm sure that in the morning—"

"Forget about in the morning. I'm talking about *now*." I didn't want my name in every newspaper, but I would be violating the patient's confidentiality if I told her mother. "Do you hear me, Doctor?"

"Yes." My legs felt as wobbly as Jell-O as I stood talking to her on the phone in the crowded ER.

"And?"

"And you have to realize that one of my jobs is to protect patients' confidentiality."

"But I'm her mother."

"But I cannot give out any information. Look, anyone can call up and say that about a patient, and I'd have no way of knowing." I wouldn't be browbeaten by her.

"That does it!" she bellowed. "I know people, and I'm making phone calls," presumably to newspapers and TV stations. "You have not heard the end of this!"

She slammed down the phone, leaving me a bit light-headed and tremulous, my throat dry as paper.

Other patients were waiting to be seen in the emergency room, and I trudged off to see them, trying to concentrate as much as possible.

In the morning, the chief resident told me I had done the right thing. The patient eventually contacted her mother. Lori was being manipulative, getting back at her mother and making her doctors—particularly me—feel helpless and abused. But there was nothing else I could have done that night.

I returned home at 4:00 A.M. and was paged again at 4:15. I had patients scheduled for the whole of the next day and shuffled through my meetings. Remarkably, I did what I had to, though it seemed to take me a few seconds longer to find the right words when I spoke, and my depth perception was gone. I felt jet-lagged, my shoes squishing my feet uncomfortably when walking. Toward the end of the day, my mind began to fade. Earlier I had thought of going jogging in the evening to refresh myself. Instead, all I was able to do was stare vaguely at the television. Lord knows what I watched before falling asleep. Joe had said that once, after being on call, he fell asleep in a restaurant over his bowl of soup. His wife had to wake him up.

Life outside the hospital seemed to drift away. A few weeks earlier, over dinner with my best friend from college, I had tried to describe the frustrations of residency. But my words failed to convey the depth of my feelings. He didn't seem to know what to say, talking instead about his job at a bank and our mutual friends, as if my job weren't a problem. I had been relieved to get away from the hospital, even if just for an evening, and return to my former world as if little had changed. But I knew that a lot had.

PART III

The Other Side of the Couch

Through the course of these experiences, residency had gotten to be increasingly stressful and painful, consuming my life. The enjoyable moments had become overshadowed by the difficult and dreadful ones. I felt myself descending into a sort of all-encompassing hell.

These experiences are hard to write about. I feel as if I am violating some taboo, a code of secrecy, not keeping such confessions within the profession but making these phenomena and feelings known. We were supposed to look and act professional—aloof and in control—at all times and not disclose that sometimes we failed or didn't have all the answers. The model our supervisors provided us was to expose the least possible about ourselves. Still, I think it is important to reveal the truth about these experiences, since the fullest, most scientific, and open-minded understanding of these processes can most benefit the profession and its patients.

It is hard to pinpoint exactly one moment when the strains of residency became too much. Bransky's death and Enrico's effort to drown himself in the bathtub disturbed me. The hospital, as part of its routine policy, had a committee secretly investigate Enrico's attempt and found that I had done nothing wrong with his care. But the mere fact that my actions had been investigated left me nervous. Despite anything I did, patients could still act in risky ways, and I'd potentially be held responsible. Though I was lucky in this case, the helplessness troubled me and made me vow to be extra careful in the future. Susan Parr's death was even more haunting. None of my patients had died while under my care, though some other residents had patients successfully suicide. Still, the potential for disaster was unsettling. Another patient's family wrote a letter complaining that when I admitted her after she had tried to kill herself, I had asked her about her insurance, which unfortunately was a strict requirement of my job and part of hospital policy. The family wouldn't cooperate, got angry that I asked, and saw me as a target for their frustration at dealing with the hospitalization. The faculty completely agreed with my actions, but I didn't like the idea of letters being written about me.

Dr. Ostrow had warned other third-year residents and me in an orientation lecture to the outpatient department that we would now be more on our own than ever before and would bear heavier responsibilities by ourselves. I was excited but also apprehensive. At the end of my second year, as an acting assistant unit chief on the fifteenth floor, I had a brief taste of struggling in the dark alone and found it trying. Ostrow had other admonitions as well. "You'll be discussing difficult psychotherapeutic issues with outpatients. It's critical to be aware of and work through your countertransference"—that is, our feelings, as therapists, toward our patients as opposed to transference, a patient's feelings toward his therapist. "Countertransference that isn't examined and dealt with can have dangerous consequences, including suicide—so be careful."

In assessing the vague and subjective factors that underlay many of my decisions, I had to rely on my fleeting impressions, though having only scant experience on which to base my appraisals and judgments.

To complicate matters, frequently the field seemed to provide little certainty and only incomplete consensus concerning many of these decisions. Senior faculty members, all knowing more than I did, continued often to disagree and to give conflicting advice. Once, at grand rounds—a weekly lecture to the hospital's entire staff—a senior faculty member presented a patient who had failed to improve. The advice of several senior psychiatrists had been solicited and was summarized on a slide listing these experts' names in Column A and their recommendations, in random order, in Column B. The audience was asked to match up the doctors with their treatments, which wasn't very difficult. The depression expert had suspected an underlying depression and suggested an antidepressant, such as Prozac. The expert on psychotic disorders had thought the patient seemed "psychotic-like" and recommended an antipsychotic drug. The lithium expert had suspected mild mood swings, and recommended lithium. Each psychiatrist had formulated the problem confidently in terms of his expertise and recommended treatment accordingly. The whole audience chuckled, but no one commented on the fact that the disagreements were profound. Many psychiatrists didn't question their efficacy, since they believed themselves objective and therefore scientific. Yet the witch doctor I had met in New Guinea had been objective, too, citing objective evidence, such as the decreasing rate of kuru, in support of his claims. When I said the rate of kuru decreased because Westerners had banned cannibalistic feasts, the Fore credited their own indigenous treatments with the success.

Moreover, many of my patients didn't get much better, and some got worse. There was often no way of knowing in advance.

I was still learning and sometimes didn't do things perfectly the first time. I had to tease out whether problems in a case resulted from my inexperience while at the same time trusting my own judgment when supervisors, who knew a patient less well, recommended tacks that didn't seem right. As a novice with little experience, I found that all of this was hard to figure out. Yet residents couldn't admit any doubts and had to act confidently at all times, even when we had to force ourselves and almost pretend. Discussions of our own fears and bewilderment weren't publicly allowed and were considered inappropriate. When Sarah was emotionally upset about having to discharge a homeless patient who didn't have enough insurance, one nurse commented, "Sarah's overinvolved with her patients. She has rescue fantasies," as if Sarah were not grounded in reality, and hence was impractical and implicitly unprofessional. Even in our T-group, we weren't supported in having doubts. It is hard to explain the atmosphere in which no one questioned and everyone just went along. It made me wonder whether there was something wrong with me that I couldn't do it.

The institution made its own demands and seemed to have a life of its own. Too often training was not about seeking the truth but about following what made the institution work best. I had anticipated entering the highest reaches of man's soul. Instead I often felt imprisoned in a dungeon of narrow-minded, callous, and oppressive professional pressures.

Supervisors were constantly observing and evaluating us. My slightest comments would be discussed for days by other staff. I had to watch my words at all times. I also had to battle with patients or their families. I wish these pressures didn't bother me but have to admit that at some level they did.

It was hard to connect this new life as a psychiatrist with my previous life and my old self. Tying patients up, for example, conflicted with my own inclinations. I had to suppress my qualms, since the profession dictated that such actions were for the greater good of the patient. It wasn't always easy to join harmoniously my professional self and my personal self, the person I was now becoming with the person I'd always been. Contrary to what I would have thought, the two didn't always fit together well. I had hoped to be able to put more of myself into my work, but it wasn't always possible. Moreover, it was difficult being criticized for being myself with patients. I had to learn what reactions each supervisor considered appropriate or inappropriate with patients. I felt obliged to fill the role of the effective psychiatrist. Yet, being a psychiatrist often meant not acting myself and having to assume a certain role and a certain stance.

Psychiatry also quickly swallowed up my time and energy. Many things I previously enjoyed went by the wayside. For months I hadn't bought or read a newspaper during the week. I used to love reading the Travel section of the Sunday paper. As a resident, I stopped even looking for it, not having time to read, much less travel, and feeling stuck, unable even to envision traveling again in the future. That part of my life felt lost, and I feared never being able to return to it. At home, some of my house plants slowly dropped their leaves, withered, and died because I didn't have time to water them. I lost touch with numerous friends. The personal rewards were also less than I had thought. Residency seemed interminable.

I had never faced any problems or stress like this before. At times I began to hate the whole field and even life itself. Like most people I had occasionally become anxious before big exams or gotten depressed over major disappointments, but mostly had had an even keel. Now, as a resident, my equanimity began to vanish. After daily strain over months, I began to feel tenser during the day and persistent, at times almost crushing dread. My confidence had been shot down too many times.

Difficult cases began to weigh on me after work. In movie theaters, thoughts about patients flooded my mind. Some patients were experiencing potentially dangerous side effects or had suicidal or homicidal ideas that I had judged to be mild; I couldn't hospitalize everyone all of the time, and institutionalization could be detrimental to certain patients. Yet there was often some risk involved in clinical decisions, and bad events could occur while I was out trying to enjoy myself for an evening.

I began to have dreams about patients suiciding or disappearing from the ER, leaving me holding their charts and trying in vain to find them. For the first time in my life I also started to have trouble sleeping. Other residents eventually told me that they had similar problems. I would wake up in the early hours of the morning worrying about patients. Decisions began to torture me at night. At one point, I couldn't shake a cold for weeks because of lack of sleep. I started glancing behind me when walking, afraid of having dropped something. At times, I felt panicky, drowning, lost in this chaotic world.

This dark hopelessness and bleak futility are difficult to convey. For the first time in my life, I felt like I was going off the deep end, as if caught in the middle of somebody else's nightmare. The intensity of these emotions and experiences was new to me. I had worked hard, trying to do well and meet expectations of parents and others, and had generally succeeded—through college and medical school and even medical internship. But this work was proving intolerably embattled and unrewarding. I couldn't stand the pressure anymore and felt barely able to remain on top of it all. Moreover, the stresses were never attributed to the ineffectiveness or the limitations of the field's available treatments. Rather, it was assumed that residents had issues or problems in dealing with patients. If only we were better, the patient would improve.

Other residents felt the same way. Anne and Sarah and about half of the residents in my group had gotten so fed up earlier that several times they talked of quitting, which had surprised me. I hadn't let myself even entertain such thoughts, though they were immensely tempting now. Abandoning the field seemed premature, given how hard I had worked to get here. It would be important to complete this process somehow and evaluate it afterward. But the pressures and blows were beginning to overcome me, leaving me at a loss and with a sense of near defeat—numbed, hollowed out, almost unable to piece together my feelings and reactions with the rest of my life.

* * *

One night I had dinner with Anne. We sat in a glass-enclosed Chinese restaurant near the medical center. Outside, a cold rain fell, smacking against the tall glass walls. I talked to her about feeling stressed-out by work.

"What do you expect? If you deal with crazy people, they act crazy," she said calmly. "Feeling hassled and harassed is a normal part of our job." She leaned over her plate of food. "Why don't you start psychotherapy?"

"You think so?" I hadn't yet thought of beginning therapy myself. I hadn't ruled out the eventual possibility, but until now, the subject had come up in conversation only in reference to others, as when Anne mentioned her own therapy. I hadn't felt the need for it before.

"I'm in my fifth year of treatment," she continued. "I'm a firm believer in it. I don't know how anyone can get through this kind of work without it. I still do neurotic things, only now at least I understand why. I know of a good therapist you can call. It's never too late to start."

The institution, I would soon observe, not only didn't support us, but in fact implicitly encouraged us to see psychiatrists as patients to handle the stress.

Initially, I had seemed to be surviving the experience on my own. Sarah had considered psychotherapy from the beginning, "for intellectual reasons," she had said, though Anne had cautioned her. "That isn't enough. You have to do it because you feel pain."

In general, I had always felt compelled to try to manage stresses on my own. Independence and self-sufficiency had always been important to me. Before starting residency, I was still influenced—though not fully aware of it—by the Puritan work ethic and a strong popular bias that having to see a psychiatrist meant there was something somehow wrong with you. Until now in residency, I had tried to get by without visiting a therapist myself. Had I become a psychiatrist in the first place because I was screwed up? I didn't think so. Rather, residency was forcing me to say and do things that I had never had to say or do before, confronting me with stresses and tensions that I had never felt before, and aspects of myself that I hadn't examined. Moreover, I was left with little alternative in resolving these problems. As a medical student and medical intern, treatments had more consensus, and led to success, praise from faculty and staff, and gratitude from patients and their families. Now none of these things were the case. Working with the mentally ill exacted a high price—potentially my own mental health—and confused and unsettled me far more than I had been prepared for. I couldn't change the structure of the educational process or the system. Consequently, to stay in the residency and the profession and survive, I would have to change myself and my reactions, understanding myself and my responses better.

Initially, most other residents didn't discuss their travails. Only later would I find out that many had reached this same state of discomfort. Over the years of my training, numerous residents and faculty would eventually admit their own personal pain in the field and need for therapy. But these confessions occurred only in private moments one-on-one, or in small groups, or as thinly disguised jests. Many would admit that they started therapy not to help them become better therapists, but because they had to, troubled by their work. Many people also entered the field because at least at some level, they were interested in exploring and grappling with their own inner lives and conflicts.

Yet, at psychiatric staff conferences an implicit assumption was that the select group of psychiatrists present were all normal and that the patients discussed were the ones who had problems—symptoms, defenses, and conflicts that could be finely dissected. Psychiatrists generally sought to appear to each other as superior to their patients, as healthy. Patients were seen as sicker because, if nothing else, they had come to us with problems. They might even have been less stressed than many of us, but their seeking us for help defined, at least externally, an irreducible difference in our relative statuses, thus defining their role as patients and ours as healers.

If I did enter psychotherapy now, paying for it would be a problem. The hospital's health insurance policy covered only a small portion of the cost. At some other medical centers, residents garnered extra money by moonlighting, working in another hospital's emergency room at night and earning up to sixty dollars an hour. My hospital forbade this practice, though some residents were rumored to do it anyway. Many residents got money from parents. Some went into heavy debt.

Another means of lowering the price of therapy was to see a psychoanalyst who was himself still in training. These sessions cost only ten dollars apiece, instead of the usual one hundred or more dollars a visit at the time. Mike had discussed this option with Steve Kasdin, who had strongly dissuaded him. "If you needed an operation for cancer," Kasdin had argued, "would you go to a surgical resident still in training? No. You would pay the additional money to be treated by a senior, more experienced physician."

"But the situations are different," Mike had pointed out. "I'm not going to see a psychiatrist for a life-threatening problem."

"The principle, though, is the same. You will probably be in psychoanalysis only once in your life. It's a critical part of your training." Mike didn't push the point. He couldn't argue with a senior psychiatrist that the problems his field addressed weren't as important. Kasdin was suggesting, however, that not all psychiatrists or psychoanalysts were the same.

At the start of residency, I had thought of myself as pretty healthy. But now, if seeing a therapist would help me get through, I vowed to do it.

When Anne heard of my decision a few days later, she chuckled to herself and shook her head. "Another one bites the dust," she said.

The next morning, I telephoned Dr. Knoedler, the therapist Anne had recommended, and made an appointment. Anne agreed to cover for me for a few hours, and I went.

It felt liberating having an excuse to leave the hospital in the middle of the day. The afternoon was sunny; the streets were reassuringly familiar after the pressures of the hospital. I took a taxi to Dr. Knoedler's office.

I pushed the doorbell and a distant electronic buzzer sounded, unlocking the door. I entered a small waiting room, neatly furnished but innocuous. Two chairs stood next to a side table on which sat a lamp and copies of *People* and *The New York Review of Books*. A generic psychiatrist's office, no sign of his personality seeping through. I sat down. A door opened and Dr. Knoedler greeted me. He was a tall man in his fifties, with a full head of blond hair, casually dressed in an Oxford shirt, without a tie. He led me into his office.

I told him about myself and explained my predicament. "Patients are troubling me," I told him. "I feel more anxious than I ever have before." He nodded sympathetically. "I don't understand why."

"I think it's probably because you're feeling angry."

"Angry? I don't feel particularly angry."

"That may be the problem."

"What do you mean?"

"It's probably hard for you to express it—as is the case with many people." I had never conceived of myself as being particularly angry, didn't have a temper, and had considered myself to be reasonably calm until then.

I decided to accept his hypothesis tentatively, for argument's sake. "What can I do about it?"

"I think you should be in therapy with me."

"With you? Why with you?"

"I think I can help you."

We spoke longer and made a second appointment. I left and realized that, though knowing almost nothing about this man, I would now be exposing my life to him and paying him for it. I was wary and somewhat resentful of this arrangement, though I routinely expected patients to enter into this same relationship with me. Being a psychiatrist didn't entirely make it easier to see a psychiatrist myself, to be a patient. I now experienced what it must be like for patients who came to see me—how alienated and uncertain they probably felt at first.

My second appointment with him was a few days later. "I'm still confused about some patients," I told him, describing a patient troubling me at that time. "I feel like I should draw limits. But it's hard and doesn't feel kind. She appeals to me to give her more." He said nothing, and sat back calmly.

"Do you have any advice?" There was another long silence. "This doesn't seem very useful."

"It appears," he finally said, "that she manages to make you feel the same way she does—frustrated."

"But what can I do about it?" I waited. He shifted in his chair.

"You need to experience what you're feeling about her more," he said after a long pause.

"I try my hardest with her, but nothing seems to do her much good."

"You're afraid you're not giving enough to her," he then said, "and you resent that I don't give enough to you." That sounded correct but still felt distant from my actual experience. I was beginning to feel like my patient, at odds with my therapist, unsatisfied with what he provided. He wanted me to stand back and contemplate the larger issues involved, as opposed to the immediate questions gnawing at me, which might provide me with more immediate relief. I appreciated this underlying principle but wanted help with my specific current problem. Insight was much more difficult to incorporate and act on than I had imagined. My patients had also disliked pursuing longer-term goals over shorter-term needs in treatment.

"We have to stop there for today," he suddenly said.

How transitory these visits seemed—mine to him, patients' to me—for forty-five to fifty minutes, brief slots of time, before wandering back out into the world again, feeling somewhat unfulfilled and empty-handed, seeking direction.

Nonetheless, sessions with Knoedler served as calming and reassuring—if only as respites during the long days and weeks. I had someone to whom to explain my predicaments who would listen and might understand. The conversations weren't effective in the larger ways I had hoped. But he was supportive when he spoke. I now had a channel in which to vent my frustrations, and was plugged in to the system, part of a giant pecking order of younger psychiatrists seeing more senior psychiatrists, who, in turn, had once seen even older psychiatrists themselves.

Also, the only person besides myself I got to see conducting psychotherapy was Dr. Knoedler—with me as the patient. Up to this point, residency had afforded no other opportunity to see a psychotherapist other than myself at work, handling various problems in a treatment as they arose from session to session. Still, it felt odd being both patient and de facto student.

Many other residents and junior faculty, I had begun to notice, also left the hospital during the day to see therapists. They slipped out through the lobby or passed me on the streets near the hospital, coming and going. Mike and Sarah, under the strain, also entered psychotherapy around this same time.

That I had to pay a psychiatrist to help me with my problems in the profession seemed not only ironic but unfair. Still, despite the expense, it's what almost all of us did.

Psychiatric treatment was much more common among therapists than among any other group of professionals I knew—pediatricians, lawyers, or architects—with the possible exception of writers. In large part, psychiatry was more personally disturbing, and the field was less supportive. Most residents entered therapy after having had to struggle with the fact that knowledge about the mind and mental illness was limited, treatments were frequently only partly successful, and faculty often didn't support and sometimes undermined residents. Another psychiatrist might empathize with us, having been through these experiences himself. Dr. Knoedler might understand these stresses better than my friends or family, outside the profession.

At least half, if not almost all of the resident group, I later discovered, entered individual therapy at some point, faced with all of these issues. Consequently, their problems can't be attributed to their individual psychopathologies alone, but to the process itself of becoming a psychiatrist. Psychiatry is shrouded in mystery—in the name of clinical efficacy. But the field's closetedness also hides the pain, adversity, and limitations many practitioners face, and the fact that there was often much we didn't know, though we had to act as though we did. These tensions and conflicts are potentially embarrassing to admit. But the situation and the field can be improved only by acknowledging and understanding the problem.

The system of seeking outside psychiatric help for ourselves had the added effect of fostering further emphasis on psychological aspects of psychiatry and maintaining the power of psychoanalysts at this and other hospitals. Moreover, the process encouraged many residents to become psychoanalysts themselves.

In fact, a significant proportion of senior analysts' patients were themselves mental health professionals. Almost the only people I knew in psychoanalysis were mental health professionals. Few other friends of mine could afford it. The system helped keep senior analysts, many of whom were supervisors at the hospital, in business themselves. A significant share of a resident's salary—at least a third before taxes—went to paying for psychotherapy.

Supervisors all asked residents, "Are you in treatment?"

"Yes," we would answer.

"Good. With whom?"

I never saw how it was any of their business, especially since Dr. Knoedler and other analysts were colleagues of theirs. Like Knoedler, residents' therapists were almost invariably on the voluntary faculty of the hospital, that is, were affiliated with the hospital as part-time, unpaid faculty members, supervising residents, able to admit their patients if that was ever needed, and gaining an academic credential. Knoedler, for example, supervised other residents in my group. The world of local psychiatrists was a small one.

Knoedler and I talked about many areas, but the major stress we discussed, at least initially, was work. On this issue he seemed to have a unique function in my life.

Being a therapist myself didn't cure or excuse me from wrestling with basic human conflicts that therapy addresses, involving fears, jealousies, anger, hopes, and dreams. Though impatient at times with the process, I eventually continued with it through residency. Did being a doctor make me a better patient? I sought a doctor's help and assistance just like anyone else, though more aware of the process than many—where it worked, its strengths, and its ultimate limitations. Being a psychiatrist made me more sensitive to issues in myself that I had been trained to see in my patients.

Some might ask how good psychiatrists can be if they are patients themselves. I think it makes us better. Everyone has personality structures and defenses that operate in the world and often lead to problems. To understand these as best we can invariably does make us more empathetic with the struggles others face as well.

Eventually, I switched to psychoanalysis and lay down on the couch. It lacked the magic I had anticipated and seemed far more straightforward.

Knoedler slowly turned out to be right in many ways, and I began to work on my frustration with residency and with, for example, patients who didn't cooperate with my efforts to help them. I had felt it was inappropriate, professionally, to be angry at those under my care. I was there to help them, to be available to them, and had to separate how I felt like acting from how I should act toward them, and also learn to use my emotions in the treatment. Most important, I had to overcome a certain reticence about my own inner feelings, resentments, and jealousies tucked away and forgotten since childhood, and not giving me any trouble until now. It was one thing to read about Freudian defenses and psychodynamics. It was another thing to see them and change them in oneself. I might never have entered psychotherapy if not forced to confront these issues as a psychiatrist. I now had to accept feelings I had dismissed but which were real and critical to acknowledge and deal with. It may sound naive to have ignored such countertransference. But throughout medical school and my medical internship, I had aspired to be a caring, concerned, and humane physician, and the model presented in the field had held that getting angry at patients was unprofessional. Yet I had to see my actual human responses, understand them, and if possible, use them. I had to try to help patients understand the responses they evoked in others.

I hadn't known myself as well as I had thought. In retrospect, I had spent much of my life trying to please others, doing the right thing—or what seemed right—which in turn made me resentful and had contributed to residency's being as difficult as it was. For each of us, the particular problems we ran into, and specific personal adjustments we had to make, were different. Eventually through psychoanalysis, I began to see and better understand the issues I faced. Perhaps these tensions had been additional, though unconscious, factors in my decision to pursue psychiatry in the first place—an incipient sense of internal conflicts as certain levels that needed resolution. In any case, I was now confronting and working on these areas.

Yet change in psychotherapy was difficult. The pace seemed slow. Knoedler offered possible insights, even if it wasn't yet clear how they would relieve the problems I faced. I observed patterns of behavior in myself that led to undesired results but still found myself doing them. It could take years to alter psychological responses, showing me how hard therapy must be for my own patients as well. The results of treatment, even after many years, were often limited compared to how much I had done as a medical intern for patients, some of whose problems were permanently cured, and what I had been led to believe I'd be able to do now. More precisely, I was being encouraged to believe that the little bit I could sometimes do to alter people's psyches over time was, in fact, significant.

In any case, therapy would assist with the stresses of training and with their psychological roots within me. But exactly how, and over how long a period of time, wouldn't be clear until residency was over.

The Unopened Fanta

Often as a resident, the issues I faced were less scientific than ethical and political. Sometimes I was even put in a peculiar role of judge, called to consult on patients for reasons primarily other than treating psychiatric illness. Residency forced me to make difficult moral decisions while relying on highly subjective experiences with patients. I had anticipated learning a science as I had learned other sciences in the past, and professors acted as if psychiatry had definite answers. Yet this specialty was still turning out to be far less straightforward than other branches of medicine. In fact, arguably the rest of medicine is more open about its limitations—how much still isn't known and needs to be researched. Now, I often had to weigh competing values within myself. The issues involved were rarely discussed, and I had to draw on some inner moral part of me—not on anything objective or taught.

"You psych?" a surgical resident asked me one day in the ER. "I have a patient for you. Cubicle seven. The name is Wendell Pauley. We want to operate on him, but he's refusing. So if you think he's competent to refuse, we'll just get him out of here."

"And if his judgment isn't intact?"

"Then I guess we have to go ahead and operate on him against his will. But that would be messy." He wrinkled his nostrils as if smelling an unpleasant odor, handed me the ER sheet, and hurried away. Surgeons were harried, no-nonsense people. My inclination was to help them out, if possible.

Cubicle seven was a narrow alcove behind a flimsy curtain. The fabric hung haphazardly, ripped away from some of its hooks. I pushed the material aside and walked to the corner where the stretcher was squeezed. A man lay rolled up in a sheet, his black glasses squatting on his thinned, hollowed face. A grizzly beard hugged the bony contours of his jaw. One of his arms twisted under him. His neck and skull tilted off his shoulders at a sharp angle, his face an inch from the blank yellow wall.

"Wendell Pauley?"

"What?" he squawked without moving his head or looking in my direction. He displayed no curiosity about who I was, what I looked like, or why I had come into his cubicle.

"I'm Dr. Klitzman from psychiatry," I said, putting on an official voice and feeling very distanced from him.

"I don't need no goddamn psychiatrist."

"Did they tell you why they asked me to come?"

"No."

"Have you ever seen a psychiatrist before?"

"I don't know . . . Maybe."

"Why was that?"

"They didn't tell me."

"Do you know why I'm here now?"

"Because my son and my daughter-in-law put me out of the house." Wendell Pauley was seventy-two and, according to his ER sheet, had diabetes and was "s/p LBKA"—meaning he was "status post," or had had a left below-the-knee amputation. His left calf, shin, foot, and toes had all been removed. A stump now bulged below his left knee in place of a leg. At present, he was refusing an RBKA, or right below-the-knee amputation, which the surgeons wanted to perform. He was about to lose his only remaining leg. He was also partially blind and partly paralyzed. The surgeons wanted me to say he was competent to refuse, so they wouldn't have to operate against his will.

"Do you know what the doctors here want to do?"

"Take my leg off."

"Do you know why?"

"Gangrene. It's a bad infection, and it can't be cured."

"So the benefit to you is . . ." I expected him to fill in the blank.

"None. The doctors just want the experience."

His response surprised me. "Why do you think the doctors suggested it?"

"They were schooled to."

"Is there *any* benefit to you?"

"None whatsoever."

"The doctors think it'll prolong your life."

"I don't believe it."

"Are you aware of risks involved?" Again, a necessary question.

"I don't know," he groaned, dismissing the question as if he couldn't be bothered. "If I don't have the procedure, I don't have any risks. I don't know if I could take the shock."

"Are you aware of any alternatives?"

"I'll die," he said definitively, with relief.

"Why don't you want the procedure done?"

"I'd be a vegetable. Look, I'm in pain all the time. I want to go out of this world in peace. If I don't have the surgery done, I'm left alone to die quietly. The surgery isn't necessary. There's no benefit I can receive from it. I *want* to die," he cried into the quiet of the cinder-block room. Overhead fluorescent lights flickered. Stainless steel equipment, reflecting back the dull light, stood parked along the walls, wedging us in. "I'm blind. I can't walk. The right side of my body is totally paralyzed. See this arm here? My right one? I couldn't move it if I wanted to. I have nothing to live for. I can contribute nothing to no one. I can't do anything for myself. I never wanted to be dependent on people. Why shouldn't a man be allowed to die if he wants? Answer me that."

For years, my goal had been to help people get better and to keep them alive. Should I now let him die? Did I as one person have the right to decide? No decision is as final. His life seemed reduced to almost an animal-like existence.

Maybe his wish resulted from depression, which could be treated. "Are you feeling depressed?"

"I've been low my whole life," he said, "though it's been worse in the past year since they cut off my leg."

"How depressed have you been?"

"I asked my grandson the other day to get me a gun." His words shook me to attention. "I'd just like to be left alone. I don't welcome dying. But I know I'm going to."

"What *do* you want?"

"What do I want?" he asked himself aloud, as if giving himself a chance to reflect for the first time in many years. "I want to be admitted here for food and shelter. But that's it. Do you understand? I don't want any needles in me. I'm sick of being stuck. And I don't want any surgery or any drugs." He also refused any medication for depression or his "nerves."

"What if the doctors need to draw blood to know how to help you?"

"I don't need your help."

"Would you like to go home?"

"Don't you dare send me home! I don't want to be there, and they don't want me. They'd just send me right back here. I just want to die." His voice rose. "Can't you see that?"

I had been trained to interpret such statements as suggestive of depression and to offer treatment, which he was refusing. Should I treat him against his will? The responses I had been taught to follow didn't make sense here.

I went back to the nursing station to read through the surgeon's note and the other papers that had been written about him so far that day.

He was a retired factory worker. His wife had died five years earlier, and he now lived with his son and daughter-in-law southwest of the city. His daughter-in-law had gotten fed up with him and this morning had called an ambulance, loaded him on board, and instructed the driver to take him to the hospital. When he arrived the surgeons saw his gangrenous leg and recommended the surgery.

But this man didn't need a psychiatrist. He needed an internist, a bath, and a shave. I would have preferred not to have anything to do with him. Nor did he want me involved.

This was not my idea of what a psychiatrist did. Who was I to take into my hands the right to decide whether unknown people could enter the final embrace of death? Psychiatry, I had thought, would be free from these dark forces of bodily decay, sickness, and dying.

I called his son, Tom Pauley, who said his father was unbearable at home. "I have my wife and kids here. Our house is small and he smells. He doesn't take care of himself."

"But we can arrange for a home health aide to come in."

"He's had them here and fires them or drives them crazy until they quit."

"But the hospital can't just take him in if he doesn't agree to treatment."

His daughter-in-law spoke up. She had been listening in on another line. "If you ship him back here, I'm going to lock the door of the house first, and the ambulance can just dump him on the street, since that's where he's going to stay. We can't have him here any longer." Their refusal to take him in seemed absurd. There must be some way to reconcile these issues and convince them. It didn't seem right just to kick him out of the house.

"Can you come in to the ER to talk to him?" I pleaded.

"There's nothing left to talk to him about," she said. "He's decided."

"What about his asking for a gun?"

"He asked my son, who's only eleven," Tom said. "But my son knows better. Nobody was going to get him a gun."

"Has he talked about wanting to hurt himself?"

"For weeks," Tom replied. "But he hasn't done anything."

Wendell Pauley seemed depressed and paranoid, thinking the surgeons "just wanted the experience." I appreciated his dilemma. But depression and paranoia could be impairing his judgment. Both of these conditions could be caused biologically by either his diabetes or his leg infection, or could be situational, resulting from his circumstances.

He might not be competent, but I didn't want the burden of surgery performed against his will to fall on me alone. I phoned the attending on call, Dr. David Katz, to discuss the case. An attending psychiatrist is present in the emergency room at all times at some hospitals, hired and paid and assigned shifts. At this hospital, no attending was routinely present—according to residents, to save money and make the faculty's life easier. Attendings took turns of one week each being on call. They rotated a beeper between them and were to be available at night to come into the ER whenever the resident on call requested. I phoned Dr. Katz and explained the story.

"Just have him put into an ambulance and taken home," Dr. Katz said.

I relayed the family's position.

"Send him home anyway. Look," he finally said. "I know this guy. I've seen him before and he's okay. He's not depressed. He's not paranoid. It's just the way he is." I didn't know if this was true or not, but doubted it. Dr. Katz lived in the suburbs and even though it was his job, I sensed that he didn't want to come all the way into the hospital on an otherwise quiet afternoon just to see this one patient.

I called the chief resident, Dr. Lou Leftow. "Katz won't come in?" he pondered. "That's a big problem. Have you read through the patient's old chart yet?"

"I ordered it from medical records, but it hasn't arrived yet."

"The patient's just sitting there now, right?"

"Yes."

"Why don't you wait and see what the old chart says. Call me back if there's a problem." I phoned medical records a second time, telling them that my request was urgent, and a few minutes later a messenger arrived with the chart in hand. Flipping through the pages, I came across a note in Anne's handwriting.

She had evaluated Wendell in the ER six weeks earlier for the same problem and found his judgment to be unimpaired. She added that he seemed depressed, but that she had spoken with his social worker, and that his wishes had been consistent for a few months. Without surgery, doctors had written in his chart that he might die within four to six weeks. That much time had already passed. Several years ago he weighed 212 pounds. He was now gaunt, skeletal, less than half his prior weight. I wrote my note carefully, and concluded that his judgment was poor but not impaired. He wasn't acutely suicidal. I decided to leave matters as they stood. Though suspicious, I had no concrete evidence otherwise, and he had refused surgery previously, when he was more clearly competent.

The surgeons decided to try to get him admitted to a chronic-care facility or nursing home directly from the emergency room. I knew that the waiting lists at these institutions could be weeks—even months—long, and was skeptical of the surgeons' being able to transfer him directly. I had also never heard of the ER being used for this purpose. Still, he was officially the surgeons' responsibility and now, after numerous phone calls and conversations, over six hours after first being called to see him—the longest I had ever spent on a patient in the ER—I staggered home and went to sleep. I was surprised the case had taken so long and was glad to be done.

Wendell remained in my head as a difficult and troubling case. Caught in the bureaucratic web of medical institutions, he had nowhere to go at the moment. It was hoped he would be sent to a nursing home to die, yet his family wouldn't even help him until then. I was curious about what happened to him, in part because the situation was left unresolved. But as a resident, I often saw and consulted on cases only once and never got to see the patient again or find out what happened. We were lucky to keep up with the patients still under our care. I wasn't attached enough to Wendell to go through the difficult process of somehow tracking him down.

* * *

A week later, my beeper squeaked in the elevator as I was up for a new consultation. We residents rotated among ourselves new assignments of patients on medical wards of the main hospital who had psychiatric problems that needed to be assessed. In the lobby, I dialed the number that had flashed on my beeper, and spoke to the secretary in the consultation-liaison office who made these arrangements. "The patient is in room L-503," she told me.

I went to the fifth floor and swung around the corner to the main corridor of L-5. The long hall was windowless and bare, built of cinder block, and lit by fluorescent bulbs behind plastic screens. I suddenly sniffed a moist, sour, and acrid scent—like rotting flesh. The odor seeped all through the hall and into the open nursing station. It reminded me of Wendell's decaying foot.

In the nursing station, I found the chart for room L-503. The patient was, indeed, Wendell. His chart said he had been admitted, "awaiting placement," but his leg had been getting worse. "The line of demarcation," a surgeon had written that morning, "has progressed to midcalf."

I phoned the surgical resident, Dr. Simon Gates, who told me, "Wendell's ready for takeoff"—that is, no other medical or surgical treatment was planned, and the patient was merely awaiting discharge. "But we want him followed while he's here awaiting placement, to see if he remains competent or if he changes his mind, allowing us to operate."

"If he suddenly isn't competent," I said, sensing that he was fast approaching the boundary, "would you go ahead and operate on him against his will?"

The surgeon was puzzled. "I don't know. Maybe. I guess so, right? I'm only doing what my chief"—his chief resident—"said. But I think we just need documentation in the chart to cover ourselves since we're not giving the guy any treatment, and since he's here in the hospital actively dying." Gates hurried off. At this point the surgeons, tired of the case, basically wanted Wendell discharged.

I read through the chart and the nurses' notes. Wendell was accepting pain medications but no others, and he still didn't want any procedures done.

On the ward, he had been given one of the few private rooms—usually reserved only for those who could afford the extra cost. I entered the alcove and then the barren, cold chamber. Though midwinter, the air conditioner had been turned on, presumably to try to clear the smell, though it only made the sour air chilly, stinging my nostrils. The overhead light was turned off, and the room was dimly lit by a single lightbulb at the head of his bed. Shivers bristled down my back. Around his gangrenous foot, fat black flies skimmed and buzzed, occasionally landing on the exposed blackened stub. The bugs sensed the moist presence of his decaying skin. I had never seen insects in the hospital before—let alone flies—and certainly none clustering around a patient or a part of his anatomy. I didn't know how they had all found their way to him through the building.

The line of purplish black dead skin had indeed crept up further into the fair-complexioned, light-haired remainder of his leg. He hadn't shaved in several days, and stiff long bristles of grizzly stubble clung to his cheeks and chin.

On a bedside table lay his last meal, only picked at, as he had trouble sitting up. The nurses hadn't assisted him in eating it. Eggs swam in fatty yellow grease, and congealed globs stuck to the corners of the plate and to his fork. A pool of spilled orange fluid was slowly drying, leaving a sticky puddle. Above his bed hung a metal triangle, dangling from a long metal beam. The contraption, screwed into vises at the head and foot of his bed, was to help him lift himself up. But he ignored it. The stark room contrasted with those of other patients. Something was missing here that was present in their rooms. I suddenly realized what—flowers or photographs or get-well cards from visitors. There was not even a suitcase of clothes, or a toiletries kit, or any other item from home. The low-wattage bulb above his head cast extended sidelong shadows through the room. The clammy, damp emptiness was eerily reminiscent of a morgue.

I flicked on the brighter overhead light. "Turn that off!" he yelled.

He lay tangled among the sheets of his bed, which looked unmade for several days. He had probably been unwilling to cooperate with the staff in replacing or straightening the sheets.

"Wendell?"

"What do you want?" His eyes stared straight up at the ceiling.

"I'd like to speak to you for a few minutes."

"Goddamn all you doctors. I just want to be left alone."

"I'd like to try to help you."

"I don't want your help."

"Is there anything you would like?"

"Just what I have: I'm finally reaching my goal of dying. And I told you all I don't want any medication, so stop trying to sneak it into me anyway."

"What do you mean?"

"I know you're putting it in the food. That orange they gave me for breakfast was heavier than it should be. I can taste the drugs in it. And they've been giving me back the same meal tray on different days." Partially blind, he could probably barely see the food. But he was also clearly being paranoid now, even though the psychiatric attending on call in the ER, Dr. Katz, had insisted otherwise. However, if I wrote in Wendell's chart that his judgment was impaired, would the surgeons—wanting to operate on him despite his refusal—go ahead? I wasn't sure.

Psychiatric medications might help him. Paranoid delusions can result from depression, though he still refused an anti-depressant. Antipsychotic drugs could help with his paranoia directly. "Why don't you want to take any medications?"

"I think I'm better off without them."

"How about a medication to help you with feelings of being scared?"

"Maybe." At some level he must have been terrified of what he faced.

I prescribed Haldol and, since he was beginning to become accustomed to me, decided to offer him the first dose myself.

"I don't want it," he told me when I brought it to his bedside.

"Being here is very difficult for you, I'm sure. This medication will ease some of the tension you feel." He took the pill.

But when the nurses offered him other doses later, he refused. I told them to offer it to him several times a day. The personal interaction might persuade him to accept.

Dr. Gates, the surgical resident, saw me at the nursing station. I felt obliged to report what I had detected and told Gates that Wendell's paranoia had become clear, and his judgment now seemed impaired.

"You mean we have to operate?"

"That's not my decision. You asked me a question about his judgment and that's the answer. I know it may not be the answer you wanted." Would Wendell now have his leg cut off because of me? That prospect was worrisome and frightening, the responsibility heavy. Doing my job forced me to say his judgment was impaired, though that determination was based solely on my interpretation of what he had happened to say to me in passing, about his orange. It would have been easy simply to say his judgment remained intact and go along with what the surgeons wanted, which was to get him off their service. But it was important that patients be carefully and correctly evaluated. Otherwise, bad management might occur, and patients at some point might not get the treatment that they needed or would get treatment that they didn't want.

My job as a physician had been to help patients. But what if they didn't want help? Wendell Pauley's life now hung in the balance. This decision was highly subjective and laden with moral issues about the value of life and a patient's right to die—topics discussed by the press recently, but rarely mentioned at the time. I wished there were a clearer basis for choosing. Some basic human elements were missing here—compassion and feeling. These halls seemed crushingly oppressive. I felt stuck in some dark, labyrinthine prison from which neither he nor I could escape. I felt somewhat protective of him in this environment and wasn't unsympathetic to his position. Wendell, though odd and frightened, wasn't completely illogical. Being professional meant protecting him, even when it would be more popular and less of a hassle to do otherwise. I would care for him, though I felt revulsion personally.

Still, I didn't know ethically and legally whether it was permissible to follow decisions he had made earlier. He had been depressed in the past, too. Perhaps after taking some Haldol he'd feel better. Could treating his psychiatric problems make him agree to the surgery?

I phoned patient services—an administrative department interested and assisting in any patient complaints about hospital staff or staff management difficulties with patients. Residents also contacted them for any problem with difficult ethical or potential legal implications.

The director there didn't know how to proceed either and referred me to the hospital lawyer. The lawyer was also puzzled but said he'd confer with associates. A few hours later, he paged me and said that though Wendell's judgment might be impaired now, we were obliged to follow his prior wishes as they were documented in the chart. He also told me to have my attending see the patient and co-sign my note. The attending on the consultation-liaison service, through which I was now following Wendell, was Dr. Danziger, whom I phoned and who came by.

"This guy's going to be a mess," Danziger said, shaking his head, as he snapped the cap of his pen back on, and rose from the desk where he had sat in the nursing station after seeing the patient with me for two minutes. "I hate stuff like this."

A few days later, I was paged by the head nurse on the floor. "Wendell Pauley just threatened to stab a nurse with a knife."

I hurried upstairs, convinced now that I was right that his judgment was impaired. I headed straight for his room. A bored plump security guard in a navy blue uniform sat on a chair outside Wendell's room. I rushed past him.

"Get away from me," Wendell said when I approached him and reintroduced myself. "*Nooo!* I don't want to talk to you."

"I heard that you threatened a nurse with a knife."

"I never held a knife to no one." He sensed I wasn't leaving. "And if I did, it was to get what I wanted. Now leave me alone."

Back at the nursing station, the nurse, Ellen Mills, was shaking in a chair. Her hair, previously tied up neatly behind her head, had now fallen loose and straggled down the side of her face onto her shoulder.

"What happened?" I asked her.

She told me that Wendell had picked up the metal knife from his breakfast when she tried to remove the tray. Wendell was hungry but had trouble eating. He didn't trust the staff to help him, but didn't want the food removed, either. He threatened to stab Ellen, then held the blade to his breast and said he was going to kill himself. Ellen had screamed. Security guards were called and arrived a few minutes later.

"How has he been doing in the past day or so?" I asked her.

"He's easily frustrated when things get busy on the floor and we don't attend to his needs right away. Yesterday at lunch he wanted me to open the can of Fanta in front of him so he could make sure it hadn't been tampered with."

I recommended that a one-to-one companion replace the security guard, since Wendell didn't seem to be aggressive and since the companion might also help him a little bit.

The next day when I went by, an aide had been assigned to him, but she was sitting on a chair outside his room, engrossed in a tabloid she was reading.

"You're supposed to be in the room there with him," I told her.

"He's just a sick old man. Besides," she added, "it smells in there." I peeked into his room. It still reeked of decaying flesh. The air conditioner was turned up even further—to its maximum setting—and now blasted in icy air. He lay with the sheet pulled up over his head, covering his face.

"Why did you hold up the knife?" I asked Wendell gently after walking into the room.

"To get someone around here to do something ... to help me more. They wanted to take my tray away."

"Given how upset you must be, the medicine I prescribed might help you."

He said nothing.

"Any thoughts of wanting to hurt yourself?" I asked, as was necessary in this situation.

"I just want to go to sleep and die. God, let me die. Why do You put me in so much pain?"

I went back and looked at his chart. The intern had written that day, "Patient refuses to be seen on rounds." I wrote a note suggesting that his pain meds be increased.

Two days later I returned and saw that he had accepted more pain meds and a few doses of Haldol—the only benefits and active comforts he was getting from the hospitalization. But the nurse still sat outside his room. Wendell didn't seem like he was about to hurt himself or anyone else and hadn't made any other threats. As long as he still had a one-to-one companion, a nursing home might not take him, probably not having the extra staff and not wanting the added responsibility. I wrote to DC, or discontinue, "the companion 'on a trial basis,'" as if it were a medication. It might get him out of here sooner. I also wrote that the staff should try to interact with him as much as they could.

He lay there in limbo.

I didn't know what would happen to Wendell. Patients usually had to wait a long time for transfer to a nursing home, as bureaucracies exchanged forms.

A few days later, I happened to be in the ward's nursing station to see another patient and spotted Wendell's chart in the bin to be sent down to medical records.

I opened up the chart, no longer gripped in a stiff metal binder, but now bent and held by paper fasteners. In the front of his record was tucked a carbon copy of an ambulance request form. Wendell had been transferred two days after my last visit to him—the quickest admission to a nursing home I had ever seen. It turned out that the hospital, under pressure from the surgeons, had made arrangements with a facility with which it had a long-term ongoing relationship. So forty-eight hours after I had last spoken to him, he had left.

I realized that I had not healed him in any way but had helped him fulfill his wish to end his life and had freed his family of him. These goals, though largely unanticipated by me, seemed right in this case. Psychiatric work differed radically from my initial impressions of helping others gain insight. Our limited ability to understand or alter others' lives often placed me in strange situations. Many psychiatrists ignored the administrative and political, rather than medical and psychiatric, aspects of patients' problems. Wendell's case was gloomy but presented important issues that arise and are often handled poorly or indifferently. Such dismissal comes at a high price.

Physicians often ignored the social and human aspects of their patients' lives. I thought of another patient, also with a poor prognosis, whom I had seen a few days earlier. "What does she have to look forward to?" I had asked her nurse sadly, shaking my head.

"Getting Medicaid so she can get out of here and go home," the nurse had replied. Medicaid was needed to pay for home health aides, who were required if the patient was to live the short remainder of her life in her own apartment, as she wished.

Standing in the nursing station now, I flipped to the end of Wendell's chart. After my last entry, an intern had squiggled a one-sentence transfer note. All it said was, "Pt. w/ DM, CHF, CVA, s/p MI, HTN, Blindness, 3 pillow orthopnea in R leg, DNR. T'ferred for comfort, placement in nursing home, and wound care."

A nursing care note then appeared. "Wound care: Betadine diluted with sterile water followed by a normal saline rinse. Air dry."

I flipped the page, to see what came next, expecting a final note, some ultimate comment or summation of what had happened, to see how the case had ended.

The last page was blank.

Chains

Psychiatry forced me to alter my ideas about many people. Situations, radically different from anything I had encountered before, turned many of my assumptions and preconceptions upside down. Residency immersed me in new worlds and led me to know intimately people whom I otherwise would never have even encountered.

Under "Reason for Admission" in the chart of Harold Daniels, a patient assigned to me a few days later while I was on call, only one word was written: "Immolation."

I hadn't encountered this term for a while. Didn't it mean lighting yourself on fire? I thought of it as something that Hindu protestors did to oppose British rule in India. I read the patient's past history. "Thirty-year-old white male with long psych history, in prison for one year, now with self-immolation. Currently on Haldol." He had been imprisoned for attacking a man on the street who he thought was the devil.

I didn't like criminals. In my neighborhood, a woman had recently been murdered on the subway when she had refused to hand over her purse to an attacker.

I shut the chart and walked down the hall of the medical unit to which he had been admitted. Outside, the morning was bright, but little sunlight broke into the ward. The patient had been assigned room L-622, bed 2, located at the end of the hall. I expected to see a frenzied and deranged criminal—tough, dangerous, and menacing. I walked into the room, which contained four beds. In one, a man lay listening to his clock radio, which was playing classical music. In the next corner, a man was talking to a woman—presumably his girlfriend or wife. Beside the far right-hand window, a man read the sports pages of a tabloid newspaper. In the last corner, a man sat quietly on a stool at the foot of his bed. He was wearing soft white cotton pajamas with light blue hospital logos printed on them in a diagonal pattern. Light blue piping wound around the collar, down the sleeves, and onto the cuffs. He had neatly cut light brown hair. He leaned over, his shoulders stooping, his head bent down below the height of the mattress. On the metal footboard, covered with fake wood-grained contact paper, a piece of masking tape read, "L-622-2 Daniels."

"Mr. Daniels?" I asked.

"Yes?" He spoke in a soft and shaky voice as he slowly lifted his head.

"I'm Dr. Klitzman." I reached out to shake his hand. He began to raise his palm toward me, but suddenly stopped halfway. Our hands had reached within a few inches of each other when his arm froze in midair. I thought it odd. Then I noticed a shiny metal chain descending from behind his wrist, arresting his hand's movement. He was handcuffed to the bed frame. Double metal rings yoked him firmly.

My arm was already mid-gesture, swinging down to intercept his. It would have been awkward to stop now as my hand swept down. I continued to reach out for his hand, bending my knees and my back and stretching to connect with him. His sweaty palm met my fingers. I bobbed his meaty hand up and down in mine, the chain restraining us. I could raise or lower my hand only an inch up or down. The links jingled as we moved. In each direction I felt a yank, a tug on my own wrist halting the momentum we gathered as our hands lifted and fell.

"I'm from psychiatry," I said.

"Hello." He nodded and looked at me with wide-open eyes, politely and patiently, to hear whatever I was going to say. He ignored his handcuffs. "How are you?" he asked me, courteously.

"Are you going to talk to him for a while?" I looked up. A prison guard was leaning along the inside wall of the room, hidden behind the door when I had entered.

"Yes," I answered. The guard smiled, glad to be relieved from his watch, and swung out of the room. "What happened?" I asked Harold.

He slowly turned back toward me after following the guard's exit and looked directly into my eyes. "I set myself on fire." He had a thin face, with big soft brown eyes and bushy brown eyebrows, and was clean-shaven. What brought this man to set himself on fire?

"Why did you do that?"

"God told me to," he said with a straight face.

Some might say this was religious, but at this point in my training, in this context, he sounded psychotic. Still, I would have expected someone agitated, incoherent, bizarre, or disheveled. He seemed very matter-of-fact, more like a shopkeeper than a psychotic criminal. "Any idea why he told you that?"

"My mother hadn't called me in several months."

"I see."

"She said she would." How little language can convey what he must have felt. His voice, calm and poised, showed no recognition that what he had done was in any way bizarre or out of the ordinary. He had probably felt abandoned by his mother and was angry. But he also had a history of schizophrenia and had much less ability to tolerate stresses of any sort.

Had something else happened, too? I phoned his psychiatrist at the prison. It turned out that Harold's medication had recently been lowered. Haldol and other neuroleptics can have long-term, permanent side effects, including tardive dyskinesia: irreversible, involuntarily quivering movements of the mouth, resembling tics, which the patient is unable to stop. Psychiatrists had recently been lowering these medications if possible as a precaution. Some patients could tolerate decreases. But others could not. Harold seemed to need the medication. In the past, shortly after his medications had been lowered at the outpatient clinic he attended, he had assaulted the man on the street. His delusions, and his acting on them when his medications were cut, pointed strongly toward the presence of an underlying biological problem.

Since his dose had been lowered, Harold had begun to hear voices in his head. In the end, a voice—loud, unceasing, disturbing, and irresistible—had told him to set himself alight.

He couldn't tell me much about himself or describe the psychological pain he must have felt. He could only act on the voices.

I increased the medication back to what it had been and requested a one-to-one companion.

"That guy really set himself on fire?" his nurse asked me. "That's crazy. Really crazy." The nurses on the ward were afraid of him and chatted more with other patients during rounds. Yet what struck me about him was his banality—how ordinary he seemed in his current interactions. It was difficult to imagine that he had committed a violent crime or set himself ablaze.

"How have things been going for you here in the hospital?" I asked him after he had been on the ward a week.

"I like it here. It's better than prison. I feel better." He smiled.

"Is God communicating with you now?"

"Not today."

"Are you hearing his voice?"

"Not this morning." It was difficult to engage him further, yet after a few days back on his medication, the voices vanished. His burns would take a few more weeks to heal, after which he would be returned to jail. We were taught psychoanalytic approaches during this rotation in consultation-liaison psychiatry—treating psychiatric problems that arose on medical wards—yet these theories weren't useful in the work we did each day. We weren't referred patients for psychodynamic issues. What took precedence were day-to-day management concerns as we ran from crisis to crisis—to cases like Wendell Pauley's and Harold Daniels's.

But Harold did increase my interest in psychiatric problems in prisons. A week later, I heard that several psychiatrists were planning to tour a city prison and I asked to join them.

Special permits were arranged to allow us to enter and leave the jail. We were told to be there promptly at 8:00 A.M. When we arrived at the prison gate, we had to wait two hours outside in the cold until the guard admitted us. He said he hadn't received official approval to let us in, though our host later said that the security department had been informed of the visit two weeks in advance.

Finally, we were admitted to the first of several outer gates and proceeded to Building 29, where the psychiatric ward was located. Along the road and in front of the building, concrete troughs were lined up, filled with dirt. But nothing grew in them, except for a few stray sprigs of clover whose seeds must have blown there accidentally.

In the building's entryway, large plastic signs were posted. "Absolutely No Weapons Permitted," one read. "Absolutely No Loading Or Unloading Of Firearms Allowed," another said.

"Come here," I heard. A guard called me and stamped my

hand with invisible ink. Only the impression from the hard rubber itself remained on my skin. No ink marks. We also signed our names with invisible ink in a thick ledger. We then lined up before another door and waited half an hour for a clerk to admit us. Behind a glass partition the clerk straightened papers in front of her. I'm certain she saw us, filling up the window before her and breathing on her glass wall, but she avoided any eye contact with us. If she had looked up at us, she'd have been obliged to acknowledge and admit us. She even stood up at one point and strolled about her room, but kept her eyes down, never lifting them above waist level.

Against the wall opposite us leaned a guard, holding a hot dog in one hand and a gun in the other.

Finally, she buzzed us in.

We were given a tour of the forensic ward—for prisoners with psychiatric problems—which had been Harold Daniels's home for several months and to which he would return after leaving the hospital. I realized how wards existed only in hospitals and prisons. The halls had low ceilings and were long and dim with little sunlight. In the door to every room was a large window, exposing the interior of each cell to the hallway. Each chamber was bare but for a sink, a toilet bowl, a small table, a metal cot, a mattress, and a sheet. Very few personal items were present. In one cell was only a box of generic butter cookies, in another a newspaper photo of a group of black men with a caption below, "The Way We Were." Some inmates had taped up glossy magazine ads of sexy women clad in skimpy halter tops. In another imprisoned patient's room a few postcards lined a desk along a wall. Another inmate had taped to the wall a picture of Jesus Christ emanating yellow rays in all directions. The painting had once accompanied a calendar, long since removed, as if it had been an unnecessary and painful reminder of days passing. Here, weeks wouldn't be marked or filled with events. Now only the picture remained, frozen in time.

Men slouched in chairs, many wearing T-shirts advertising various products. Several men wore shirts for Newport cigarettes with green letters, reading "Alive With Pleasure." But these wearied, preoccupied, and tense men seemed similar to patients at the hospital. Many had probably not been in control of their actions.

We left the cell block and walked back down the stairwell. On one landing, a group of staff huddled closely, peering through the window on the door. Inside, a riot squad was lined up in six rows, ten men across. Black helmets, much larger than their heads, added to their height. The visors were shut down in the front two rows to protect the officers' faces. In the rear rows the visors tilted back and up. On the stairwell door graffiti was scratched vertically in the yellow paint: "KILL-3."

I felt sad thinking of Harold, vulnerable and confused, in this environment. He had not interacted with me like a criminal, but as a person, a human being, and had been in prison because of mental illness and psychiatry's failure to treat his problem more effectively. Better psychiatric medications might help him and others in the prison ward. My role as a psychiatrist suddenly seemed small as he had been shuttled from one institution to another. He had shown me how little we understood about mental illness and its ability to incite behavioral disruption and even assault, and how seemingly tranquil, soft-spoken people can commit violent acts. All criminals were not what I thought.

Moreover, my hospital, though derided as a jail by Nancy Steele and others, and resembling a prison in some ways, was clearly not nearly as oppressive. As bad as the hospital might be, it seemed far more pleasant and calm. I left the prison building glad to step back out into the sunshine beneath open blue sky and clouds, and relaxed in the car once we drove off the grounds.

Two days later, I went to visit Harold again on the medical ward. Walking down the hall, I noticed that the guard wasn't standing at his doorway. I turned into the room. Harold's bed was now stripped, the footstool where he used to sit, chained to his bed frame, was in the same place. But Harold had been discharged, sent back to the prison. Despite all I could do, he had returned there. The hospital for him had been a respite, a temporary escape, offering freedom from without, and from within.

Heaven

The most vulnerable patients, affecting me the most in many ways, were children. Child patients, more than others, showed me the importance of my work—how much I was needed and could potentially do. The simplest actions—requiring the least medical or even psychiatric expertise, and only basic common sense or human feeling—could help them enormously.

Residents received some lectures about working with children, who, compared to adults, are generally less able to deal with or articulate their feelings or what ails them. I didn't think I knew much about child psychiatry, as the patients I had treated thus far had all been adults. Yet adults faced psychological and social problems throughout their lives stemming from interactions in their families while growing up. I anticipated liking this branch of psychiatry, working with parents to help them with their kids.

We evaluated children, assessing if treatment was needed, by meeting with them and their parents two or three times in a special child outpatient clinic. My first patient there was Michael Gálvez, a seven-year-old. First, I met with his mother, Juanita Gálvez. She was a short woman in tight jeans, a T-shirt, and dirty pink slippers edged in frazzled gold brocade. She spoke in broken English with a Spanish accent.

She told me a little bit about her son, then looked at me and added, "Sometimes I hit him hard."

"You hit him?"

"Sometimes I use the end of a cord."

"How do you mean?"

"An extension cord. I take it and whip him with it," she said matter-of-factly. I was concerned. Was this child abuse?

Child abuse had not yet received the major attention in the media that it soon would as the result of a few well-publicized cases. At the moment, I couldn't draw on anything that had been taught to me but had to rely on my own intuition, connecting occasional stories in the newspapers with what I was newly seeing in a case. I made an appointment for her to come back.

Who was I to criticize how a mother interacted with her child? I realized I was now a professional, invested with authority to do so, based on what my role required, and my own sense of right and wrong.

"Should I report this?" I asked my supervisor, Dr. Richard Liff. He was a child psychoanalyst, used to much more polite and mannered problems than those confronted here at a big city hospital.

He lifted up the edges of his bottom lip, stuck his chin forward, and raised his eyebrows. "Well, I guess so."

"How do I go about that?"

"I don't know. Why don't you ask Dr. Berman?" the head of child psych.

"If the mother's confessing this to you," Dr. Leon Berman then told me, "she's asking for help. We're legally responsible. We have to report it to the state. Contact the child protection team."

"How do I get ahold of them?"

"I don't know. Try the hospital switchboard."

"What do I tell the mother?"

"That you're talking to other people because it seems she needs help and is asking for help in handling her son." It sounded deceitful to say that and not tell her the full story—that we were reporting her to the state.

"I'm also not completely sure it's abuse," I told Dr. Berman. "I'm just concerned."

"That's okay. If there's even a question of abuse, the state wants to know. They'll do their own investigation."

The child protection team consisted of an older pediatrician, a child psychiatrist, a social worker, and a younger pediatric fellow, Dr. Ilene Braverman, to whom I spoke. "Bring the mother with the child when they come to see you again," she told me. "And remember—bring the child."

"What's the procedure?"

"We notify the state and then take care of it. You don't have to do anything."

Still, I felt bad exposing Mrs. Gálvez to all of this, based on what she had, in embarrassment, told me.

"There are some other doctors I would like you to speak with," I told Mrs. Gálvez the following week, uncertain how she would respond, "since it seems you could use, and would like, some help."

"Other doctors?"

"They're concerned."

She nodded sadly.

"Is that okay?"

"Yes," she said. "I whipped him again just the other day. And broke a broom." She grinned meekly. "When I use an extension cord it doesn't break." She tittered nervously.

"We'd like to call an agency to help you, too," I added.

"Okay," she said, looking down. She accepted my reporting her more readily than I had feared, or could have imagined.

We walked downstairs together to the pediatrics section of the ER, where Ilene Braverman had told me to bring her. When we got to the busy ER, Mrs. Gálvez started to cry. "They're interested in helping you to try to deal with Michael better," I reassured her.

She held a crushed ball of Kleenex and pressed it against her eyes. "I know." She wiped her eyes and blew her nose into the tissue and then continued down the corridor.

"We'd like to talk to Michael and do a physical exam on him," Ilene told her. "If you wouldn't mind, have a seat here in the waiting room."

Mrs. Gálvez sat down. Michael stood between her legs, one of his hands holding her thigh. The rest of us—the child protection team and myself—gathered around a black phone on a gray metal desk as Ilene dialed the state capital. Mrs. Gálvez looked down at Michael. I tried to catch her eye but she didn't want to glance at me. The phone rang unanswered. Then Ilene was put on hold. "It's hard to report someone," she said to me quietly, "on a Friday afternoon."

Someone finally answered the phone. Ilene gave her name and phone number and hung up. "They're going to call us back," she announced. "In the meantime we can go ahead and examine Michael."

My beeper started squeaking, and I went to return the page.

Ilene took Michael off to the examining room. But when I returned to the waiting area, Mrs. Gálvez was gone.

"Where did Mrs. Gálvez go?" I asked the secretary seated at the reception desk, busy ruffling papers.

"Who?"

"Mrs. Gálvez."

"Oh, she said she's going off to the cafeteria for coffee." Several minutes later she still hadn't returned. Had she run away? I decided to go to the cafeteria myself for coffee and also to make sure she was there. I hurried down the hall and perused the dining room: patients, families, medical staff in white coats, janitors in dulled blue uniforms, gray Formica tables, pale green fiberglass chairs. But no Mrs. Gálvez. She wasn't there. My heart raced. Where had she gone? Maybe the serving lines. But she wasn't there either. I hunted along the edge of the dining room, scanning the room more vigilantly than before. Still, no Mrs. Gálvez.

I wandered back to the ER, and told Ilene that Mrs. Gálvez was gone.

"At least we have Michael here," she said. Almost as a hostage, I thought.

Forty minutes later, Mrs. Gálvez reappeared. She had stepped outside to smoke a cigarette.

Ilene filed a report with the Bureau of Child Welfare. Both Mrs. Gálvez and her son were referred for further evaluation and treatment through the child protection team, who would take over and monitor the case. I had been shocked at Mrs. Gálvez's openness but glad Michael would now be hooked up to the necessary services. I went to say goodbye to Michael and his mother. She dried her tears, shook my hand, and thanked me. I was glad to have been able to detect and prevent a case of child abuse, which might have otherwise continued. I had done my job but would never see Michael again, which saddened me.

Getting a patient connected to the right services was often not easy.

The following week I was assigned a new patient for evaluation—seven-year-old Timmy Maguire.

"There's something not normal about my son," his mother, Louise, told me when I met her for the first time. "He's hard to handle at home. He's klutzy, always falling down, and can't even blow his nose right. I have to tie his shoes for him. He's never had any friends, and he still wets his bed. He doesn't care about school and has no ambition in life."

The list of problems was long. Some of these items could be of concern, though others seemed odd, possibly reflecting her issues more than his.

She complained that he was always slow—at toilet training, at talking, at walking. But when I asked the dates when he reached these developmental milestones, they were all normal.

She had brought him briefly to a psychologist last year but had then stopped. "It's hard raising three kids and being single," Louise confided. "I don't have time for anything.

"I don't know what's wrong with Timmy," she continued. "He doesn't seem happy. The only thing he cares about are video games. My two daughters are fine—so far." She tapped her knuckles on the side of my desk to "knock on wood" for good luck.

Louise was tall with long blond hair, wore purple eyeliner and deep red lipstick, and had long gold fingernails. She was wearing a bright orange skirt and a violet blouse, and carried two Bloomingdale's shopping bags.

She had gotten divorced from her husband, John, a year earlier. They had only gotten married after she was pregnant with Timmy. After their second year of marriage, John had been laid off. "He stayed unemployed, and after a while he stopped even looking for work. Some days he wouldn't even get out of bed unless I dragged him out. He started drinking, too. Finally, after two years, I just left him. Now he works in a factory in Jefferson City. I've had a few dates with different guys since the divorce, but nothing steady."

"Does Timmy see his father?"

"On weekends. But that's a problem, too. I don't know what John does with him and his sisters. Timmy once mentioned that his father had taken him to a bar. I don't know if it's true but it scares me.

"Anyway, Timmy started wetting his bed after the separation. Last year, the psychologist suggested giving him blue stars for when he doesn't wet. With thirty, he could buy a video game."

"Did the system work?"

"Sort of."

"How come the therapy stopped?"

"I didn't feel it was doing much good. Last week, though, he began to worry me again. He started talking about dying.

He was playing with his two sisters and said, 'Watch me jump out of the window.' So I decided to bring him here. Only it's very far to get here. We live in Pineville, to the west, and it took me over an hour from home. But I've heard this hospital is good."

The following week she brought Timmy with her. "This is Dr. Klitzman," she said slowly, bending down, lowering her head to talk at his level. He retreated closer to her, leaning against her leg, and wrapping his arms behind her. "He's going to talk to you while I wait out here." He shifted his weight from one foot to the other.

"Hello," I said, bending down and holding out my hand for him to shake. He stuck his thumb in his mouth.

"Shake the doctor's hand," Louise told him. Reluctantly, he removed his thumb from his mouth. A coating of saliva glistened. His hand lowered in the air and would have dropped to his side if I hadn't intercepted it. He looked up at me. His eyes were blue-green, as clear as polished emeralds, and reflected back unblemished light. He had short black hair and big round eyes.

"My office is over here," I said, pointing behind me.

With hesitation, he started to step in my direction.

"Go on," his mother urged.

He followed me into my office and sat down. I shut the door.

"I'm a talking doctor," I said. He looked at me, then down at the floor. His white Keds sneakers didn't touch the ground. His one ankle, hooked behind the other, ticktocked back and forth in the air. "Do you know what that is?"

He slid off the cushion to stand up. He was wearing Oshkosh overalls and a white shirt with thin red stripes.

"Where's Mommy?" He looked worriedly toward the door.

"She's sitting outside. She'll come back in a few minutes. Why don't you sit back down?" I reached out to guide him back. He closed his sweaty palm and fingers around my thumb and I led him back to the chair.

Dr. Berman had given us a few suggestions on engaging children.

"Let me ask you a question," I said. Timmy's eyes shifted about restlessly.

"If you could be given three wishes, what would they be?"

He put his hand to his mouth, thinking.

"That I don't wet my bed . . . That I have all the Nintendo

games—I want Zeldor and Ice Hockey—and I want Great-Grandpa to come back alive."

His last response surprised me. "Tell me about Great-Grandpa."

"Great-Grandpa woke up in the hospital, and I saw him before he died." He strung the words of this sentence together as if repeating something he had heard. "But I know where he is now."

"You do?"

"Yes," he answered matter-of-factly.

"Where?"

"He's in Heaven-Paradise." Timmy climbed up onto the seat of his chair, stood on his tiptoes, and stretched his arm as high as it would go, pointing with his index finger at the ceiling. "Up there!"

I motioned for him to sit back down.

"What do you know about heaven?"

"God's there. It's a nice place. They have video games, and my sister says you can go on rides and don't have to pay a quarter. But," he reflected, "I don't know. I want to go to heaven to see how big God is."

"Do you want to die?" He looked at me, not understanding. "Do you want to hurt yourself?"

"No."

"Do you feel sad sometimes?"

"About Great-Grandpa."

"What did you like about your great-grandpa?"

"He used to give me cookies."

"Your mother tells me that you said you wanted to die."

"I was just tricking. I said I was going to jump out the window."

"Did you want to?"

"No way. I was tricking my little sister Patty. She's stupid."

"Are you sad most of the time?"

"No." He was surprised I asked. "Just when I think about Great-Grandpa."

"Do you know why you're here?"

"For a checkup ... I'm going to get it in the arm." I assumed he meant a vaccination.

"Do you know why you're here seeing me, a talking doctor?"

"I've been wetting my bed." He looked down, embarrassed. "I never know why I do it."

"How do you feel about it when you do it?"

"Sad . . . but I'm going to get a quarter for not wetting."

"How are things at home?"

"Sometimes my mother hits me." He looked down at his lap again. His small legs stopped swinging. "Because of something. I get messed quickly." He meant from wetting his bed. To help him I would need to understand more about what was wrong.

"How's school?"

"Sometimes okay. Sometimes not."

"What's not okay about it?"

"Sometimes the teacher makes me stand outside the room." His eyes moistened.

"How come?"

"Because I spill stuff. But," he added, "not on purpose. I don't mean to."

"What do you spill?"

"Crayons, glue, paper . . . it just happens."

I asked him if he remembered any of his dreams.

"Sometimes I dream that Great-Grandpa isn't dead yet."

I felt bad for Timmy, and thought he was trying hard and seemed perplexed by the problems he was having. He was a cute kid, and reminded me of myself when I was his age—curious, alert, and active. Therapy, I thought, could help him, and rescue this likable and engaging boy before it was too late.

I scheduled another appointment for the following week.

Later that day, Dr. Berman called me to ask if I could present a patient that Friday in Child Psychiatry Case Conference. Usually, a patient was presented who was being evaluated and had been seen two or three times in treatment.

I mentioned Timmy. "But I've met him only once."

"It doesn't matter. It sounds interesting."

"But I don't know if they'll complete the evaluation and want to be treated here."

"That doesn't matter either."

I phoned Louise, who agreed to come with Timmy. "Can we schedule another meeting before that?" I asked her. As complete an evaluation as possible would make the conference more useful.

"No. I can't. My mother's birthday's on Wednesday, and on Thursday I have to bring the car in to be fixed."

I also tried unsuccessfully to reach Timmy's father.

I phoned the psychologist who had treated Timmy in the

past. "I couldn't get a real handle on the case," she said. "The mother kept refocusing on something else. Initially he came in for bed-wetting. I recommended that he clean up the mess himself and go back to his own bed, which seemed to help. The mother changed jobs a few times. They'd miss every few appointments. She'd claim their car would break down or something. The parents used the kids as go-betweens, always quizzing Timmy and Patty about what the other parent was up to, and relaying messages back and forth. I spent a lot of time with Timmy going over the divorce. He had a lot of fantasies about his parents getting back together. I tried to tell him that he wasn't to blame."

"Did treatment help?"

"He stopped wetting his bed. But they dropped therapy—right after I suggested that the mother come for separate appointments to see me individually. She said she didn't have time, and then stopped bringing Timmy. She said she couldn't afford it any longer. It's a shame, because Timmy could really have benefited."

I hung up the phone, disheartened and disillusioned. Timmy had been in treatment. It *had* helped him, but in the end his mother had stopped it—not a good sign.

I also phoned his teacher, Elizabeth Fromson. "Academically, Timmy seems extremely bright. He has a good vocabulary, but he's only in an average reading group because of his problems. He's easily distracted and gets disorganized. His desk looks like a bomb's gone off in it. He always makes a mess and never sits still, but shifts around all the time, putting his head down, then draping himself over the chair, putting one leg over the back of it or squatting in the seat. He has a hard time connecting to other children. Other kids stay away from him, because he displays a lot of negative behavior—throwing his arms around other boys and kissing them. He says 'I love you' to anybody. He's a good kid but needs a lot of TLC, and it gets him into trouble."

I called Louise to confirm that she'd come to the conference and asked her to arrive a little early. But at noon, when the conference was about to start, she wasn't there.

"They said they'd come," I told the audience of child psychiatrists, social workers, and other residents.

"Why don't we start anyway," Dr. Berman said. "And you can give us the HPI," the history of present illness.

"Timothy Maguire is a seven-year-old white male in first grade at Chestnut Ridge Elementary school in Pineville, who lives with his mother and two younger sisters . . ." The format sounded stiff and removed.

I presented his "developmental milestones"—when he first walked, when he first spoke. When I was done and went into the hall, to my surprise, Timmy and his parents had all arrived, including his father—a short, balding man in a lumber shirt, jeans, and a denim jacket.

Dr. Berman interviewed them together. Mr. Maguire seemed very concerned about his son as well.

Afterward, I led the family out into the hallway to thank them, make sure they were okay, and set up an appointment to see Timmy the following week.

Back in the conference room, Dr. Berman turned to me. "There are many things you need to find out. Why did the parents divorce? And how did they meet in the first place? When did he first say 'Mama'? What did he want? Do we know when he first crawled?" My presentation had included his age at all of the other major milestones. "Do we know what his Apgars were?" Apgar scores, given to newborn children, reflect biological stability outside the womb. "Apgars are important," he continued, "the first of many graded tests we embark our kids on. What are his fantasies? How is he doing academically? Is there a question about whether to leave him mainstreamed?"

I repeated some of his teacher's remarks.

"Why does Timmy like video games?" I thought to myself: "What's to wonder about? What does any child, or anyone for that matter, like about video games?" To me—who had occasionally played them—there was no mystery, though to Dr. Berman, in his early sixties, there was.

"Did you call his pediatrician?"

"I tried, but he didn't return my call."

"Talk to him. Make sure there's nothing else going on that the mother didn't tell you. You should also meet with the father. Where is he working now?"

"I don't know."

"You should ask. How long was his great-grandfather ill?" I didn't know. He was close to the boy and had died and Timmy missed him. Apparently that wasn't enough.

"What did the other therapist think of the mother?" a social worker asked. "The mother seems borderliny." "Borderliny" referred to borderline personality disorder, and was often bandied about as an adjective, though ill defined.

I had only met with Timmy once. He wouldn't continue here for treatment anyway—Mrs. Maguire had repeatedly reminded me that our hospital was too far. There might not be any treatment spots available in the clinic, anyway. Dr. Berman's questions, though of interest, were in this particular situation mostly academic—teaching points. But a process had been started. Once conferenced, as it was called, a whole slew of questions was raised, regardless of their practical relationship to the particular case. Further questions were suggested. Then there was silence. There was a lot to find out. It could take weeks. And there was always more we wouldn't know.

"But I'm most concerned that she won't follow through with treatment," I said.

"Well, get the information you need first."

"Shouldn't we hook him up with treatment, though, as soon as we can?"

"No. Do a complete evaluation first." The outcome of the evaluation—that he needed treatment—was clear. But we would go through with a full, though unnecessary, evaluation.

"But they may not come back."

"Do it anyway. You never know."

"But they live outside of our catchment area," meaning that we might not have any treatment spots to offer for him in my case. "I'm wondering whether it makes sense to foster a further relationship with me, when it will be difficult enough for them to develop one with the doctor who eventually treats him."

"See what you turn up first."

The conference taught me about how to put together a coherent presentation about a child, but I was still concerned about Timmy, and wasn't sure whether it had or would help him.

The following week, Louise left a message that she had to miss our appointment. We scheduled another meeting, but she didn't show up or even call to cancel. I dialed her work number.

"Howard Johnson's Motel," someone answered. I recognized her voice.

"Ms. Maguire?"

"Yes?"

"This is Dr. Klitzman."

"Oh hello, Dr. Klitzman," she said, as if nothing were wrong.

"I had understood that we were going to be meeting today."

"Oh, I couldn't make it. My work shift changed."

"I see . . ." To ask, "Did you think of calling to cancel?" might be too blunt and rude on the phone. "Are you interested in continuing the evaluation?" I asked.

"Oh yes," she said enthusiastically. "Only, well, it's just that your hospital is a bit far for me. But I do want to come."

"It's up to you. If you decide to have Timmy treated it can be somewhere else. But he can really benefit from treatment. I think you should finish the evaluation in the meantime."

"Okay."

But they missed the next appointment as well. I called Louise and left a message. When she didn't call back, I tried a second time, eager to try to help him. "Oh yes, Doctor," she said, unperturbed.

"I understood we had an appointment," I said once more.

"I couldn't make it. The electrician was coming that day."

"It helps to call!"

"I had planned to but didn't get around to it."

"Are you interested in completing the evaluation?" I also repeated.

"Well, it's kind of far for us."

"It would help Timmy to be in therapy again. If not here, then somewhere else. I'd be happy to give you the names of other clinics or psychiatrists closer to you," I said. "Or you can go back to the psychologist you saw."

"No. I didn't like her," she said. "She didn't do Timmy any good."

If I were meeting with her face-to-face, I would have challenged that statement and confronted her with my sense that she was running away. But it was this very confrontation that she seemed to be avoiding by not coming to see me. Dr. Ostrow had said never to make an interpretation to someone who wasn't in treatment with us. But here I felt something was called for. "Look," I finally said, "it strikes me that it's been very hard for you to get Timmy into therapy. Your concern for him is very good, but it's important that he gets what he needs."

"I know what you're saying," she said. "You're right. This time, I'll follow through." I gave her names of psychiatrists near their home and she said she'd bring him.

"If there's any problem or anything else I can do, please give me a call."

I never heard from her again.

Dr. Berman said that since our relationship had ended, it wouldn't be appropriate for me to call her to encourage her or pursue the issue with her further. My evaluation of Timmy was over. "Too bad the mother didn't follow through with the eval," Dr. Berman said in passing. But even if Mrs. Maguire had finished the evaluation, she might not have allowed the final treatment to go on. I had wanted to help Timmy, even if in some small way, and hoped for his sake that he got into treatment and stayed. But I would never know and could do nothing else about it. I felt engaged and concerned for him, but ultimately helpless. There was only so much I could do.

Timmy was getting further lost in the chaotic shuffle and swirl of events in his parents' lives. It was unclear where he and his problems fit in the flux. His troubles resulted partly from the tumult around him. His relationship with his great-grandfather must have been one of the stabilizing influences in his life—probably why Timmy missed him dearly. Now his great-grandfather was gone, unreplaced. Treatment just might help—at least an adult would again be in his life on a regular basis in some form. But this was not to be had—at least not now.

This experience was humbling and sad for me. Timmy yearned for attention. At some level Mrs. Maguire was trying, but was perhaps just too overwhelmed. Yet now was the time to catch problems, before it was too late.

A psychiatrist could help him—once he arrived at the psychiatrist's office regularly once or twice a week. But the larger "systems" issues—his parents' problems—gaped open before us. Psychiatric treatment was but a Band-Aid given the larger social and economic problems affecting his life: his parents' divorce, his father's unemployment, and his mother's difficulties settling herself down, trying to work and support three kids.

Psychiatry was in many ways limited—not because it was unable to address psychological conflicts but because other problems loomed. I kept seeing and learning this lesson the hard way. Though I tried raising these limitations at the conference, the attendings discussed what they knew and were good at: further questions to ask the patient and his family when they came back. But once again we had little or no ability to treat or solve the larger problems. As a result, the patient never returned. All our discussion, possibly helpful in other circumstances, was for naught. Psychotherapy, as one tool for change, can be effective, but sometimes isn't enough by itself.

Psychiatrists often blamed the patient or the family for failing the treatment rather than discussing the ultimate limitations of the tools we had, or even of ourselves. Sometimes our expertise didn't work because we needed to adopt a wider perspective to glimpse beyond what we'd been trained to see, and take in the whole.

When treatment didn't work with adult patients, I usually could at least assume that the patient, as an adult who had managed to endure until that point, had some basic skills to continue to get by. At worst, the patient could perhaps bring him- or herself to the ER to get treatment, if needed. Not always, but at least there was a decent chance of such a fallback. But with children, the case was different. Children were at the mercy of somebody else—usually their parents—and if treatment didn't work or if they missed sessions it might be due to their parents, not themselves.

The last note in Timmy's chart remained mine, documenting his mother's failure to finish the evaluation and describing how he would benefit from treatment if it could be arranged.

I don't know if it ever was.

Yellow and Red Balloons

Through these experiences, I was becoming part of not just a particular hospital's residency program, but an entire profession. Psychiatrists as a group, I began to learn, differed from my preconceived notions in many ways.

This broader level of membership became apparent to me in the middle of residency, when I was able to attend the annual meeting of the American Psychiatric Association, held in San Francisco. There, outside the hospital's walls, other aspects of the profession became clear.

I had rushed to finish my duties before leaving the hospital the evening before and looked forward to getting away, to hearing lectures from the nation's leading psychiatrists, and to seeing the cutting edge of the field—the latest scientific advancements in understanding the mind and the brain.

I arrived in the city late at night and early the next morning strolled out to the convention center. Across the street from the center in the middle of a square, a huge hot-air balloon brightly painted in yellow and red stripes bounced in the light breeze. Large letters read "Asendin," the name of an antidepressant medication. The balloon was the drug's logo, appearing in the company's psychiatric magazine ads.

In the conference hall, I joined a long line of psychiatrists from around the world waiting to register and was handed a plastic bookbag with handles and shoulder straps, packed with ten pounds of research abstracts, schedules of proceedings, and lists of commercial exhibits. I headed back to the hotel a block away to pore over these.

Roy spotted me in the hotel lobby. "Want to have a drink?" he asked.

"Sure."

We ordered gin and tonics and ate from a black bowl of cocktail mix. I had never had a drink with him before. "It's nice to get away from the hospital for a few days," he said, popping some of the nuts into his mouth. "But it was murder arranging coverage for my patients. Everyone wanted to get away at the same time ... Shelly!" he suddenly called out, spying Shelly Tarr strolling through the lobby. As a faculty member in the outpatient department, she specialized in research on anxiety disorders. She was tall, with long, straight black hair.

She sauntered over now, carrying two shopping bags.

"Want to join us?" he asked.

She plopped down her glossy packages. "I've spent the entire morning shopping," she said.

"What did you buy?" he asked.

"I found some nice shoes." She removed a box from its plastic sack, lifted off the lid, and displayed black leather pumps. "I never have time to buy shoes back home. I'm so busy all the time. I checked in here, switched my room, and went out shopping. Originally, they put me on the top floor of the hotel. I never stay at the top of these places, though. I mean, what if there's a fire?"

"So do you always change rooms?" Roy asked.

"I haven't been in a big hotel like this for a while," she said. "The last time was actually the night before my boards. That hotel was right next to the airport, and I heard landings and takeoffs all night. The next morning at my boards I was a nervous wreck."

We talked about some of the symposia, finished our drinks, and left.

In the lobby elevators I kept running into other psychiatrists I knew, just like at the hospital. I returned to my room and lay down for a moment with the bag of conference proceedings and brochures and information booklets about the hotel. The hotel occupied an entire city block and consisted of wings extending out from a central axis. The complex included hundreds of rooms with beds, in addition to restaurants, a gym, a laundry service, a barbershop, meeting rooms, and offices with copiers and fax machines available. It, too, was like a hospital—all-containing, all-encompassing. You could stay in the building for weeks and never leave. Yet one could check out of a hotel when one wanted, which was not always the case in a hospital. A psychiatric hospital seemed somewhere between a prison and a hotel.

The next morning I headed to the main convention hall to hear some lectures. One was on neurotransmitters—chemical messengers in the different portions of the brain. I spotted Anne going into the auditorium and we sat together. A petite woman with long silken blond hair in a white blouse and pink skirt discussed her research and showed slides. She announced that to analyze neurons, she had killed two hundred mice and extracted and ground up their brains. Anne leaned over to me. "What," she whispered, "is a nice little girl like that doing killing all those mice? You wonder what makes people study the things they do!"

After the presentation, we wandered out into the hall and on to other lectures. At each, psychiatrists milled in and out, many listening for a few minutes to decide if they were interested in staying longer.

I tried to see and hear the people whose journal articles had impressed me. Now, after one and a half years of psychiatry, I could stand back and pick and choose specific areas rather than feel overwhelmed by the whole field. But the biggest crowds at this convention and at subsequent ones I would later attend flocked to hear nonpsychiatrists. Each year, writers and artists were invited—Stephen Sondheim and James Lapine discussing the shared creative process, Tom Wolfe and Mordecai Richler talking, respectively, on the cultures of the United States and Canada.

One of the most subversive sessions was held in a quiet back room where the theories of the late French writer Michel Foucault were discussed. Though the room was typical of others, the discussion here challenged those in all the hundreds of other rooms of the convention. Foucault had criticized what Western medicine and psychiatry had termed normal and sick. He questioned whether we could determine what mental illness is. Weren't diagnoses merely categories we applied to behavior we didn't like or couldn't understand?

The questions were interesting and deserved to be posed, but I found myself feeling that no good answers were given—certainly no clear alternative to replacing psychiatry as a field. Psychiatry's diagnostic categories might be relative, yet I had by now seen how some individuals were subject to thoughts and behavior, troubling to themselves and others, that the profession could sometimes alleviate. The power psychiatrists subsequently assumed over these people's lives could be questioned. But psychiatry, though imperfect, served some purposes better than anything else currently available.

After sitting through several lectures, my brain felt numb. Objects seemed flat. I took a break and ran into Mike in the hallway.

"Hey, have you seen the exhibits yet?" he asked.

"No, I haven't had a chance."

"Let's check them out. I hear you can get all kinds of free gifts."

Spread through the hall were huge promotional exhibitions by the largest drug companies that manufactured psychiatric medications. Each corporation had built an island of carpeting with well-padded, fabric-covered chairs and high-tech design lattices arching overhead. Plastic signs illuminated from behind spun around, advertising the company and its latest leading drugs that I placed in patients' bodies each day. One exhibit consisted of columns and arches of rough gray cardboard painted to look like stone. A large yellow sign read "Anxiety" in four-foot-high orange letters. Several young women milled about along the side of the exhibit wearing white Styrofoam Panama hats with shiny red, white, and blue paper bands wrapped around the crowns. The women, all with neatly cut, straight shoulder-length blond hair and uniforms of navy jackets and skirts, looked like cheerleaders at a political rally. A clean-cut salesman in a fresh-pressed suit behind a counter smiled eagerly as he unfolded pamphlets and brochures in front of a potential customer. The company representatives looked like they could have been selling expensive new cars.

Three long lines of psychiatrists wound away from another exhibit. The front person on each line was speaking on a white telephone.

"What's that?" I asked Mike.

"Free telephone calls. You can call anywhere in the country for free. The drug company pays."

"Anywhere?"

"That's right."

The line seemed too long to bother waiting, and we strolled on.

Another drug company supplied free Styrofoam cups of coffee. People milled toward the urns, empty cups in hand to be filled with fluid to keep them awake for a few more hours of discussions.

Across the area were stretched cushioned seats, each occupied by a weary psychiatrist, bags of brochures, books, and free gifts dropped on the ground by his feet or piled on his lap. The sitters looked like tired travelers in a railroad station waiting for a much delayed train, none about to give up his or her place any time in the near future.

The companies also distributed to us gifts and glossy brochures with expensive transparent color drawings of cross-sections of the brain. They gave out handsome gray pens, with the brand names of antidepressant drugs emblazoned on the side. Bronze Prozac paperweights lay neatly on thick squares of cotton, wrapped in navy blue gift boxes. Free coffee mugs had the names of different drugs glazed on their sides. Asendin mugs depicted the drug's red and yellow balloon flying up the side of the cup next to the handle. Another company's mugs displayed a squiggly black cartoon of the brain. One exhibit brandished a six-foot-high illuminated cross-section of a skull. Yet how little we really knew about the brain or about the details of how these drugs worked or the mechanics of some of the chemicals' longer-term side effects. How odd to think that my hard work with patients was supporting multinational corporations that made handsome profits. Drugs were often emphasized to the exclusion of other approaches to assist patients. Perhaps if drugs weren't as expensive, there'd be more funding available for other kinds of mental health facilities and resources. I had conceived of my job as assisting patients, not as supporting corporate giants, earning money for them. Patients might be aided in the process, but it was still shocking that someone was making profits off of them and their disorders.

At another exhibit, a crowd of psychiatrists flocked around two white egg-shaped modules with speakers built in the walls. A California stress-reduction company made videos to alleviate anxiety. Psychiatrists sat in each module with their feet up, watching a television screen of an ocean shore, the surf rolling before an orange and violet sunset, white crests gently cascading and disappearing over each other.

We stood in line. Each seated psychiatrist in his suit, with his legs stretched out before him, head thrown back, and his fingertips pressed together, looked as if he were listening to a psychoanalytic patient on a couch. Neither psychiatrist was about to budge, and they ignored the twelve of us standing in line at each chair. After about twenty minutes without either line moving, Mike and I gave up.

Ahead lay the largest crowd, surrounding a platform on which two metal contraptions sat, looking like machines from dungeons of the Spanish Inquisition.

Brown metal straps were molded to form a chair with strips descending down and forming baskets for each leg. A psychiatrist was seated in each machine, one strap wrapped around his skull, another rising up over the back of his scalp and forward down his nose, a third traveling across his head like the strap on a pair of earmuffs.

Each apparatus was contoured to the shoulders and back and resembled a human cage. The grillwork positioned the body while measurements were taken. Over the top were various metal attachments. It looked like an electrocution chair.

"Have Your Phrenology Done," a sign read above the exhibit. The contraptions were nineteenth-century relics once used to measure skull dimensions, thought by psychiatrists at the time to indicate and predict a wide variety of personality traits from intelligence to potential for violence.

What amazed me was how unabashedly the crowd now gravitated toward these devices. The theory that bumps on the skull correlate with behavioral traits has been dispelled as a myth, yet obviously still possessed allure. Even today, psychiatrists generally attribute severe mental disorders to biological abnormalities, though the exact mechanisms and details of these deficits haven't always been fully understood, and treatments are often suboptimal. The notion that psychiatry could quantify vague concepts of mentation still appealed—even if, as in the case of phrenolgoy, scientific grounding was wanting. There is an enormous need to structure and order mental states and make them tangible, even if the theories involved are incorrect.

The next day, the front page of the main local city newspaper showed a large photo of the two chairs in its coverage of the conference. The idea of making abstract emotional states concrete captivated others besides psychiatrists. The paper displayed nothing of the scientific findings presented, only these robotlike machines in human shapes.

PART IV

Cutbacks

Unfortunately, only limited resources were available for helping many of my patients. Sometimes what patients wanted conflicted with what the hospital or I could provide. Many psychiatrists responded to the frustration of such problems by merely distancing themselves from the patient, and I felt a lot of pressure to do the same. It was all too easy to become wary of those under our care.

Yet patients occasionally became victims of the hospital's policies. Sometimes, in pushing for the patient's best interests, I had to stand up on their behalf and fight the institution itself.

"Just see him once every month or two for fifteen minutes to give him a refill," Betsy Coover, the director of social work in the outpatient clinic, told me as she assigned me an extra new patient. My caseload was already overbooked. "In four months we're terminating him from the clinic."

Gene Blango was being given to me for medication backup. For twelve years, he had been seeing a social worker, Louise Montgomery, for psychotherapy. However, she was retiring and because of cutbacks would not be replaced.

He wanted to continue to see a therapist, which he had found helpful, but the hospital forbade it because of money. He would have to find another clinic—even though he lived only a few blocks from the hospital, and had no health insurance. He didn't want to go.

"It sounds like he's being dumped on you," Anne later said to me when I told her about the case. "Typical of this place."

I met with Gene for the first time in Louise's office. He had a long history of vague problems, mostly depression and low self-esteem. When younger, he had finished two years of

237

college and had worked as a librarian at one point. But anxieties had gotten in the way. For a few years now he had been unemployed. He had been seeing Louise once a week and received antidepressant medication, meeting a psychiatrist for a prescription once every month or two. I would merely continue his medication.

Gene Blango was a short man of Portuguese descent with light brown hair. He wore a navy blue sport coat, wrinkled, but smoothed out over his body, and a striped tie, wide as was the style several years earlier, and also creased where it had been folded. He seemed to be trying to preserve some small amount of dignity.

I wrote a prescription for two months and told him I'd see him again at that time.

"You know they're taking Miss Montgomery away."

"I know and am sorry to hear about that." I handed him the prescription and got up to go.

"Wait a minute," he said. "Can you tell me what the side effects are?"

"Didn't your other doctor go over them with you?" He had been on the medication for four years.

"No."

"I think he did," Louise interrupted.

"Well . . ." He paused. "I don't remember. Can you tell them to me again?"

"Okay." I listed the most commonly encountered side effects: "Dry mouth, tiredness, blurry vision, and dizziness, particularly when you stand up."

"Any others?"

"Some. But they're rarer."

"Like what?"

I was concerned about telling them to him, since he was anxious already, but listed several others.

"I've been having chest pain."

Chest pain could indicate a cardiac problem, and was important to evaluate. "How long have you had it?"

"On and off for years, but it has just returned after being absent for a while and has been worse than before."

"Have you talked to your internist about it?"

"Not since it has come back."

"Will you?"

"Okay."

* * *

A month later, I met with him again to give him a refill.

"Are you sure this is the best medication for me? I've been feeling more depressed lately."

"My understanding is that the medicine has worked better overall than others you've been on in the past. Besides, a pill can't change everything. Talking about what you're feeling with Ms. Montgomery is important, too."

"But she's leaving soon. Plus, the pain in my chest has gotten worse."

"Have you told your internist, Dr. Summers?"

"No."

"Why not?"

"I forgot."

"Oh brother," I thought to myself. I asked him about it, but it didn't seem to be a genuine cardiac problem.

He was putting the burden of his chest pain on me and wasn't doing his part.

Afterward, I phoned his internist.

"It's nothing new," Dr. John Summers told me. "He's been having pain off and on for years."

"You've worked it up?"

"Countless times. It's never anything."

"He says it's been worse the past few months."

"It hasn't been a few months. It's been years. You can get him an echo"—that is, a cardiac echo. "But it would upset him more than it's worth. The outcome wouldn't change the treatment."

At the end of my next meeting with Gene, the same thing happened, and he tried to engage me as long as he could by talking about the medicine.

He now had only two sessions left with Ms. Montgomery. He called Dr. Gillis, the director of administration in the hospital, to complain that he wasn't being assigned a new therapist.

He also called me and left a message, which I returned. "I can't speak with you now," he told me. "Can you call me back in fifteen minutes?"

It was 7:00 P.M. I was ready to go home. "Can it wait until tomorrow?"

"Maybe—maybe not. Fifty-fifty," he said, almost as a threat.

"Why don't *you* call *me* back?"

"No, please call me back, Dr. Klitzman. Please."

I called him back later from my home. "What's up?" I asked.

"I just want to go over the side effects of the medications with you again."

"But we've gone over all of them."

"I forgot them." He seemed nervous. His memory had been fine when tested.

I was getting angry. "Why did you say this couldn't wait until tomorrow?"

"Well, I didn't want to be dishonest."

"But it seems that it could wait."

"Side effects I may be having are important."

"But we've gone over them before. I'm wondering how this relates to your feelings about Ms. Montgomery leaving."

"No. My side effects have nothing to do with her."

It didn't feel right to snap at him. He was, perhaps, not fully in control of his behavior.

Gene was rousing conflicting emotions in me. He was trying to draw me in because Louise Montgomery was leaving. But while he wanted to engage me professionally, he also acted nonchalant and entitled to my attention. He was getting me angry, making me resent helping him. I was left having to resolve the tension between my professional duty and my frustration with him even though I knew he was transferring part of his distress onto me as a way of dealing with it himself.

As a medical backup I was involved in only one aspect of his care but responsible for all of it. If the case were straightforward, there would be no problem. But often, having two caregivers fragmented the treatment and had disadvantages. It was set up for convenience and cost. Yet Gene's psychotherapeutic issues were relevant to how he behaved with me.

I answered his questions as briefly and firmly as possible on the phone, told him we could talk about it further when we met, and was glad to hang up.

Two weeks later, Louise Montgomery left. Gene called Shelly Tarr to complain that he couldn't possibly afford both a psychotherapist and a psychopharmacologist. She decided I should continue to see Gene for medications until I finished the year in June. "Just see him once every month or two to give him a prescription. Don't meet with him for more than twenty minutes or maybe half an hour if you absolutely must."

But it became clear that he needed someone to talk to as well.

I spoke to Betsy Coover, the director of social work, about getting him a replacement for Louise.

"Just tell him he has to see someone privately."

"I don't think he can afford it."

"We don't have any slots available for him here. We have to save money somewhere, so we have to make cutbacks. It's as simple as that. There are other clinics in town. Let him hook himself up with a clinic elsewhere. In June we'll terminate him. That's the only dispo," or disposition, "we can give him."

"How can you drop me from the hospital?" he asked me at my next meeting with him. "I've been coming here for twelve years! This place is like a home to me. I feel safe here. What gets me through the week is knowing I can come here." He reminded me of one particularly frail patient of mine who would come to the hospital waiting room every Wednesday at four o'clock—the time of our usual appointment—even on the weeks when I was on vacation, since merely being inside the building calmed and reassured her.

Gene called Dr. Gillis again to complain. Gene phoned me more often, too, and started calling Betsy Coover every day. He was too invested in the hospital after all these years.

"Okay," Shelly finally told me on Monday. "I see this isn't working. He can be followed here, but only in group. The group therapist could also give him medications." An extra patient in group therapy didn't require any additional time from the therapist. Individual one-to-one therapy would take up an extra forty-five minutes of a therapist's time each week. But in a group, six to ten patients could be seen together in a single hour. Dr. Ostrow had said there were specific reasons for recommending group as opposed to individual treatment. Gene would do better in individual therapy, given his need to establish close connections to the therapist, as opposed to the broader, diffuse feelings he would have toward the group as a whole. Yet residents often cited group therapy as a "dumping ground" for patients when slots with individual therapists weren't available.

"But I don't want a group," Gene said when I told him the plan. "I want my own therapist!"

Gene called me up a few days later to ask for a refill. I told him that his last prescription included one. If the pharmacy didn't have a record of it, he could call me back but should just leave a message that the pharmacy needed a prescription phoned in.

He called back but didn't leave a message, other than that he had phoned.

"Yes," he said, when I returned his call. "You were right. The pharmacy had a refill for me."

"Good," I said, ready to hang up. He was silent, waiting for something. "Anything else?"

"Mrs. Coover says I can't get medication at the hospital anymore."

"You'll get it in the group," I said to end the conversation.

"Can't I just ask you something else?"

"Okay, what?"

"Is the quality of care not as good if I get my medication in group?"

"The group doctor is very good."

"But isn't it not as good?"

"You'll have one therapist instead of two."

"But I want two."

"People usually just have one." I finally got off the phone.

I walked into the hall and saw Betsy Coover. "You wouldn't believe Gene Blango," I said to her. "He just called me—twice." I told her briefly what had happened.

"Don't even talk to him. Just tell him he has to wait until his next meeting with you and refuse to speak with him further. I practically have to hang up the phone on him when he calls." Her approach, removing herself from him, seemed somewhat insensitive, but that was what staff seemed to do, and I could understand her inclination.

The leader of the group to which Gene was referred, Dr. Nick Seligman, met with him and decided Gene could come to the group for therapy. But Gene's medications were still an ongoing issue, and to have them discussed each week wouldn't be fair to the other members of the group. Shelly Tarr told me I should continue to give him medications until June.

Gene joined the group. But after a handful of sessions, he stopped going. I was left as the only one seeing him.

My last meeting with him—the last time he would be seen at this hospital—was scheduled for the first week in June. He complained of more chest pain, headaches on one side of his head, odd "spells," and other problems, all of which I thought were somatic, bodily sensations that can occur as part of depression. Still, I had to ask about each ailment to make sure it wasn't new or the sign of a significant medical problem. As soon as we finished discussing one complaint, he'd suddenly raise another.

Finally, when our half-hour session was over, he added, "I'm so down I've been thinking of killing myself. I've been thinking of buying a gun." I couldn't believe he was bringing this up at the end of our last session. It would have to be evaluated. "What are your thoughts about that?"

"That I want to do it."

"What percent chance do you think there is that you would act on these thoughts?"

"I don't know. I've been thinking about it for a few days. Also that if I jump from my apartment—twelve stories—it would probably work." He spoke calmly, as if calculating a physics experiment, and then looked down sadly at the ground.

"Why are you waiting until now at the end of the session to tell me this?"

"We were talking about other things before."

He might be exaggerating. But he also seemed genuinely distressed.

I spoke with Betsy Coover. "You'll have to meet with him again." She sighed. "Maybe we'll even have to change our plan. I'm not a happy woman this afternoon."

According to hospital policy, Shelly Tarr, as the attending, also had to see him, since he said he was suicidal. "Now I see what you've been saying all along," she told me afterward.

He finally said he'd be able to come to the ER rather than hurt himself, and I told him I'd meet with him again next Monday.

"So if I'm suicidal I get to have an extra session," he concluded. "Now I see what it takes."

"That's not the message I want to communicate." I had to write an extensive note, detailing what he had said and justifying why we were sending him home anyway and not hospitalizing him. Instead of twenty minutes, all of the conversations, consultations, and documentation had taken two and a half hours. I was angry and fed up and felt taken advantage of.

I was behind schedule and had to hurry to a local travel agent to pick up airplane tickets for a trip before the office closed. At the travel agency, I sat down on one of a row of bright red vinyl chairs. Dusty cardboard signs of foreign cities and resorts dangled in the air around me. I could barely breathe, filled with anger at being caught in the middle, essentially having Gene assigned to me because the hospital wanted to cut back on staff to save money and didn't care about how patients fared as a result. He, on the other hand, was trying to hold on to me as tightly as he could. The competing demands tore at me. I had the image in my mind of sticking a pin in my face. I was angry and couldn't accept it, enraged about getting an extra patient who was bothering me and with whom the hospital wouldn't support me. Professionally, I had to be available to help him though he frustrated me. I felt I couldn't reject him.

At the time I felt he was purposefully making things hard for me. I was trying to help him, while he irritated me, taking time from other things I wanted or needed to do. Only in retrospect do I see that he was trying to get what he needed and realistically probably couldn't stop his actions.

I realized that something was wrong in the treatment. I had only wanted to make it through to June when he would be out of my hair, but he was putting pressure on me. I would have to rectify the problem.

Before starting my residency I had thought I dealt with problems pretty well. In my daily social interactions, I did. But now, in new situations, I had to confront my anger and frustration at people. I couldn't just walk away; I had to mobilize my resources, not by just fighting in return, but by sitting back and trying to understand my feelings.

As a response to all of these pressures, I felt the desire to become more detached. There was comfort in saying and doing things with patients that sounded or looked or felt "psychiatrist-like." I had told myself that I would avoid that stereotype, yet was now finding it necessary to respond to patients based primarily not on my personal feelings but on how I felt a psychiatrist should or would respond. Many of the sayings and actions and tones of voice of psychiatrists had long rankled me. Psychiatrists can be stiff and formal and can hide behind their theories and their sheer professionalism. Although there is not always sufficient scientific support for this behavior, the reasons psychiatrists acted removed now became clearer.

I met with Gene again, now realizing what I had to do. I couldn't just go along with Betsy, Shelly, and Dr. Gillis in their plan to drop him. They wouldn't like my supporting the patient, but it felt right. I would be terminating with him in a few weeks, but it didn't feel appropriate leaving him in the lurch.

I phoned Gillis and explained the situation. "Look, he can't handle being terminated very well," I said. I also phoned Shelly and Betsy. In the end, they agreed. He was assigned to another social worker as an extra patient. Another resident would soon be assigned as backup.

The issues were not at all clear until the end. I had to learn that he wasn't just being a pain in the neck but really couldn't handle a situation the hospital was putting him in. It was my discomfort, which I could barely articulate at the time, that made me realize that something was wrong in the treatment and had to be changed. I was learning that in caring for a patient I might feel internal unease that I needed to be aware of as a sign that something was possibly awry. It was painful for me, personally, to stand up against an unfairness in the system, but I had gotten him what he needed.

He is being treated in the clinic to this day.

No-goodniks

I was seeing how my supervisors were sometimes wrong about cases and how it was important to trust my own judgment— particularly with outpatients whom they never met.

This became ever more critical with patients who were assigned to me for long-term, insight-oriented psychotherapy in my third year of residency. I was looking forward to conducting outpatient psychotherapy: helping patients through talk alone, and assisting them in gaining insight into their problems. This approach is largely what had attracted me to the field in the first place. Based on Freudian psychoanalytic, or "psychodynamic," principles, modeled on the "talking cure," insight-oriented therapy was psychiatry at its most "artlike." I assumed the patients would be higher-functioning, more like my friends and myself. In addition, outpatient work was more representative of how most psychiatrists spend the majority of their professional lives. I assumed the tasks would be easier and more interesting.

For these long-term cases, we were assigned supervisors, voluntary faculty members, most of whom were psychoanalysts in the community. Ordinarily, these supervisors never saw the patients. It would be awkward to have a supervisor there in the session with the patient. Instead, I would tell the supervisors each week about my sessions, and the supervisors would then give me their opinions. I looked forward to sitting back with experienced psychoanalysts, discussing my meetings with patients, interpreting the meanings of dialogue and dreams. But this system had its potential drawbacks. Supervisors could miss important aspects of the person under our care that we forgot or didn't know to mention; and they could also be very rigid in their application of Freudian theory, which has increasingly been criticized by many both inside and outside of psychiatry for being unscientific and ineffective. Back in medical school, I had once asked a professor if he had any advice for beginning a residency in psychiatry. He offered only one comment: "Lie to your supervisors."

"What do you mean?" I had asked him, perplexed.

"Tell them what you think they want to hear. You can always do what you want with the patient anyway." I had been surprised and puzzled, as that didn't seem very appropriate or scientific. I couldn't imagine why he was saying this and didn't feel inclined to follow his advice. But his remark stayed in the back of my mind.

In addition to supervisors, we had classes on long-term psychotherapy in which we read psychoanalytic articles. Some of these classes were very interesting, but others were highly abstract and theoretical and not very helpful. They focused on different therapy-related areas—one of the most frequently discussed being the importance of fees. Patients attached particular meanings to the bills they received from their psychiatrists, which could be important to address in treatment. But the attention devoted in repeated classes also seemed the result of psychiatrists as professionals wanting to arrange to get paid, and not wanting to feel guilty about it. The value of the service provided—psychodynamic psychotherapy—was controversial. Even the director of the hospital, Dr. Farb, had once told us, "Psychoanalysis is the most labor-intensive practice in all of medicine, the most expensive one in psychiatry, yet the one that has been least shown to be effective."

The first long-term insight-oriented psychotherapy case assigned to me was Isabelle Dupree, a medical student.

She came to my office for the first time right after a long day of classes. She had been sitting in a lecture hall for eight hours, as I once had in medical school as well.

"So what do I talk about in here, anyway?" she asked.

"Whatever comes into your head."

"Just like that?"

"Yes."

She pulled back, and squinched her eyebrows down, surprised. "That's it?" She was short, had a round face and auburn hair, and was simply dressed in jeans, a white T-shirt, and scruffy gray sneakers.

"Yes, that's it."

"Well, I don't feel sick or ill," she said.

"Why are you here?"

"I get nervous in school when I have to speak to my teachers or in front of a class or take exams." She had gotten so anxious in medical school that she had taken a leave of absence last year after a few months and now thought she'd try school again, with therapy to help her. "So how exactly is seeing you going to help me?"

"By helping you understand what makes you anxious."

"Isn't it obvious?"

"Not necessarily."

I had to teach her how to be a patient. This coaching occurred with almost all patients who were in psychotherapy for the first time. We had roles and I had assumed she knew what to do as a result of popular cultural knowledge—novels, movies, TV shows, and magazines depicting psychiatrists—but she didn't and so had to be guided.

My second long-term case was Anita Connors. Another resident had evaluated her and thought she was depressed and would benefit from insight-oriented therapy. Anita was twenty-eight, tall and slender, with long blond hair that dangled down to her waist. She had a slight Boston accent, having grown up there, straight, white, perfect teeth, and cool gray eyes. Her family was Irish Catholic.

The first day I met her she wore black and white tiger-striped glasses, a black skirt, and a purple blouse. She had on a suede jacket with a pattern of two dogs' heads looking at each other: one in black on a white background, and one in white on a black background.

She had been a political science major at Boston College and now worked as a paralegal at a law firm that served as counsel for the hospital. She was therefore eligible for free psychiatric treatment. She lived with her mother and three sisters in a suburb, Mountville, which was outside the hospital's catchment area.

"What brings you here today?"

"My boss."

"What about him?"

"He told me to come."

"Why is that?"

"I had an affair with him. He's one of the junior partners in the firm. I love him. He had said he'd leave his wife for me. But now he won't."

Her problem, dealing with a relationship, sounded similar to those of friends of mine. An acquaintance of mine had also recently had an affair with her boss, and I knew it was a difficult situation from which to extricate oneself since the roles of employee and lover became confused. At last, I thought, here was a higher-functioning patient, someone to whom I could relate more readily and be of help. Many of my friends were also lawyers or had been paralegals, and I had a sense of the high pressure of large corporate law firms, as where Anita worked. I was excited to have her as a patient, relieved not to be dealing with far more severe mental illness. She seemed bright, and her problems were ones with which I could identify. My session with her was a refreshing break from the more oppressive emergency room and medical wards. The pace seemed calmer, the risks less, the stakes not as high.

Because she had been assigned for long-term treatment, we met twice a week. Over the next few weeks, we discussed her situation. She and the junior partner, Joseph Arnaud, had gone out two months earlier, though for less than a month. They had been working late together on a legal brief, had dinner, and then spent the night in a hotel room. It was the first time she had ever slept with a man. He told his wife he had pulled an all-nighter at the office. Over the next few weeks Anita invited him out several times and twice he accepted. But then he decided to end their liaison. The case they had worked on together was completed. She kept suggesting they go out for a drink, but he repeatedly refused. When she wanted to have lunch with him, he also said no. When they were assigned to work together on another brief, he arranged to switch cases. "Every time I see him," she told me now, "even walking down the hall, every time I hear someone mention his name, I cringe."

I asked her about her background and her childhood.

"I don't remember much about growing up."

"What do you recall about it?"

"It was fine."

"Fine?"

"Yes."

"What comes to mind when you think about it?"

"Nothing."

". . . Anything?"

"We used to live in a big apartment in Back Bay with my grandfather, who was ill. Then we moved to Wellesley."

"How was that for you?"

"I told you. Fine."

"What were your parents like?" I was surprised how difficult it was to get her to talk about herself. I had imagined that it would be easier, that patients would be very willing to talk about details of their lives—closer to what's seen in various films.

"My dad wasn't around much. He worked in a downtown Boston bank and was rarely home." I waited for her to elaborate but she said nothing.

"How did you feel about that?"

"My mother basically raised us—my two older sisters and me."

"Did you miss your father?"

"No." Her dad had died a few years ago while on business in Chicago.

Over several weeks I tried to get her to distance herself from her boss, but she saw him in the office and thought about him daily. "Have you considered changing firms?" I asked.

"Of course. But I can't."

"Why not?"

"There's nowhere else to go."

"What do you mean?"

"This firm is very powerful. We get lots of interesting cases. I'd lose everything if I went elsewhere."

"How so?"

250 In a House of Dreams and Glass

She reeled off a list of other law firms. They all did less real estate work, or more corporate work, or were too WASPy or snobby for her, or weren't prestigious enough. They were all either too big or too small. People worked too hard there, or the work wasn't as interesting. They were rumored to be laying people off, or had recently expanded too rapidly and were disorganized as a result.

"It sounds like you really just don't want to move, even though it means continuing to be near Joe."

"If I found the right place I would."

"What else makes it hard for you to move?"

"I just can't find a new place."

"It sounds like you're having trouble giving him up."

"Fuck you." I was amazed at her response. I had hit a nerve.

We continued to speak every week, but she refused to try to leave the firm.

"Why do you think you're so attached to him?" I asked.

"Because I love him and he said he would marry me."

"But you only went out with him a couple of times."

"That doesn't matter."

Even after several weeks, she wasn't interested in reflecting on her responses. "What are you hoping to get out of treatment?" I asked her one day.

"Joe said I should get professional help. So here I am." She crossed her arms.

"I can't help you unless you want to be helped."

"I want to be helped," she said casually, without genuine commitment.

"I wonder if you think Joe will come back to you if you're in psychotherapy."

"You never know."

"But you can't depend on that as a reason to be here."

"I'm not."

"But is that your expectation?"

"He's the one who should go see a shrink—not me!"

"But the point of *your* being here is to try to understand your role in what's happened."

"But he's the one who rejected me."

I just couldn't get her to reflect on what had occurred.

She had never seen a psychiatrist before or doctors much, never having had any medical problems in the past. She was wary.

* * *

The following week we had to change a session. She took her appointment book out of her bag. The book was held in a pink plastic binder decorated with a drawing of a little girl in a blue and white plaid gingham dress carrying a red watering can to sprinkle flowers at her feet. Beside the girl stood a tree and behind her a red wooden barn. The picture seemed out of character for Anita.

"I see there's a drawing on your appointment book," I said.

"Oh, it's just something I have."

"Tell me about it."

She looked at me as if I were nuts. "What's to tell? It's old, and I haven't had time to buy a new one." She shoved it back in her bag.

"How do you feel when you look at it?"

"It's just a lousy picture."

She wasn't engaging much in the treatment. I spoke about the problem to my long-term-therapy supervisor, Dr. Elman.

"She's coming to sessions?" he asked.

"She doesn't miss one."

"And she comes on time, right?"

"Yes."

"That's something," he said. "She pays?"

"She gets free coverage from her firm."

"That's not critical. That she comes is enough. Just continue to see her and let the transference sauté. I once treated a patient—an eight-year-old—who wouldn't engage in the process at all. He wouldn't even talk. One day he started picking threads off the seat cushion and off his clothes—little tiny threads. So I started doing the same, picking off little threads and letting them twirl down, and we got a game going and then he started to talk." He was a child psychiatrist who had recently moved to town. He had never supervised adult patients before but wanted to be affiliated with the hospital and was assigned to be a supervisor. Nonetheless, he was far more experienced than I, and I trusted him as I had been schooled to do. "With your patient," he continued, "just try saying things and see what happens. Float balloons by. Maybe she'll respond to them. You can see."

"It seems you have a hard time talking in here," I said to Anita at our next session.

"I talk."

"But you don't seem interested in standing back and exploring your feelings—for example, about the situation with your boss."

"I tell you all about it."

"Does Joe remind you of other people in your life?"

"No."

"How about your father?"

"No way."

"I'm so fucking mad at him," Anita announced a few weeks later, "I could kill him. And I may do just that. He told me he'd get a divorce and marry me, and now he won't. I gave him my virginity and got nothing in return. I swear I'm going to murder the bastard!" She shook her fist in the air. "I'm going to kill him!" Her pupils narrowed to tight black points in her overcast gray eyes.

"Do you think you could control these impulses?"

"I didn't yesterday."

"What do you mean?"

"I chucked an ashtray at him in his office after hours."

"And . . . ?"

"He ducked. It smashed against the wall and shattered. I'm going to strangle him!"

"I understand you're angry at him. But it doesn't make sense to get violent at work like that."

We continued to discuss her anger at him for several sessions.

"That's it. I'm going to go home and turn on the gas," she told me a few weeks later. Joe had told her never to talk to him again.

"It sounds like you're very angry at him."

"I just feel like killing myself. That's what I'm going to do."

"Do you think you can control those thoughts?"

"No. I've had enough of all this. I swear to God I have. I'm going to murder myself. That'll show him!"

Hospital policy stipulated that for legal reasons, attendings had to see patients whenever there was even a question of suicide or homicide and we weren't hospitalizing the patient—given the cost of lawsuits by families of several patients, not seen, who later killed themselves. But I wasn't sure if Anita fit these critera. Still I decided to phone the attending on call, Dr.

Morowitz, to let him know the situation, just in case. "If that's what she's saying," he said, "then I'd better come down and see her."

She told him she'd calm down.

Anita often was angry or depressed and met some of the criteria for a personality disorder. There are people with whom nobody gets along and about whom everyone says, "He should go see a psychiatrist." That meant me. Dr. Kasdin once said to us, "In neurosis the patient feels miserable, but everyone around him thinks he's doing well. In a personality disorder, the patient thinks there's nothing wrong with him, but everyone around him complains and thinks there is." Anita had a personality disorder. The tumultuousness of her relationships, first with Joe Arnaud and now with me, suggested borderline personality disorder, which I had previously encountered as a diagnosis in Nancy Steele. For outpatients, the treatment usually recommended is psychotherapy, in part because we have nothing else to offer that might be effective. Compared to other psychiatric disorders, personality disorders are less severe by many standards—many patients are able to work, often successfully. Yet treatment of these conditions depends not on a drug but on interactions with a psychotherapist. Unfortunately, psychotherapy is not always very effective.

"I wonder if she's not right for this kind of treatment," I said to Dr. Elman at our next meeting. Though I had initially wanted to engage her in the treatment, she wasn't being amenable.

"Since she isn't benefiting much," I said to him, "what do you think of my perhaps cutting back from meeting with her twice a week, or even considering changing her to supportive therapy?" In supportive therapy, defenses are supported, and the therapist just helps the patient get by. In insight-oriented therapy, based on psychoanalytic principles, the therapist tries to get the patient to gain insight into his or her problems and to develop new, more adaptive defenses instead of supporting defenses already used.

"You may be right, but you have her as a patient now," he answered. "You might as well continue with her and try to deal with her resistance. See what happens. What's to lose?"

I would soon have to divide up some of my long-term therapy cases among new supervisors. Each new supervisor would assist with two cases. I decided to balance the issues and problems posed by my patients. Some patients required more in-depth psychological supervision than others. There were many more intricate issues to understand on some, since I discussed more areas with them. I wanted to pair up the patients evenly, to have about the same number, intensity, and importance of issues to discuss with each new supervisor, and decided to split up Anita Connors and Isabelle Dupree, and have each new supervisor handle one of these two cases and one of my other ones. I met with my first new supervisor, Dr. Roberta Winkler, and told her about Anita Connors and another patient named Meg Reese, presenting each. I mentioned the others, but she said she'd prefer the first two.

A while later I met with my other new supervisor, Dr. Larry Schoen. I discussed my cases, told him my plan, and suggested he supervise me on Dupree and a patient named Tim Kennedy.

He asked to hear more about my other cases.

"No," he said after hearing about them. "I will supervise you on Dupree and Connors."

"But I thought of pairing up Connors and Reese with one supervisor, and Dupree and Kennedy with the other. Plus, I'm thinking of cutting back or even closing the case with Connors."

"I think Dupree and Connors are the patients I can help you with the most."

"But it makes things less balanced with my other supervisor."

"But from what you've told me, *I* am interested in Dupree and Connors." He was in his late fifties, chubby, with horn rim glasses and balding hair, once light brown, now gray. He was a member of the most conservative psychoanalytic institute in the region, strictly Freudian—more Freudian, it was said, than Freud himself.

"But I've already discussed Connors with my other supervisor."

"You've only recently started with your other therapist—I mean supervisor, right?" His slip was interesting, confusing therapist and supervisor. It showed how some faculty members often saw residents as patients, inferior to them in both rank and category. They saw us as nondoctors.

"I discussed it with my other supervisor," I said, "yes."

"Then it shouldn't matter. *I* will supervise you on her."

"But I don't think Connors is good for this kind of treatment. She hasn't benefited much."

"But *I* can help you with her and turn her around. You should be interested in that. Aren't you?"

Though wary, I couldn't say no. Our session was over, and he got up to go. My original plan would have worked better for me, but my supervisors' preferences just didn't coincide. Supervisors were there for my benefit to help me in the work I was doing. But at the time, I didn't want to antagonize them, in part since their evaluations were important career-wise. Later I would realize the gravity of my mistake.

I escaped from my small office to check my mail in the basement. Dr. Roberta Winkler happened to be standing in the lobby. "Say, by the way," I said, "I think I'm going to switch around the patients from the way we first set it up."

"Oh?" She cast me a quizzical eye.

"Yes, I just met with my other supervisor, and *he* wants to supervise me on Dupree and Connors."

"But I thought *I* was going to supervise you on Connors."

"Well, yes. That's what we had said. But I'm trying to fit together what we spoke about with what he wants."

She looked at me with a more distant analytic gaze. "Well," she said, "this will be the first issue that we deal with in *your* supervision." With that, she walked away.

Now I felt like I was off to a bad start with both of my supervisors, but I went along with Schoen's wishes since he remained adamant and was, after all, my attending.

Every week, Dr. Winkler met with me. After six months, which proceeded smoothly without any major incident or much expression of conflict or emotion, she gave me my midyear evaluation. All it said was, "I'm still getting to know Dr. Klitzman. But he had difficulty dividing up his patients for supervision initially." I thought this comment was unrepresentative and unfair, especially since it was her only one.

After a few months, Isabelle Dupree began to think about dropping out of medical school, wanting to do research instead. I sympathized with her frustration: although generally I liked medical school, I found it wearying at points. "I keep having a dream," she said, "of finding myself in some large place like a shopping mall and not fitting in. That's the way I feel in medical school."

"For her to leave medical school and a lucrative career in medicine," Schoen said, "would be crazy. Really crazy. Lunacy. This is real pathology. Get her to talk about her past and her family."

I tried to trace her current problems to her past, as Schoen suggested, and to have her talk about her anger and frustration with medical school, about growing up, and about being here. But she didn't want to talk about other things and kept returning to her anxiety. Recent studies have showed that anxiety can result from biological causes. But Schoen believed that her anxiety was caused by psychodynamic problems. "Just keep raising these issues with her," Schoen said. "Sometimes psychotherapy involves having to hit a patient over the head fifty times with a sledgehammer."

I pressed her and repeatedly tried to trace her current problem to her past.

"What were things like for you growing up?"

"I felt comfortable in my family."

"Yes . . . ?"

"I don't see how that relates to me now."

"It may relate to the problems you're having."

"I don't have a problem; just some anxieties."

"What makes you anxious?"

"Exams."

"What does it feel like for you to take an exam?"

"I am terrified by the possibility of failing."

"These sessions all sound the same," Schoen said. "Flat. Isabelle's putting you in the place of demanding from her, as she feels everyone else does, too. I want you not to talk."

"Not to talk?"

"That's right. Say nothing to her. Be silent. Then whatever she says is a free association that we can interpret."

I tried his technique.

She sat and said nothing. I waited for her to talk. Seconds passed. Then a few minutes. Five minutes . . . ten minutes.

She finally spoke. "Aren't you going to ask me something?"

I said nothing.

"Why are you just looking at me and not saying anything?"

Still I said nothing.

"You used to be more helpful."

"How do you feel when I don't speak?" I finally asked her.

"Shrinks *usually* don't say anything."

I described the session to Schoen the following week. "You said something!" he complained. "You shouldn't have said anything to her at that point."

* * *

"Aren't you going to ask me something?" she asked again at our next meeting. I sat three feet away, facing her in my tiny office, looking at her, saying nothing. "Why aren't you saying anything?" I nodded at her but kept my mouth shut, trying not to appear a complete fool. "Why are you looking at me if you're not going to say anything? This is so unhelpful. I heard shrinks do this—say nothing. But it sucks. Well, I guess we can talk about the exam I have tomorrow. It's a final."

"Ah!" Dr. Schoen declared the following week when I presented the session to him. "See: she made a free association!" That was straining the definition. "Continue not to speak anymore," he reiterated, "and see what she says."

"What's happened to you?" she asked, bewildered, at our next session. "Why don't you say anything? You used to be supportive and helpful, and I liked that. Can't you do that anymore?" She asked me other questions that I just had to sit through without answering. I felt I had to follow Schoen's instructions and give his technique a chance to work. But it's very hard to sit with someone for forty-five minutes and say absolutely nothing when they plead with you to speak and want and need you to talk as they painfully wrestle with stressful problems that they are paying you to help them with. Isabelle became increasingly frustrated that I wasn't talking and, confused, began to say less herself. She started to resent seeing me. She started arriving late, canceling sessions at the slightest excuses, and missing many. Once she came thirty-five minutes late for the forty-five-minute session, because she had decided to go home first to change her shoes and remove her high heels. She started telling me that her boyfriend, a first-year law student, thought her seeing a psychiatrist was silly.

Still, Schoen told me not to speak when she came to sessions.

Psychoanalytic psychotherapy wasn't straightforward or always very effective. Schoen was following psychodynamic principles, yet no one in the hospital, except for Dr. Farb in his one offhand comment, ever discussed the fact that psychoanalysis had never been proven to work and was now being heavily challenged, and often abandoned. Psychoanalysts had often been wrong in the past, using their techniques for various illnesses for which they were later found to have low or no effectiveness. The success rate of psychoanalysis has never been adequately investigated. In fact, many psychoanalysts, now with many fewer patients, are busy relearning how to prescribe drugs.

Schoen's dictum didn't fully make sense in the context of Isabelle's treatment. She was struggling to get through medical school with its grueling rigors and demands, and she sought some support, a chance to allay her anxieties by talking about them and getting some feedback. Schoen didn't want me to give it. In the immediate stress of the first crucial year of medical school, she essentially wanted supportive treatment. Schoen wanted to give her psychodynamic treatment. I was caught in the middle. He was displeased I wasn't giving her what he wanted. She was mad I wasn't giving her what *she* wanted. Schoen and I disagreed fundamentally about the case: first, how "crazy" it was to consider leaving medical school, and second, whether she should be provided the kind of supportive, more interactive therapy she wanted. He wanted me to let her drift in a long process of less tangible "exploration" in which I became more and more silent as she sought more and more from me.

Only later would I hear Dr. Ostrow say that sometimes supervisors aren't right for particular cases and that the chemistry isn't right, though he never defined why, or said how one distinguished issues that needed to be worked on with supervisors from those that indicated that the chemistry indeed simply didn't work. At the time I thought it best not to make waves and to try to resolve the issue on my own. Still, I was seeing that a difficult aspect of becoming a psychiatrist was figuring out how one stood with regard to patients and supervisors, and how much to align oneself with each.

"She's failed the treatment," Schoen concluded a few weeks later. "I don't think she should be in treatment anymore. She's a no-goodnik. I would drop her. Terminate her."

"Treatment might be helpful to her in a more supportive way." I told him that therapy was helping her survive each hurdle of the first year of medical school, which she hadn't been able to do the previous year.

"Well, then you aren't doing the treatment right with her." I knew I was, but that she didn't want this kind of treatment. I had been forcing his approach on her. She was being blamed as a no-goodnik. Then, I was being blamed for not doing the treatment correctly. Schoen felt that he was right and that the patient—whom he had never met—was bad. But he had no direct evidence, and my experience with the patient indicated

otherwise. He acted confident about his psychoanalytic principles. Many friends and acquaintances had told me of bad experiences they had had with psychoanalysts who, after several
years, hadn't helped them very much. I now understood better
how that could happen. It seemed very rigid and unfair of
Schoen, when his approach wasn't working, to blame the patient, and after that, me.

However, I remembered observing this same pattern in
Papua New Guinea when Satuma, the witch doctor, had
blamed patients who failed to improve on his treatment, which
I knew to be ineffective against the kuru virus. Moreover, like
Satuma, Schoen remained confident, though to others looking
on from outside, the treatment wasn't effective. Their views
were different, but the two men had important similarities.
Each operated in a closed system: there was no way someone
inside the witch doctor's world could have known that he was
wrong, no way to disprove him. Satuma cited empirical data—
the fact that some patients got better—that seemed to support
his argument. He also had answers to objections raised against
him. Everything was explained, but was incorrect.

A resident had to be careful politically. Such skills weren't
taught. A resident either had enough savvy to survive the complicated social and political dynamics of a mental hospital or
didn't. Business schools offer lectures, seminars, and courses
on how to manage people and time, and view institutions from
a systems perspective. Residency did not. I was continually
amazed to see how much of what happened with patients
wasn't science but was based on social and essentially political
interactions within the hospital. If this were a law firm or a
corporation, such considerations would be expected to play
prominent roles. But in a psychiatric hospital, following the
model of medical science, I would have expected such factors
to be far less important than they were in fact proving to be.
Sociologists in the 1950s and early 1960s studied psychiatric
hospitals and concluded that group processes, such as issues in
the social hierarchy of the hospital, exerted important roles on
patients' treatments and care. Their scholarly tomes have been
largely forgotten. The research was never once mentioned or
referred to in our courses or supervision. In the hospital's library, the books themselves had been weeded out and relegated
to storage, rather than being left taking up space on the shelf.
Yet what surprised me was how relevant these perspectives remained. Organizational factors continued to play important

roles, not necessarily following the specific patterns found in the past, but present and powerful nonetheless. I wasn't prepared for how political residency in this field was. An introspective turn of mind wasn't enough.

Schoen seemed to be relying on his position of authority, and in response I needed to appeal to a higher figure.

I went to speak to Dr. Morowitz, who coordinated long-term cases, and was affectionately called by residents Dr. M. His door was wide open. As I entered, he stretched his arms out, put his hands behind his head, and leaned back. "Nice tie," he said.

"Thanks. I rarely wear it. An attending once told us never to wear red ties. They may be too stimulating for patients."

"That's ridiculous. I wear red ties all the time." He was also wearing red suspenders and a blue-and-white striped shirt. He was nicknamed Santa and was considered very atypical of the hospital. "What's up?" he asked.

"I'm having some problems with a supervisor on a case."

"Have a seat. Tell me about it." His office was crammed with antiques, a nineteenth-century ceramic model of a human head with phrenology markings of personality traits inked across it, old bookcases with glass-paneled doors, and simple wooden furniture from earlier in the century. I told him about the patient.

"Tough case," he said. "She's difficult, isn't she?"

"Yes."

"Well, try to work it out between you and your supervisor," he said. "But I see there may be a problem here. It sounds, though, like you're doing the right thing with your patients. Just try your best."

I decided to continue to see Isabelle for the moment. Schoen might disagree, and his stubbornness and criticism were getting to me as he attacked my instincts. I felt anxious about it. But continuing the treatment seemed to be in the patient's best interests, and I decided to persevere.

Several of my other cases did well. Tim Kennedy, who had rejected four previous therapists, had stayed in treatment and was dating more and got a promotion at work. Meg Reese had done well, too. But with Isabelle Dupree, I remained caught in the middle, though still trying to help her.

Anita Connors also remained more entrenched than I would have thought. Talking about her problems was not making them go away.

Anita started complaining of feeling more depressed, and having trouble sleeping and low energy. Antidepressants often help patients in psychotherapy, too, and Schoen suggested starting her on one. I prescribed nortriptyline, beginning as usual at a low dose of 10 milligrams per day. When I increased it slowly to 50 milligrams, she said she felt less depressed but began to complain of feeling tired, saying she had trouble staying awake at work. This dose was still comparatively low. She seemed fully alert and awake during my meetings with her. But as she was adamant, I lowered the dose back to 25. Still, she complained of fatigue, and I lowered her dose even further, back to 10 milligrams a day, which she said helped her, and lifted her mood. The dose was the lowest I had ever prescribed on an ongoing basis. Since she occasionally complained of lethargy on this dose as well, I decided to check the blood level, which turned out to be zero.

She kept complaining of tiredness, however, worse than while off the medication. But as she said the drug made her less depressed, she and I decided to continue it. In the meantime she finally found and started a new job at a large corporate law firm that also assisted the hospital legally, but mostly represented financial institutions and worked with securities. For the job she needed to have experience with banking and with several complicated computer software packages, which she told her new employers she knew. Unfortunately, she didn't. She assumed she could learn whatever she had to on the job, but the skills turned out to be too difficult, and she had to ask questions frequently. She also didn't like her boss, a bald man who reminded her of Joe Arnaud. She started arguing with him when he corrected her or asked her to work faster. After three and a half weeks without much improvement, he told her the job wasn't working out and asked her to leave.

"It's on account of your goddamn medication," she berated me. "If it weren't for that drug tiring me out all the time, I could have worked faster."

"But you said the medication made you less depressed."

"It also made me tired all the time."

"But you never seem tired when you're here."

"I'm tired in the morning."

"I've prescribed nortriptyline to many people who take it before they go to bed as you do, and I have never heard that."

"But that's what *I* feel! My body's very sensitive to drugs. I know when it's in my body and interfering with me."

I was skeptical of her claim of fatigue from the drug.

It is easy to say, "Just help the patient." But with borderlines it was often difficult. One had to incur their wrath. Moreover, I felt like I was engaged in combating, not healing her. Her affair with Joe now definitely over, she started getting angrier at me.

"Why not stop her medicine?" Dr. Schoen asked.

"She says it's helping her."

"Does she seem any different?"

"Not significantly."

"Her level is zero. Why prescribe a patient a medication when the level is zero?"

I told her at our next meeting that it didn't make sense for her to be on the drug.

"But I want to take it."

"It doesn't seem to be doing anything, though."

"It is."

"Do you feel less depressed?"

"Yes."

"How is your sleeping?" She sat staring at me, silent. "Well?" She pushed back her long blond hair and glared at me. "How is it?" She sat with her arms laid down firmly on the chair's armrests, refusing to speak. "Are you going to answer the question?"

"No."

"Why not?"

"Because I don't feel like it."

"How come?"

"Because you won't give me what I want. I'm not going to answer you unless you give me the goddamn medication."

"You seem to want to fight with me. I think it's important to try to understand what makes you so angry about this."

"Just give me that damn medication! Don't you dare stop it! That medication is food to me." She refused to think about how she felt. I left her on the medication for the moment.

A few days later, I was finishing a patient write-up due that afternoon when I was interrupted by a rap on my door.

I opened it. Anita stood before me. "I'm here now!" she declared. "Can we start early?" She was standing in the doorway, her feet planted right on the threshold. Her face must have been almost touching the door when she knocked. Our appointment wasn't for thirty minutes.

"We have to wait until the usual time."

"Why?" she asked indignantly, refusing to budge. "I am here now."

"I have some things I have to do first." I had to complete some paperwork. My time was tightly scheduled. She wanted me to operate according to *her* agenda and timetable.

I met with her at our usual time.

When our session was over, I was finished for the day and escaped outside, glad to be done. Cars were running along the street as they always do, and people were walking unperturbed along the hard pebbly sidewalk—all of which somehow reassured me after the stormy fog that filled my head from dealing with Anita.

Now unemployed, Anita complained even more. She remained continually in crisis. Disruptions occurred in her life one after the other, but she avoided focusing on any one issue and wouldn't stand back and look at the overall pattern when I pointed it out to her. She wanted help now and talking about the issues and her past, as Schoen had told me to have her do, didn't feel helpful to her.

People came to me at the times they were their most upset, angry, and depressed—not at their best, most healthy, or well-mannered moments. After all, what else is a therapist for? But this role was far more trying than I had anticipated, especially when left alone, often without much support or even agreement on how to treat these problems.

"You're just a job to her," Dr. Schoen said to me. "Nothing more. She just wants to fight with you." He leaned back in his chair. "I'd terminate her," he said without much concern. He had insisted on supervising her and on my not stopping with her earlier, but now he wanted me to close the case. Suddenly, he didn't want her as a patient anymore. I had been right that psychodynamic, insight-oriented psychotherapy wasn't the appropriate treatment for her. Finally, he agreed with me.

Only now, I was even more involved with her than before, and her life was in more turmoil than earlier: she was unemployed, was now on a psychiatric medication, and was more upset than she had been earlier. "Should we drop her now in the middle of her looking for work?" I asked Schoen.

"Her job search could go on for years. What are you going to do—continue to see her until she has a job? She could quit it or be fired and you'd be in the same boat all over again. At the moment she's not getting much out of therapy—that's the thing that concerns us. Plus, you're finishing the year in a few months anyway and this way you won't have to pass her on to someone else to start with all over again. She's just not psychologically minded," Schoen said.

"What do you mean?"

"She's not able to benefit from psychotherapy." The term seemed tautological. He viewed it as an a priori category. But one's "psychological-mindedness" usually became apparent only after being in psychotherapy, and in the end referred to whether one benefited or not. "Just drop her," he concluded.

Could we just discard patients and forget about them? No one ever said so. Schoen felt he was justified in doing it. But dropping Anita abruptly felt awkward at the present time. She had come to me for help and still seemed troubled. I had long felt she wasn't right for this treatment but wondered whether we had any kind of ethical obligation toward her to put together an appropriate alternative plan, rather than suddenly get rid of her. Does a psychiatrist have any kind of longer-term commitment to his patients, once he's said he'd try to help them?

"She may not want to stop the medication," I said.

"She can be seen much less frequently than twice a week for that."

There was only so much I could do to change someone's personality and how that person interacted in the world. She was sending her résumé around and was busy interviewing for jobs. I hoped she'd find one soon.

"I'm not sure how much you're getting out of treatment," I told her at our next meeting.

"What do you mean?" she asked, insulted.

"The purpose of this is to explore your inner feelings about things, and it's not clear how interested you are in doing that."

"I tell you many things. I've told you all about Joe and me."

"But this kind of treatment is for exploring how you feel about these things."

"Well what about my medication?"

"We can meet less frequently for that."

"But seeing you is very important to me. You're the only person I can talk to about all these issues in my life. I can't talk to my family about them, and I don't really have any friends. Why can't I come if I want to? You're the most important person in helping me get by and survive. I can't believe you're saying all this. What am I going to do if I don't see you? First you don't help me the way I want, and now you tell me you won't help me at all! It's just not fair."

I didn't know what to make of her not wanting to stop. Initially I had wanted to engage her in treatment and she was reluctant. Now I wanted to close the case and found that she wanted to stay. Our roles had reversed. The lines of conflict with a patient clearly could shift radically in the course of treatment—particularly with borderline personality disorder patients, notorious for confusing and manipulating the feelings of therapists. Such patients manage to transfer anxiety and conflict onto the therapist. The patient's pain may decrease, but the therapist's rises. Nancy Steele had given me a sense of these issues on the ward. But now I was the only one dealing directly with Anita. She lived and worked outside the hospital, giving me less control over her environment and making these issues more personally difficult.

Could I drop her if she didn't want to be dropped? At some level, satisfying my desire to get rid of her left me feeling somewhat guilty. She provoked me to want to reject her, yet if I did, I would be acting out of frustration—as well as out of professional concerns—which troubled me.

"She says she wants to come," I told Schoen later. "She seems motivated."

"No she's not. She just wants to torture you and make your life unpleasant. That's not the same thing."

In retrospect, Anita opposed whatever I said. Perhaps it was a mistake that the hospital had given her free treatment. She didn't pay and consequently devalued the therapy and acted entitled to it in some way. Her expectations were that somehow seeing me would get rid of her problem. Unfortunately, she needed to do more of the work in treatment, which was often hard and which she didn't want to do. However, psychiatry didn't have a better treatment to offer.

She quickly received and turned down one or two part-time job offers, wanting full-time work—dragging out the period of uncertainty and turmoil in her life.

She confused me because she wasn't behaving according to what I thought were basic, if unstated, rules of psychotherapy:

that the patient would cooperate and try to get better as much as he or she could. It was also assumed that the patient would tell the truth about how he or she felt. Otherwise, how could therapy function? Sociologists have described a social contract, the doctor-patient relationship, that follows such principles. Both doctor and patient try as hard as they can to work together. Yet Anita wasn't abiding by this arrangement. She wanted me to do my part and help her but didn't want to do her bit and cooperate as much as possible. As a result, I found myself required by my job to try to assist her, but I felt berated at the same time. She generated conflicting emotions in me, making my life painful. My job was to care for her, but I felt angry and taken advantage of. She left me with my head spinning, feeling turned inside out. She'd trap me one way or the other. I felt I couldn't win.

She put me at odds not only with my supervisor but with myself as well, eliciting a tension between my personal and professional responses. Once again, I was left having to fight against myself and my anger—often for my own emotional equilibrium and survival. I felt bad for her, but she also attacked me. She looked and acted toward me in ways I had to understand and separate from my own sense of myself. There are difficult patients in the world and they are often left to residents to treat in psychiatric hospitals. Senior psychiatrists are able to choose patients they want, and more difficult cases are usually under residents' care in hospital clinics and inpatient wards.

At parties or when residents got together after work, a major topic was, invariably, borderlines. Residents complained about these patients more than any others. I remembered asking Mike at one such gathering, "How are you?"

"I have this horrible borderline," he had answered. "She swallowed a bunch of thumbtacks when I wouldn't give her a pass. We had X rays taken every day, and we watched, nervous as hell, as the tacks went down her stomach and into her intestine. It turns out she had wrapped them up in masking tape so she knew she'd be fine. But we were on pins and needles for days. It was horrible. I can't stand borderlines. They drive you crazy." I initially had thought it peculiar and a little unkind that residents would scoff at patients. But I now saw the impetus; treating Anita was difficult and stressful.

We identified only one other group of patients by their diagnosis—schizophrenics—for whom, similarly, only problematic treatments were available. By comparison, there wasn't even a word for the group of patients who had anxiety disorders. "Manics" was almost never used as a term. We wanted to be caring, but borderlines, knowing this, often took advantage of it.

Anita kept fighting with me. It might not have been something that she consciously wanted to do, but it's what she ended up doing and wasn't prepared to stop.

I decided to confront her with the conflict I was feeling. "When you're here you berate me," I told her the following week.

"That's only when you do things wrong."

"But this pattern is important to examine."

She pouted and crossed her arms. "You don't know what you're talking about."

"Yes I do." I had to defend myself at every turn.

The following week she sat down and announced, "If I get a full-time job somewhere else, I won't be able to come twice a week, or maybe I just won't be able to come at all. It's a long way from my home." She spoke as if it were a threat.

"I wonder if your talking about backing out of treatment now is related to my bringing up the topic of termination." She also knew about the system of residents' rotations and that I was finishing the year in a few months. She was aware that if she stayed in treatment she would be starting anew with an incoming resident.

"Maybe I just won't be able to come anymore. That's all," she replied.

"But I wonder how you feel about our seeing each other less or even possibly terminating."

"If I can't come, I can't come." I couldn't get her to talk about how she felt about this issue, though I suspected that she wanted to reject me before I left her. She wanted to quit first.

We had to update Shelly Tarr periodically about our patients' progress. I told her the plan to terminate Anita. While Schoen was a Freudian psychoanalyst, Shelly was an expert in psychopharmacology, specializing in the treatment of anxiety disorders.

"The patient's on an antidepressant, right?" Shelly asked me.

"Yes."

"Then you can't just drop her in the middle of treatment.

You have to make appropriate plans for her—either taper the medication and see how she does or arrange a referral."

"I got a job in West County," Anita said at our next meeting. "I won't be able to come here as often as now. Do you have Saturday hours?"

"No." She knew my week went from Monday to Friday. Psychiatrists, by convention, don't ordinarily see patients on other days.

"How about nighttime appointments?"

"What time were you thinking of?"

"Eight-thirty."

She knew from previous discussions about meeting times that I wouldn't be able to see her then, but she wanted to feel that I was being uncooperative and not accommodating her.

"We'd be meeting only occasionally—for medication, if you're interested in continuing it."

"How often?"

"To start, maybe once every few weeks."

"*Maybe* I can do that for a while," she said. "But I'll have to see."

We started once every three weeks.

"How about Prozac?" she asked at our first such meeting. "I want to be on *that* instead."

"But it has never been completely clear how much the nortriptyline has helped you."

"Maybe you just put me on the wrong drug. Maybe you didn't know what you were doing." Her swiftness to attack irked me.

"I know what I'm doing and thought it might help." I had to fight back.

"Why not give her the Prozac," Shelly suggested, "if that's what she wants?"

"She's not interested in Prozac," Dr. Schoen told me when I met with him later that week. "She's still just interested in pestering you. I wouldn't give it to her."

I told Anita no.

A few weeks later, she said, "I spoke to my internist, who said he'd prescribe Prozac if you call him and tell him to."

Shelly said, "Why not call him if she's asking you to?"

"Shouldn't she see a psychiatrist?"

"If she can't, she can't. What are you going to do?" She shrugged.

"Don't call her internist," Schoen said. "What would you ordinarily do?"

"Recommend a psychiatrist."

"Why do anything differently here?"

"Because she . . ." I paused. "Wants it?"

He shook his head. "No."

"Dr. Tarr said I should call him," I added.

"There's no reason to."

"So are you going to call my internist?" Anita asked at my next session with her.

"No."

"Why not?"

"If you are interested in continuing medication, I think you should see a psychiatrist."

"Why should I pay to see a psychiatrist when my own doctor can write a prescription as well as any goddamn psychiatrist?"

"Because it's a psychiatric medication."

"I can't afford to see two doctors when I can just see one instead."

"You can go to a clinic where the fees won't be high."

"Like where?"

"You could go to West County Hospital."

"Are you kidding me? That snake pit? It's a complete dump. No fucking way." West County was not in as nice a building as our hospital, but it could provide the basic treatment, the medicine she needed.

"There are other clinics."

"The treatment won't be good." She was making things difficult.

"Some clinics provide good service." She was in a clinic now.

"If you won't call my internist, then give me a prescription for a year's worth of nortriptyline."

"I can't do that either."

"Why not?"

"Because if you take it, you need to be monitored."

"Nothing will happen to me."

"You never know."

We had only a few minutes left.

"Let's just deal with the medication for today, just for the moment. Then we can discuss the future again next time. I need to take your blood pressure." I measured it when giving prescriptions since it could drop from the medication, leading to dizziness and dangerous falls. Blood pressure had to be gauged both sitting and standing because it could differ. I took it now, first with her sitting, as usual.

"Okay, stand up please," I said, stepping back to give her room.

"No."

From my ears I removed the rubber earpieces covering the ends of the stethoscope.

"No?"

She sat and crossed her arms and legs tightly.

"I'm not getting up."

"Why not?"

"Because you won't do what I want."

I cursed to myself, feeling like I was dealing with a recalcitrant child.

"I can't give you any medication unless you stand up."

"You do what I want! Do you hear me? If you don't, I'll hit you with a lawsuit!"

"I'm not going to give you the medication if you're not going to take it properly."

"If you don't give it to me, I'll kill you. Do you hear me? I'll kill you," she screamed. Her gray eyes were fixed, cold, and unwavering. I didn't think she would do anything. But I had never had a patient, or anyone else for that matter, threaten to kill me to my face before. Her demands were becoming increasingly absurd and thereby easier to reject.

"Our time is up."

"I'm not going until you give it to me."

"You have to."

"I'm not. I'm going to sit here until you hand me a prescription the way I want it."

"Look, Ms. Connors. I know you're upset. But there are reasons why I'm doing what I'm doing. Anyway, our time is up."

"Tough."

"I understand that what you want—"

"It's not what I want. It's what I need. Without it I'll lose my new job."

"But it's not even clear how much it's helping you."

"I think it is."

"This treatment isn't working."

"That's your fucking fault. Not mine."

"Look. I have another meeting to go to. I'd be happy to talk to you about these issues further another time. In the meantime, I gave you a prescription for two weeks' worth." We had set up another meeting in two weeks. "We can talk about it again next time."

"You'd better do what I say then."

"We can talk about it," I said, wanting her to leave my office before I was even further delayed for my next appointment. Reluctantly, she agreed to go. "I'm thinking of firing you," she said as she left, even though the hospital would undoubtedly not have reassigned her to someone else here. Still, she wanted to threaten me. The meeting had continued an extra twenty-five minutes.

Later, Schoen said, "I would have simply called hospital security and had the guards escort her out."

"She wouldn't have willingly gone."

"Just calling them might have motivated her. Or security might have had to carry her out." Schoen sat with tense lips, never cracking a smile. I felt alone, not fully supported in having to deal with her outbursts and threats. Initially, this was my long-term, "insight-oriented" therapy case that I had wanted to terminate and that he had insisted on supervising, and for which he now advocated the use of physical force.

At the time, her pushiness took energy. At every turn and roadblock she set up, I had to decide how to proceed, and then balance her wrath, Schoen's rigid judgments, and Tarr's distant but equally definitive proclamations. I was caught between all three, the only one in contact with each. Anita must have been feeling a great deal of pain to be inflicting it on me to such an extent. At some level, she was very unhappy. But she wouldn't cooperate with the treatment I was trying to provide. Some patients, like Jimmy Lentz during my first night on call, couldn't cooperate because of their illness. Anita, I believed at the time, could potentially control her outbursts by an act of will if she wanted. But I couldn't get her to bend.

At my next meeting with Anita, I thought of a compromise and said, "If your internist calls me I'd be perfectly willing to speak to him."

"You'd better not tell him about my affair with Joe that

started this whole thing! You only tell him to give me medication."

"I'll make my recommendations as I've told you."

"You'd better be careful what you say!"

No matter what I told him, she might get angry. I decided to obtain a signed consent form as was officially required, giving me permission to speak to someone else about a patient.

"If you want me to speak to him, you need to sign this consent form." I filled out our names and handed the page to her across my desk, setting a blue Bic pen beside it.

"Fuck you," she yelled. She picked up the paper, skimmed it, and then ripped it up, tearing it sideways and then lengthwise into small square shreds that she stuffed in her palm and flung into the air, casting them as wide and high as her arm stretched. They fluttered down, showering like snow all over my entire office, my swivel chair, and me. Then she picked up the pen and hurled it past my head. The plastic smashed, leaving a splash of blue ink on the wall. She leaped up, reached for the door, banged it open, and stormed out, screaming, "I'll never see you again!"

The wind from the door scattered the white confetti along the floor in an eddy.

Why was I doing this? She made me think she wanted help, then turned around and abused me. Professionally, I couldn't say, "Leave me alone." She was in a tantrum with me, like she had been with her boss. But she would never listen to this interpretation.

For a few days I attended a conference in another city. She still occupied my mind, though. While away I had a nightmare of being chased down a dark street. Though asleep, I felt compelled to try to speak. In my dream, I struggled to open my mouth and groaned, "Ahhh," just to hear the sound of my voice, to prove to myself that I could still speak out, and wasn't wholly helpless. I woke up shaken. I didn't remember ever speaking in my sleep before. I felt tortured, threatened, but unsure what else could be done. Roy and others always warned us about borderline patients: "Just don't let them get under your skin." Still, I was surprised that she had. I called Mike, who was covering for me.

"Anita Connors may call you for more medication or another prescription," I told him. "But she has enough until I get back." She had made a point of writing down his name and number.

"Don't worry," Mike said. "I'll take care of it."

She never called him.

"I'm surprised she hasn't made your life more miserable," Dr. Schoen said on my return. I was surprised he didn't see that she had. At the time, I was afraid to tell him just how much she disturbed me and the fact that I had had a nightmare related to her. I feared he'd think me inappropriate or unable to handle this case.

"I think it's because I rolled out the big guns in the beginning," I said, "and had Dr. Morowitz see her."

Dr. Schoen sat there, distant, nonchalant, calm, intellectually speculating about her, while she caused me grief. "It's only a job," I told myself, but I was still vexed.

When I met her again, she said she was being moved to a different department at her law firm, and her schedule would change and become tighter. The job was keeping her busy, but she liked the work. In any case, she would no longer be able to come to see me. We scheduled our last three sessions.

She missed the first of these.

The following week, she left a message to cancel our four o'clock appointment, which would have been our second-to-last meeting. The brusqueness of her action surprised me. I felt somewhat dismissed by her, but I also heaved a sigh of relief. An extra hour was now free—forty-five minutes plus ten minutes for writing up notes from the session. But at four o'clock the front desk paged me. "Miss Connors is on the phone," Gina told me. "She says it's an emergency."

"Okay—put the call through."

"I just want you to know that I can't get out of bed today," she said. "I'm depressed and not feeling well. I can't believe you said I can't be on the medication anymore."

"I didn't say that. I recommended you see a psychiatrist."

"That's all I need! I'm so depressed I could kill myself. Is this what you goddamn doctors are paid to do?"

"If you want to come in and talk about these issues, we can."

"I'm too depressed to come in." She yelled at me further on the phone. I tried hanging up, but the call took thirty minutes in all, two-thirds of our appointment time. I felt abused. She didn't sound depressed as much as agitated. Certainly she was unhappy. But she still wanted her problems automatically solved by me and wouldn't acknowledge or cooperate with the terms of the treatment.

I now had one last appointment scheduled with her.

She arrived twenty minutes late for the forty-five-minute session. After over a year, this was to be the last time we would ever see each other.

"Well?" she demanded as she sat down. "Did you call my internist?"

"I didn't say I would."

"You have to call my internist and speak to him," she said.

"If he wants to talk to me, he can call me." I tried to change the subject and ask her about how she was doing and how she felt about our meeting for the last time.

"Things are the same. I went out on a date with another paralegal," she said hurriedly. "So you won't call my internist?"

"What for?"

"To tell him to prescribe the medication."

"No. If he wants to, he can, but I do not recommend it. Our time is up in a few minutes," I added, "but I want to wish you the best of luck."

"Then call my internist."

"As we discussed before, I cannot. If he wants to call me, I'm willing to speak to him."

"You doctors. You're all a bunch of assholes!"

She got up, collected her belongings, and stepped toward the door to exit. I stood up as well and faced her.

She hadn't thanked me for our time working together, or wavered in her sheer insistence that I had failed to give her what she wanted. Nor had she acknowledged that she hadn't cooperated.

I had thought that by now things would somehow resolve themselves, that as in novels and movies, there would somehow be a neat ending. She would come around; I'd be able to bring closure to the situation; she'd realize that she had acted inappropriately and at least apologize, which even Nancy Steele had done; or some larger cause would become apparent as to why the case had been so trying. But none of these occurred. She continued to feel cheated and angry. Dr. M. later told me, "You have to accept that patients may be enraged when they leave sessions or terminate."

Clearly, psychiatric issues were not always readily resolvable, resulting in good endings. The rest of medicine had made me used to resolution, but mental illness was far more ambiguous. In medicine, patients and their families routinely were grateful for my efforts. But psychiatry was different. "She wants to keep you on the hot seat," Dr. Schoen had once commented. She might not have been conscious of this desire, but this was the effect she achieved. She transferred onto me the distress that she couldn't deal with herself.

In some ways, what was happening with her made sense. She wanted more than I could give her and wouldn't accept what I offered. In the end, she was about to leave me before I would have to leave her at the close of the year. After Joe Arnaud, she wouldn't allow herself to be rejected again. She had decided to save face, and maintain her pride. She had chosen to pursue her freedom and end treatment when she wanted, but as a result wouldn't improve further. Intimacy no doubt frightened her. She now had to try to reject and destroy whomever she got close to, rather than let down her guard.

I suspected that at some level she knew that treatment had helped her. Except for the last three sessions, she never missed an appointment or came late. She often looked relieved when she arrived. Occasionally a smile slipped out. She had often seemed glad to see me, though she never admitted that or acknowledged what I meant to her.

Moreover, in our time together the treatment had some accomplishments. She had ended a relationship with the junior partner that had caused her pain, hadn't physically harmed herself or him, and had started dating again. She had changed jobs, finding and starting a promising new one at a different law firm, and was settling in there. She had tried psychotherapy and pharmacotherapy to see what they might do for her.

But she acted unsatisfied with these changes. Some might say the treatment was a success: she hadn't gotten any worse, and I had seen her through a difficult period. Perhaps over a few years, if she had been motivated to stay, she might have made further progress in these areas. But the brutal fact was that success in psychotherapy was often elusive or only partial. Progress could be painful and slow.

I had also learned from the experience certain lessons that might help me with future patients. My job wasn't always personally gratifying, but it was part of my continuing education and would allow me to go on and assist other cases further. Anita had taught me a lot about personality disorders—to be on my guard and not get too emotionally involved.

I had had to alter my expectations concerning treatment. Though realistically the field can't remedy everything, patients all come wanting to be helped, and psychiatrists act, at least initially, as if they can alleviate almost anyone's mental problems. "Your primary goal in psychotherapy should be understanding the patient, not changing or curing them," Dr. Ostrow had once said. He had even recommended conducting one therapy in which all we would do would be to get a detailed history of the patient. I wasn't sure if that was to help us or the patient. Now I grasped why his expectations were only to understand the patient—because often, that was all we could do. To hope for too much could leave both patient and psychiatrist frustrated.

Psychiatrists believe that helping patients understand themselves will alleviate symptoms. Unfortunately, the approach doesn't always work as hoped. From my experience with Anita I was learning to take a professional stance: there were patients like this, and I would try to help them. They might remain troubled, but I would continue on, and if one case didn't work well, go on to the next one, anyway.

A patient's improvement could also cost me a small bit of my own equanimity. The rest of Anita's life had gotten better, but she had channeled her rage at me. She didn't want to feel I had helped her. I learned that patients can be assisted but would sometimes take me through fire and brimstone in the process. This case left me feeling stunned and angry, my nerves raw, with nowhere to vent my frustration except in my own psychotherapy.

It is difficult to write about this case, as it wasn't more of a success. I fear opening myself up to criticism. But these cases occur. Psychiatrists are often accused of being somewhat distant or of being ineffective. As professionals, we generally try our best but unfortunately can't always succeed. I could attempt to forget these events and pretend they didn't happen, but they illustrate issues that are important to understand.

Psychotherapy, though touted in our society as a veritable

cure-all, doesn't always work well. Some patients don't accept the way it operates, and it may just frustrate them more by making them hungry for a solution.

How did most psychiatrists deal with these issues? What does the profession do with patients who don't do well? I saw how psychiatrists blamed patients for "failing the treatment," calling them "resistant" or accusing them of not being "psychologically minded." Psychiatrists also distanced themselves. In my conversations with Schoen, he had begun to act indifferent toward Anita, at first implicitly and then explicitly rejecting her. I saw some psychiatrists, rather than admit that anything might be wrong with their theory, framing of the problem, or attempts at solution, conveniently interpret their failures as their patients' fault.

Psychiatrists pursued psychotherapy themselves, partly to deal with these issues. We then occupied the position with our therapists that our patients did with us. Treatment helped us to understand that we were not as inadequate as patients implied, and we passed on frustration with the field's limitations to senior psychiatrists, who believed that psychotherapy could work if only we understood aspects of our own reactions better. We told ourselves that patients' anger didn't reflect any failing of us as professionals or anything about us as people but was merely patients' transference, to be analyzed.

Conducting psychoanalytic psychotherapy disappointed me in some ways. It was painful and difficult being insulted, being put in a position at odds with my supervisor—all symptoms of the patient's diagnosis of borderline personality disorder. Even senior psychiatrists had trouble with borderlines. Dr. M. later told me, "I never schedule two borderlines back to back." I now felt that outpatient psychotherapy was not how I wanted to spend the majority of my professional life. It was far more draining than it seemed, and there were other areas to devote my energies to instead, even if they didn't pay as well. Initially, I thought that my career would focus on psychodynamic treatments and that other approaches and activities in the field would engage me less. But I was changing my mind. I would still continue to practice some psychotherapy and when it was successful, would appreciate it all the more. But I had also seen that all was not fair in love and war, and in the combination of the two known as psychotherapy.

Suddenly, the picture on Anita's yellow appointment book of

a young, innocent girl made sense. She was in many ways a little girl, lost in an adult world she couldn't understand. She was screaming for help, yet was disappointed with the assistance she got, invariably unable to give her the simple purity and innocence she sought.

When Anita was about to leave my office for the last time, thoughts along these lines passed through my mind. She stood before the door, ready to exit for the last time. "Goodbye," I said, offering her my hand to shake.

"Bye," she repeated bluntly but without lifting up her hand from her side.

My hand remained outstretched. I didn't retreat. Only with hesitation did she reach up and shake it—cursorily—before whipping around on her heels and exiting.

I never saw her again.

I was glad to have the extra time free. A weight had been lifted from my shoulders. I felt like a rubber ball that had been squeezed and dented, and was now released and was slowly expanding back to its earlier size. Over the remaining weeks, I used the extra time to work on a research project I started, allowing me to read important background material and learn research skills that would help me in my future work. Also, in the now long late-spring afternoons, I occasionally took work home with me and left the hospital a little earlier to go jogging first.

I never found out what happened with Anita. I hope she is doing well, but suspect that until she can better understand her feelings and need for others, she'll never fully be at peace. I had tried to make her understand that feeling close to others and even dependent on them shouldn't be humiliating or threatening to her. But she wouldn't accept these notions. In the end we went our separate ways. We each did what we had to do. Still, I often find myself thinking of her and wish that wherever she is, she's okay.

I was continuing to treat my other patient, Isabelle Dupree, who was surviving the first year of medical school. But Schoen wanted me to drop her as well after I finished the year. He now wanted me to get rid of both the patients on whom he had supervised me. Near the end of my time with him, he gave me my evaluation. "You didn't treat Dupree properly," he said.

"I've tried to be sensitive to her needs."

"You didn't just say nothing enough as I suggested."

"I tried, but it didn't work."

"You listened too much to the patient's words."

"Yes?" It wasn't clear what was wrong with that approach.

"Try to focus on ... ah ... ah ... what she hasn't said."

"I tried that, but it didn't lead anywhere." He thought there would be a key, a magic statement or approach that when uttered by me would radically alter the case and the stresses she faced. But there was not. Schoen's working assumption was that therapy was a strict science with clear right and wrong ways to do things. Yet others would disagree with him and argue that therapy was also an art.

"We can agree to disagree," Dr. Schoen said. He wasn't going to back down. "And I think you should drop her from the clinic, and not pass her on to another resident." I felt, though, that therapy had helped her get through the year, despite his criticisms.

His lack of compassion crushed any humanity and humanism out of the work. His rigid theories, his belief that he was right and I was wrong—though he had never met the patients—all felt absurd.

It didn't feel right dropping her. Deep down I knew that treatment could benefit her. "I think it would help if you met her yourself and saw," I suggested.

"Well, I don't know if I have time for that. I can only come here a few hours on Wednesdays," the day of grand rounds, when he was required to be here anyway. In fact, the hospital mandated that supervisors come on another day as well, which he didn't do.

"I'll see if she can come then," I said. He agreed. "It's a complicated case," I added.

"All cases are complicated. You just didn't follow what I said."

Dr. Roberta Winkler gave me a glowing evaluation, based on my handling of my other patients.

Dr. M. said about Schoen's evaluation, "Don't worry about it. Sometimes the chemistry between a resident and a supervisor isn't right. It happens."

My own therapist, himself a supervisor at the hospital, said,

"You had a bad supervisory experience. Big deal. It sounds like a mosquito bite."

Dr. Schoen came to meet Isabelle Dupree. "I feel very strongly," she said, "that medical school has been very painful for me. I don't feel comfortable there. My life has been hard. It hasn't been easy. In my family, things were safe, comfortable. Outside, the world is full of snakes. I feel out of place, threatened, like I don't fit in. Constantly. Even in here, with you, Dr. Klitzman, though it's been better lately. I've told you about my recurring dream of being in a shopping mall. I'm not sure medical school is the right thing for me. First year has been extremely stressful for me and I'm not sure it's worth it in the end."

"What did you think?" I asked Dr. Schoen afterward.

"What do *you* think?" he quickly asked me back.

"I think therapy's been difficult for her. She's not without ambivalence, but she can potentially gain from it."

He nodded, then suddenly glanced at his watch. "Oh, I see I have to run."

"Any other thoughts about the meeting?" I asked him.

"Very poignant," he said tersely. He then walked out of the room, saying nothing else about the interview.

He called a few days later. "I have to cancel our supervision this week," he said. "I might be able to meet with you later in the week. If not we'll meet next week."

But he canceled the next appointment as well, which would have been our last. I never met with him again and never had a chance to find out what else he thought about the patient other than the two words he had uttered at the end of our meeting. I felt that his two cancellations were an admission that he didn't know *what* to think now, that the case was much more complicated than he had argued or imagined, and that he had been wrong in thinking I hadn't handled the case right. The "very poignant" quality of the patient overturned his belief that the patient was "flat" and incapable of psychotherapy, and that I was wrong to try to engage her. In short, the mere fact of the patient's poignancy suggested that Dr. Schoen—not I—had missed much of the case. His cancellation of our last two sessions—virtually unheard of among psychotherapists, who are quick to interpret such behavior—prevented us from ever discussing the case again, and tacitly indicated and perhaps implicitly acknowledged his guilt.

Those who most talked about and professed the importance of feelings—the psychoanalysts—were often the coldest and least feeling toward their patients and supervisees. They might analyze their own feelings, but they often didn't acknowledge or support them in others.

Isabelle continued in treatment. I referred her to a resident beginning her third year, Jane Pomeroy.

Isabelle did well and eventually completed medical school, helped by therapy.

If Anita disillusioned me about psychotherapy, Isabelle showed me how important the work could potentially be.

But the experiences left a bitter taste in my mouth. I had nowhere to respond to Schoen's unfair and inaccurate statements. He had run before he would have had to apologize for, revise, or amend his assessment of the case and his inaccuracies (and, though less important, the evaluation he had written), or even discuss the case and the issues involved. I felt haunted by the experience, caught in between, and saw how difficult and personally painful being a psychiatrist could be, particularly if questioning a supervisor.

Afterward, Anne said, "I've learned to have my supervisors meet my patients right in the beginning. That way, the supervisor gets a better understanding of the patient." I was wary of asking a supervisor to see a patient, thinking it suggested an inability to handle problems alone.

A few weeks later, after graduating, a resident one year behind me, who also had Dr. Schoen as a supervisor said, "He's your typical, cold, wooden, inhuman analyst. I almost fired him. We just didn't get along."

I felt Dr. Schoen was wrong on both of my cases. Yet I had learned critical lessons. Psychotherapy and supervision were complicated arts, with pitfalls and logic of their own, and didn't always proceed in the expected ways.

Differences of opinion about patients were often wide. I expected flexibility in psychotherapy but, finding sharp disagreements, was often forced to take strong positions with supervisors and patients.

Again I saw the importance of following my own instincts with patients, particularly those I knew best, by standing up for what I felt was right and doing what made the most sense, not necessarily relying on others' theories. I now understood what had motivated my medical school professor's advice about lying to supervisors. I hadn't followed his suggestion and had gotten caught in the middle.

I saw Dr. Schoen only once again. Several months after finishing residency, I was waiting at a bus stop. He was crossing the street carrying a pile of dress shirts to bring to the dry cleaners.

I spotted him first and didn't shift my gaze. "Hello," he said curtly.

"Hello," I said broadly, stepping toward him, leaving the bus stop to greet him and shake his hand. But he didn't stop. He swiftly hopped up the curb onto the sidewalk and kept striding, his hand hiding beneath the pile of shirts, not deigning to reach toward me. He tightened the corners of his mouth in an icy grin, which he dropped as he passed. His face then hardened as dark, heavy lines on either side of his mouth fell from the corners of his lips. He hurried on. I watched him as he disappeared down the block. He never turned around.

Harmony

During each year of residency, we had only one opportunity to criticize or comment on the faculty or administration in public—and that only by using humor. Otherwise we had to keep our grievances and complaints to ourselves. Every year the residents staged an annual Christmas Show. The show was part of the annual departmental Christmas party that residents were responsible for organizing.

"How typical," Sarah said, "that the residents put together the Christmas party for the faculty and administration, rather than them putting it on for us." The residents had to finance the party, charge admission, haggle with caterers, reserve a space, rent stage lights, speakers, and microphones, and buy props. Attendings balked at the price of tickets that paid for the show and the dinner that followed. Every year a few supervisors refused to pay. In contrast, the Department of Medicine paid for a black tie dinner for all medical residents every Christmas season. In psychiatry, some faculty, such as Shelly Tarr, never bothered to attend the Christmas party, though they had once been residents themselves and presumably involved in such an event. Shelly seemed to think the comic show too frivolous, a waste of time.

In the early fall, residents began seizing upon anything funny that happened at the hospital. "That would be great for the Christmas Show," we eagerly told one another. Everyone called it "The Christmas Show," though most of the residents and faculty were Jewish. There was a "Holiday Bazaar"—a fund-raising sale arranged by the OT department and put on by the patients, very few of whom were Jewish. Patients sold arts and crafts they had made and held an auction of prizes donated by neighborhood businesses.

Three years before, the residents, disgruntled with the residency program, had decided not to hold a Christmas party. The residents complained that they felt alone and unsupported. As a result, the administration had introduced more changes than ever before or since. Meetings at 9:30 were instituted every other Thursday with Dr. Farb or Dr. Peter Robins, the director of education, as a way for residents to air and discuss problems.

Last year, Lou Leftow, who wanted to be chief resident this year, had sung a song devoted exclusively to the chairman. He sang to the tune of "Sir Joseph's Song" in Gilbert and Sullivan's *H.M.S. Pinafore:* "He analyzed so carefully that he became the chairman of the faculty . . ." Lou had two backup singers, and in three-part harmony they suggested that Dr. Farb was narcissistic and controlling. Lou had a beautiful tenor voice. The whole audience laughed and applauded. One could say anything one wanted—criticisms one could never utter directly—provided it rhymed and was in three-part harmony. Dr. Farb was a brilliant man and any hospital director, having to implement decisions that are often unpopular, could easily be criticized.

A few weeks later it was announced that Lou had been chosen as chief resident.

To plan the show we began meeting at Anne's apartment.

"Ideas?" Anne asked. Each year the show consisted of a series of skits, spoofs on the faculty and on the hospital.

"Why don't we make Dr. Kasdin Muammar Qaddafi?" Sarah suggested.

"Or we can do psychiatry through the ages," Mike said, "and have medieval psychiatry, and Spanish Inquisition psychiatry, with Kasdin as the psychiatrist."

I was astounded to hear other residents' biting criticisms and frustrations that until now we had each kept mostly to ourselves or discussed only with the other residents with whom we felt closest. We all now sat at Anne's, making jokes about the faculty and laughing together as we had never done before as we munched on chips and drank beer. It was the closest that we had worked together outside the hospital and the most fun we had had as a group. The meetings were excuses for parties as we wrote a script.

Only a few of us volunteered to act. Many residents were too shy. Several male residents volunteered to do technical work on the lights or build the sets.

"Who wants to be in charge of the booze?" Mike asked.

"Do we have to have booze?" Anne asked.

"Are you kidding?" Mike said. "The most important part is making sure all the attendings have a few drinks beforehand."

A dress rehearsal was held the day before the party. The band consisted of a hodgepodge of residents who played musical instruments—one guitar, one overly elaborate drum set, and three flutists. One woman sang in an operatic voice. The flutists drowned her out.

"Shouldn't we maybe have just one flute?" I asked Anne, pulling her aside.

"It's a long story. Don't ask. It's *very* political."

"How are you, Dr. Klitzman?"

I was standing at the cocktail party. "Hello, Dr. Swire." He was a senior analyst, one of the attendings on the fourteenth floor. He called all of the residents "Doctor," seemingly out of respect. In fact, it forced us all to call him "Dr. Swire"—we couldn't very well call him by his first name in return—promoting a strained formality between the residents and him.

Sarah sang a folk song, as another resident accompanied her on the guitar.

Mike acted in a skit as the DOC. Six plastic toy telephones—bright red, yellow, green, blue, orange, and pink—crowded a small grade-school desk. Ding-a-ling, one rang.

He picked it up. "This is the doctor-on-call. May I help you?"

Ding-a-ling-a-ling, another phone rang.

"One moment," he said to the caller as he picked up the next receiver, which was ringing. "Doctor-on-call. What? You're home and about to kill yourself? . . ."

Another phone rang. Ding-a-ling-a-ling.

"Hold on one moment please, my other phone is ringing . . ."

"Doctor-on-call . . . No, we have no beds available for transfer . . ."

Ding-a-ling-a-ling. He was holding three receivers in his hand, all midconversation.

Ding-a-ling-a-ling . . . Ding-a-ling-a-ling . . . Two more phones were ringing simultaneously now, which he picked up and added to the pile in his hand. Another phone rang.

In the end, he swept all the phones off his desk, leaped up, and stormed away.

The audience laughed and cheered.

The skits moved on to the events of the final year.

Sarah was in the ER. Patients were lined up waiting. Joe had volunteered to play a drug abuser coming to the ER to get drugs. He dressed in silver reflecting sunglasses, a leather jacket, and metal chains looped around his neck and off his shoulder like a sash, while smoking a cigarette.

Another resident had dyed her hair blue and green and wore purple glasses. Sarah walked up to her.

"Hello. I'm Sarah Gould. How can I help you?"

"I'm borderline and I want to be admitted to your hospital. For life." She filed her nails as she spoke.

"But I don't think you need to be here."

"If you don't admit me, I'll go out and kill myself."

"Don't kill yourself."

"Then let me in."

"No. But please don't kill yourself."

"I'm going to."

"Oh no. Please. Please don't do it." Sarah got down on her hands and knees. "I beg of you, don't."

"Maybe I'll just cut my wrists."

"Oh no, no. I'll do anything, anything. Only please don't do that. I'll get blamed." The passion with which the skit was staged, and the heartfelt laughter with which the audience responded, showed that I was hardly alone in having concerns about these patients.

"Or maybe I'll shoot myself." She took out a gun and bumped the barrel against her temple, ready to pull the trigger.

"No. No."

She shot the gun.

The child psychiatric residents sat on the floor imitating the child psychiatric faculty as children. Dr. Berman was shown in lederhosen and a bow tie. Sarah imitated one of the female faculty members and wore a short frilly dress. They played with toys but started fighting over them. Dr. Berman, as the male, and now the director of the program, hoarded all the toys from the girls.

One skit depicted consultation-liaison psychiatry. "Here's the patient, Dr. Danziger," Jessica, a resident, said. A body lay on a stretcher under a sheet.

"Mr. Jones?" the resident said to the patient. "Mr. Jones?" Jessica shook the patient lightly, then said, "He's dead! He must have died overnight. What a shame. Well, let me see," she said consulting her clipboard, "if there are any other patients we can talk to."

"No," Dr. Danziger said, "that's okay. We can talk to this patient anyway. It's useful to learn how to speak to as many different types of patients as possible."

"But Dr. Danziger—"

"I'm Dr. Danziger," he started, addressing the patient, undaunted.

"But he's not going to respond!"

"If a patient doesn't respond, it's always important to address why. It could be resistance that's important to analyze and comment on.

"It seems to me that you're not responding. Am I correct?"

In another skit, one attending was shown always falling asleep during rounds.

We worked very hard to have the faculty enjoy the show, as

if, even as we satirized them, we wanted to please them and earn their praise.

The faculty all said this was the best Christmas show yet. Every year they said that. We didn't think that was the case, and I doubted that the shows were improving. Rather, it seemed that their memories of past ones faded and they were struck afresh each year by the talent they saw.

PART V

Green

At last, having survived through all these rotations and experiences, I was about to change my position in the hospital. The first change was the choice of a selective.

Not until the final year did we have elective time, which we would be able to use to chart a course for ourselves within the profession. We were encouraged to choose a project that interested us and apply for selectives. We would propose an elective—such as a particular research study or particular administrative or clinical rotation—and Dr. Robins would approve some of our projects, granting or denying us the time to do them. We were told to choose what we wanted to study. "Doing research is hard." Dr. Desmond, one of the instructors in our research course, said. "It always takes twice as long to do half as much as you thought you would get done. Therefore, I very strongly encourage you to choose what will really interest and engage you the most, to get you through the difficult times."

I chose to study social issues in psychiatry. After reading a book by Susan Sontag, I was inspired to develop a research project conducting descriptive, in-depth interviews to study the range of people's attitudes toward HIV infection, exploring beliefs, metaphors, and meanings of the illness. I was excited about the project, which would connect psychiatry with social issues such as stigma and cultural responses to plague. Other residents sought areas in which to do research, from psychobiology to psychoanalysis, child psychiatry, substance abuse, and schizophrenia.

"What's your selective going to be?" Dr. Robins asked me when I went to speak to him about something else. I told him.

"But what are you going to measure?" he asked.

"Measure?"

"You have to measure something."

"But sociological research is often descriptive, not quantitative."

"Well, what are you going to measure then?" He, who as a psychoanalyst had never done any quantitative research or measured anything scientific in his entire professional career, was insisting that trainees measure something rather than be able to do work that was descriptive, as all of his had been.

I was concerned and spoke to Dr. Desmond, who reassured me. "I'm on the research selection committee," he told me. "And I like what you're proposing and others on the committee will, too."

It turned out that only those residents whose projects measured something and conformed to the interests of a handful of prominent faculty members had their selectives approved. Projects that were more innovative—studying psychiatric education, using video, or investigating cultural or social issues or AIDS—were almost all refused full-time support. Though initially we had been told that we were doing the selecting in deciding our projects, in the end it was the faculty who chose which of us would have our projects approved and be given time to do them.

I went back to Dr. Desmond, who said, "In the end Dr. Robins made all the decisions."

I then went back to Dr. Robins, who claimed, "I didn't make the decisions; the committee did."

"But that's not what I understood from Dr. Desmond."

"No, the committee gave me a list of names they had compiled." I was confused.

In the end, I was given half time for a selective. Some residents got no time, others full time.

Still, in choosing our projects we found ways of becoming more knowledgeable in particular areas within the profession and integrating ourselves into the field further.

Another change occurred in my final year of residency: I was given administrative responsibility. As a medical student and as a junior resident, I had been the low man on the totem pole in the hospital hierarchy. In that capacity, I had rotated through the full spectrum of situations in which psychiatry is practiced—from inpatients to outpatients to consultation-liaison on medical wards, and from adults to children.

I would now be returning to inpatient wards where I had started. Only now I would be supervising other staff and residents, helping to run a ward as Greg and Roy had when I was a second-year resident. The tables would now be turned.

I had been wary of the politics of the institution and the importance of power in clinical care—the fact that much of psychiatry involved the use of authority. But I would now have administrative authority myself and wondered how I would perform this role, having to change my position and sense of myself as a psychiatrist yet again.

I was assigned to be an assistant unit chief on the sixteenth floor.

"Are you going to run community meeting?" the head nurse, Valerie Henders, asked me on my first morning there. The unit chief, Dr. Eliot Higgens, was a psychobiologist and was not very interested in the social interactions on the ward. He never attended community meetings and left it up to me if I attended them or not or ran them. How could it be a community meeting, however, if the most powerful part of the community—the doctors—weren't even there?

"Yes," I said. "I will run them." The first community meeting was scheduled right after Monday morning rounds.

At the meeting, I introduced myself and Todd Spitzer, a fourth-year resident, as well, who was starting as a therapist on the floor. He would have clinical responsibilities while I would handle administrative tasks. He was a tall Chicagoan with whom I hadn't worked before.

I welcomed new patients and said goodbye to old ones. "Is there a patient agenda?" I asked.

"The toilet in my bathroom doesn't work," one patient, an older man, said. "There's no seat. How are you supposed to use a toilet if there's no seat?"

I wasn't sure what to say and turned to Valerie beside me. Her brown curls and large glasses obscured her eyes. She avoided looking at me and said nothing.

Another patient, a younger man, spoke up. "At least you have your own bathroom in your room. *We* have to share."

The nurses remained quiet.

These weren't the issues I had anticipated being responsible for.

Afterward, in the post-community meeting, I asked the nurses why none of them spoke up.

"Did you want us to talk?" Valerie asked. "We didn't know if you wanted us to speak or not."

"Of course," I said. "You've known these patients far longer than I have, in some cases almost a year. You should feel free to speak. I'm sure you have ways of running this meeting, as well."

"We don't. It's up to the assistant unit chief. And you didn't say anything about it." I suddenly realized that I was in charge of some things and had discretion, but was also alone at the top.

"How have you worked it in the past?"

"We talk. But we didn't know if you wanted us to." I had never heard of a community meeting where nursing staff didn't talk.

Many of the patients were treated by junior faculty who didn't carry beepers. If an emergency came up with one of these patients, the nurses would try telephoning the therapist. But if the junior attending wasn't sitting in his office, he could not be reached. The nurses had repeatedly requested that these therapists carry beepers and had always been refused.

"You carry the beeper for us," I was told by one of these junior attendings, who had just finished his own residency.

Yet it seemed to me that they, as the patients' primary therapists, should be responsible for the problems that arose with their patients. I had my own beeper and was available for emergencies as well, if needed, in any case. But the therapists knew their own patients best. I spoke with the chief resident and the senior faculty, who agreed with me. But the junior attendings still categorically refused.

One of them, Dr. David Katz, even threatened me. "I don't know what your plans are for after your residency, but if you want to stay on at this hospital, you'd better carry that beeper!"

"But Dr. Gillis," the director of administration in the hospital, "said that it was your responsibility to carry the beeper."

"No he didn't," Katz told me. "I spoke with him myself and you're wrong."

"But he did. I just spoke with him." I rechecked with Dr. Gillis, who confirmed what he had said to me previously and told me that if I *wanted* to, I could volunteer to carry their beeper, but that it was their responsibility, not mine.

In all this discussion, which felt like high diplomacy, I was astonished that these attendings weren't interested in being available for their patients. These therapists obviously knew their patients best, and care rendered by a covering physician in an emergency can easily be less optimal than that rendered by a patient's primary therapist. The question of why these therapists weren't interested in knowing about problems that arose with their patients was not mentioned in this debate. In the end, I had Gillis himself phone the junior attendings, who reluctantly agreed to carry the beeper. The nurses were enormously grateful, as they were now able to contact patients' doctors when emergencies arose. I was pleased the system had gone into place and knew it was best for the patients, but I was shocked at the degree to which political negotiations played a role in a mental hospital and was exhausted by all the effort.

At the following year's Christmas Show, David Katz and the other attendings were shown strolling off for the day at noon to play tennis, practicing their forehand swings and abandoning their patients on the ward for the rest of the day.

Each day on the ward, I led morning rounds.

"Miranda Glebe and Charles Zimmerman were found together in her room on her bed," Valerie announced on my second Monday morning.

"I'll make an announcement about the unit policy in community meeting," I said.

"What is the unit policy?" Cathy, one of the nurses, asked.

"There's to be no physical contact on the ward," Todd, the other resident, said.

"What about kissing someone hello or goodbye?" Mark, another nurse, asked.

"No physical contact," Todd said. "A lot of these patients don't know the difference between what's too much and what isn't."

"What about hugging someone goodbye?" Valerie asked.

"No physical contact is allowed."

"Patients can't hug each other?" Cathy asked.

"Who are we to stop it?" Mark said. "They're grown adults. They're going to do what they want when they're not here anyway. And hell, they could do whatever they want on pass, and we'd never know about it. We're not their parents, after all. If we think we can enforce social restrictions, we're kidding ourselves. We can't stop them."

Some of the other nurses looked disgruntled. But the community meeting was to start in a few minutes. We all pushed our chairs away from the table and got up.

* * *

"Is there a patient agenda?" I asked in the community meeting.

"Yes," a patient said. "The only fruit we get are green apples. They're sour, and I'm sick of them. Can't we get something else?"

"Speak to the dietitian who comes around every week," Valerie said. "I will speak to dietary, too. If enough people complain, maybe something will get done. Maybe."

"Yeah—right," Cindy, a patient, smirked. "Typical."

"Any other items on the patient agenda?" I asked.

"The shower's broken," another patient said. "Parts are missing. When is it going to get fixed?"

"The parts are getting thrown out," Valerie said, raising her eyebrows. "They disappear."

"Oh, so now it's the patients' fault?" Cindy asked.

"I'm not saying who's disappearing them," Valerie retorted. "But I will speak to housekeeping about it."

There were no other items on the patient agenda.

"I want to remind everyone," I said, "that unit policy prohibits any physical contact on the ward."

"Can't we kiss someone goodbye?"

"No."

"What about shaking hands?"

I was puzzled. "Shaking hands is part of normal social discourse," I said. "The intent of the policy is to prevent physical contact beyond that."

"Can we hug each other?"

"No." Todd's dictum was stringent in practice. But some of the patients wouldn't know where to draw the line. For their sake, if for no one else's, the policy had to be defined rigidly and vigorously. I knew the rule would be broken. Personally, I felt that was okay at times. Who was I, after all, to say that someone could not hug or kiss their mother goodbye if she visited? Todd would later comment, "Borderlines, particularly, are notorious for arguing with you about these things, nitpicking, trying to undermine your authority." I had no choice but to defend this law, though it felt restrictive. Todd sat there silently, letting me be the one to disarm the challenges and wrath. He was paged out and seemed glad to go. He never returned to the room.

I was left alone upholding the norms of the profession, which felt not kind but necessary.

"Our time is up," I finally said.

"This place sucks," someone said.

We all got up to leave.

"The policy isn't very popular," I commented to Todd, who was standing back in the nursing station.

"You have to be firm," he said, "and draw limits like that or they'll try to find loopholes." But to uphold this rule was to incur patients' and nurses' ire and to be seen as being a restrictive authority figure, which I had always been wary of myself. I tried at least to be nice about it and to hear and respond to people's criticisms. But the institution strongly shaped how we were perceived by others. I had to accept that part of my role entailed having staff angry at me and had to tell myself they were not angry at me personally, but at the decisions I had to make as part of my position in the institution.

"I still don't see what's wrong with hugging a patient goodbye," Cathy commented.

At morning rounds the next day, Miranda was said to be still holding Charles in the hall. The topic of physical contact reemerged. The discussion continued heatedly. Finally, Eliot Higgens, the unit chief, who came to rounds once a week and was present that day, spoke up. "These decisions are based on clinical grounds. If a psychotic woman becomes pregnant from a co-patient who has AIDS, as a result of their physical contact, we haven't done anyone a service. We've made things worse for someone."

"For three people," I thought.

But with Dr. Higgens's comment, the debate finally ended.

The Heat

Summer wore on. Thick muggy air wafted through the hospital and sank into the hallways. The only air-conditioned rooms were the East Lounge, the doctors' offices, and the nursing station. None of the patients' rooms were air-conditioned, and few patients had family members who brought in spare fans from home. The door to the nursing station now remained shut at all times to maintain the coolness. Doctors stayed in their offices more, and the patients all huddled in the East Lounge. I was worried that the patients would get along worse now, forced into close confinement. I expected hostility and fights. But instead, to my surprise, they cooperated more and got along with each other better. I suppose they realized they had to, given the heat. The patients all sat quietly in the lounge during the day, reading to themselves, knitting, playing cards, watching TV, or staring off vacantly into space. They tolerated and accepted each other more than I had ever seen on a psychiatric unit.

But tensions still simmered. "We have two patients being admitted to the hospital," Wendy in the admissions office told me a few days later. "An elderly couple—man and wife."

"Both?"

"Yes. They're both depressed. Can you take them on your floor?"

"Let me talk to Valerie."

Valerie was puzzled.

"The question is," Valerie said, scanning a chart of patient beds she had untacked from the nursing station bulletin board, "would we put them in the same room or not?"

"Let them room together," Mark said on overhearing our conversation. "Why should this be any different than a home? We want to make them comfortable, don't we?"

It didn't seem right to me. I thought it best if they were separated. This wasn't a home. It would confuse issues on the ward, where celibacy still reigned, at least officially. This decision was difficult to make and wouldn't necessarily be popular. But patients wandered into each other's rooms, often unexpectedly and at odd hours. The couple was to be here primarily as patients, not as spouses. Most important was appropriate treatment, not just their convenience, the idea of which the nurses liked. In the end, I had the couple put on different floors. I realized that I now had authority over staff as well as patients.

My decision turned out to be right, since one of the couple's problems was fierce, incessant fighting, often violent, though we didn't know that at the time.

* * *

Not only did I have to rely on my own judgment more, but I also had to defend and enforce it. I felt frustrated, always having to fight for what seemed right.

"What brings you here today, Mr. Wilkins?" I asked a new patient late in the afternoon the following day. He was assigned to the ward's intern. But as with all new admissions to the ward, I had to meet him, and form my own clinical impression.

"Voices."

"Voices?"

"I've been hearing voices." Don Wilkins was a tall, muscular twenty-eight-year-old. His fists were clenched, his eyes fixed, unwavering, glaring with fiery intent. The muscles around his eyes tightened, too. His shoulders were thrust up and forward underneath a lime green tank top. Tight black-and-white striped Spandex shorts descended down his thighs. He wore white high-top basketball sneakers. When I had introduced myself to him, he had shaken my hand only with uneasy hesitation. I would have been apprehensive and frightened to meet him in the street.

"What have the voices been saying?"

He stared at me with uncomprehending, preoccupied eyes, like a bull about to charge. I feared he might attack me and eased half a step back toward the door to exit quickly if necessary. He seemed suspicious as to why I had asked him this question. He was paranoid, had schizophrenia, and had been hospitalized twice before.

"Kill," he said in a surprisingly quiet voice.

"Kill?" I swallowed hard.

"They're telling me to kill . . . people."

"Anyone in particular?"

"No."

"Do you think you would be able to control these thoughts?"

"Sort of."

"What do you mean?"

"I don't know if I could."

I nodded, trying to show understanding and support for his honesty, and stay calm and not reveal my utter terror.

"Is there any chance you might act on them?" I was surprised I managed to get the words out. He hesitated. "Is there?" I had to know.

"Yes." At this point, after dealing with Jimmy and other

patients, I had a clearer sense of my role and what had to be done.

"If you had to say, what percent chance is there that you might—from zero to one hundred percent?" We had been taught to ask this question to help gauge patients' potential for violence to themselves or others. It was reassuring if the patient said zero—that is, that even if he thought of doing something, he knew he wouldn't. Violent fantasies are very hard to get a fix on.

"Seventy percent."

"That you might act on them?"

"Yes."

"While here?" My forehead had broken into a sweat, but I tried to remain cool and conceal my fear.

"Yes."

"Do you think you'd be able to let the staff know first?"

"I don't know." His mother had brought him here after he had been menacing at home, brandishing a knife. "I don't think so."

I walked him back to the nursing station and ordered Haldol for him. Cathy poured it into a cup as she prepared the medications for other patients. He stood at the counter of the nursing station and took a small sip, then set the plastic cup back down. Most of the drug remained on the bottom. "I've had enough."

"You have to finish it," Mark said.

"No I don't. I don't want to."

Mark was at a loss for words as he stood face-to-face with Don. Cathy stood next to Mark. The intern stood behind her. I stood behind the intern. The doctor on call entered the nursing station on his 4:30 rounds and now joined us. On Don's side of the counter, in the hallway of the ward, several patients began to collect around him and watch. Some of the patients were on his side. Some were angry that the staff wasn't controlling him more.

"Why won't you take the medicine?" Cathy asked him. She held a gallon-sized can of generic grapefruit juice from which she had been pouring out glassfuls for other patients to take with their medications. He looked around and saw that he was surrounded. He reached for the cup and chugged the remaining fluid. We all sighed in relief, and he walked away.

He calmed down slightly but remained tense, on the edge of agitation. The intern was frightened. Other patients in poor

control of their behavior could say or do things that might
provoke him. Or he might erupt without provocation. I didn't
think he'd do anything. But having a staff member there
might be a buffer and a shield and might help him, and would
certainly lower the risk. The DOC was worried about him as
well, and together we agreed to continue him on Haldol and
put him on maximal observation for the night. I went to tell
the nursing staff our plan. Cathy was sitting in the back room
of the nursing station copying orders.

"I don't know about putting him on MO," she said, her
voice shaky, almost cracking.

"Why not?"

"I don't know. Don't we usually use it with patients who
are suicidal?"

"That's because we have more patients who are suicidal
than are homicidal. But if he's just come in here and is potentially dangerous, we shouldn't take any chances." I remembered Roy repeatedly saying, whenever nurses balked at
having to care for a difficult patient, "They don't really want
to work in a psychiatric hospital. What do they think goes on
here, anyway?" This patient was troubling, but I didn't have
a choice.

I wrote the order and signed it.

The next morning, Valerie pulled me aside. "We don't put patients with homicidal ideation on MO."

"Why not?"

"We just don't."

"But it's not like there's a policy."

"The staff said you didn't take their thoughts into account.
You didn't listen to them."

"I did," I protested. "I listened, heard what they were saying, and put their opinions into the hopper. But the decision is
not like that concerning a pass which I may want to give for
eight hours and you might want to give for one hour. There,
we can compromise and give it for four hours or require that
the patient be accompanied. This isn't a democracy. In the end,
I'm the one who's legally responsible."

"Well, the staff felt threatened having to sit with him." This,
finally, was the problem. "That staff tells me that you didn't
feel comfortable going over the DOC's head. But the DOC
isn't assigned to our floor. You are and you should know our
policy."

"That's not it. I agreed with the DOC that Mr. Wilkins should be on MO."

"It's not just that it ties up one of my nurses for an extra shift!" she added. For MO, she had to arrange for one of her nurses to spend the shift just with one patient and sometimes work overtime. Valerie was often against MO. But as Mike later commented when I told him about this conversation, "It's your ass on the line, not theirs." The senior hospital administrators had no problem with residents putting patients on MO. Dr. Farb once mentioned at a 9:30 meeting, "All the MO in the entire hospital for the year still costs but a fraction of the millions of dollars involved in a lawsuit if one of our patients commits suicide or homicide while here."

The burden of executing the decision fell on me.

In retrospect, I see that my actions were right—that MO had kept Wilkins safe. Increasingly, I was seeing the need to stand up for what I believed and accept that while my perceptions were valid, my decisions might be controversial and opposed. My agenda and the nurses' often conflicted and had to be negotiated, often with me asserting my professional status as a physician. After all, I wrote the orders. Such political issues are expected in a business or large bureaucracy but are surprising to see this pronouncedly in a medical science center.

After two days on medication, Don felt calmer. He walked around the ward and began to talk to a few other patients.

At community meeting, the other patients were still scared. "The staff is taking a calculated risk with us," one patient, a former fireman, said. "I've seen murderers and killers before, and I hope the staff knows what it's doing." He looked directly at me.

"This isn't a security institution," Valerie said. "It isn't a prison."

"He's in pain," a young black woman said. "I'm his friend and I know he's not feeling too good. Anyone who's not his friend shouldn't force themselves to be with him. If you like him, talk to him; but if you're afraid of him, just stay away."

"Nobody here really cares about him," another young woman said. "Except his friends. Nobody really wants to help him."

After two more days of medication, Don began to experience side effects and stopped it. I started another medication to control the side effects, but he refused it and the voices returned, telling him to beat people up.

The following morning the nursing station was abuzz when I arrived.

"What's happened?"

"Wilkins eloped." At 7:00 A.M. Cathy had come to work, inserted her key into the lock in the stairwell door, turned the bolt, and opened the door to enter the ward. Don, hearing her from the hall, had suddenly raced over and barged through the narrow opening, hurling her to the ground. He had flown down the stairs and out.

He was potentially dangerous, having talked about assaulting people. I was nervous about him and decided it would be best to call the police. He had taken a few doses of medication to calm himself down, but I was still concerned. An operator answered 911 after a single ring. I introduced myself and breathlessly explained the situation, including his potential dangerousness.

"So you have an EDP?" the woman asked in a gruff voice.

"A what?"

"An EDP."

"What's that?"

"An emotionally disturbed person."

"Sure. An EDP."

"Name?"

"Donald Wilkins."

"Age?"

"Twenty-eight."

"Physical description?"

I told her.

"Any idea where he might be?"

"The only address we have for him is his mother's," which I gave her.

"Okay."

"That's it?"

"That's it." They didn't want to know more about him—his diagnosis, treatment, or history, or what he had said.

"Is there anything else I should do?" I asked her.

"No. If we find him should we bring him back to you?"

"You can, but he should probably go to a state mental hospital." I also phoned his mother and told her.

* * *

We were late starting rounds.

"Are you hurt, Cathy?" Valerie asked.

"No, I just scraped my knee, my elbow, and my ankle." She tried smiling.

"Is that all?" I thought to myself. Her modesty and dedication despite her injury amazed me.

"I think we should put up bigger 'Elopement Risk' signs on the door," Valerie said, "just to make sure visitors can see it."

"I think we should get a new lock," someone said. "This one is loose sometimes."

"I think we should get a better-*designed* lock," Mark suggested.

"And we should get the door replaced," Valerie said. "And have one with a window, so you can see if someone's there.

"You contacted the police?" Valerie asked me.

"Yes."

"Thank God." She sighed.

No one said directly that they were upset or worried about Don Wilkins or felt helpless about what he might do. These feelings were not allowed for discussion and had to be dealt with in other ways—indirectly, through suggestions of things that could be done, or simply on our own.

A few minutes later, community meeting began.

"I want to welcome the new patients," I said, greeting them individually. "Also, Mr. Josephson is leaving."

"Yes," he said, "and I'd like to thank all the patients because they're the ones that helped me here." The patients all applauded. "Oh . . . ," he added, "and I guess some of the nurses were helpful, too." He didn't mention the doctors.

"Do you want to say what your plans are?" I asked him.

"I'm going to visit my sister in Hawaii."

"How about your plans for psychiatric follow-up?" Patients almost always omitted future psychiatric treatment when initially announcing their post-discharge plans.

"Oh, yeah. I'm going to go to a day program and see my outpatient shrink."

"I also want to announce that Mr. Wilkins eloped today," I said.

Patients gasped.

"He eloped?" someone asked.

"Yes. He left." Some of the patients knew. Others didn't.

"You should get a door with a window," one patient said, "so you can see if anyone's standing there."

"Last night a bunch of us were talking here in the lounge," another patient said, "and he came in to hang out with us, but the group broke up right away. I hope he didn't think it was because of him."

"Maybe if I hadn't snubbed him at breakfast," someone else said, "he wouldn't have gone."

That the patients felt part of the community and jointly responsible moved me. "I'm sure there were many things he didn't like about being in the hospital," I said to reassure them.

"Everything feels like it's falling apart here," another patient complained. "There's nothing to hold everything together."

"That's not true," Valerie said. "Every patient has a multidisciplinary treatment plan, which has input from nursing, social work, OT, and the doctors, and unifies everyone's treatment plan."

"But that feeling," I told the patient, sensing that Valerie had missed the point of the patient's comment, "is something you should discuss with your therapist as well." When I had started on the wards, the nurses knew far more than me. I now saw their limitations.

In the post-community meeting, Todd said, "Could you believe Josephson's thanking the nurses? He didn't want to thank the rest of the staff," Todd continued, meaning the doctors. The nurses said nothing. No one talked about Don's eloping or mentioned the patients' concerns about him. We each felt nervous and overwhelmed.

A few days later a nurse called the ward from Rivershore State to obtain information about Donald because he had just been admitted there. I was glad to find out that he was safe and hadn't hurt anyone, but also amazed to see how much my concerns about other patients subsequently admitted had already begun to push my worries about him to the back of my mind.

The following week, Valerie was going away on vacation. She would be gone through Labor Day weekend, when the unit chief had planned a party for the staff at his summer house south of the city. "Before I go," she said, waving to the blank wall, "I'll post a big sign so people can list what they're going to bring to the party."

At community meeting that week, I welcomed new patients and said goodbye to old ones. "The only staff announcement is that our head nurse, Valerie, will be going on vacation for two weeks."

"Yes," she said, "I will be away until September tenth."

"Rhonda, the occupational therapist, will also be on vacation," I continued. My own vacation would be starting the following week. It seemed like many of us would be away. I decided to announce my vacation then, too, to give patients time to get used to the idea, so the absences wouldn't hit them unexpectedly. They might as well get all such news together and be able to respond. "I will also be going on vacation," I said, "leaving one week after Valerie."

There was silence.

"I want to talk about the phone," a patient finally said. "My friends call me up here and I never get the message."

"Yeah," another patient said. "Certain people are always hogging the phone. When I want to call someone I can't."

"If you ask the person maybe they'll get off," Valerie suggested.

"Yeah, right," a patient muttered sarcastically.

"I don't see why they don't have more phones here."

"I think it's good that everyone's working out the problem with the phone," I said, realizing that the patients were trying to take control of a problem themselves. "But does anyone have any thoughts about Valerie's vacation or mine?" These issues were underlying the conversation.

"When do we get a vacation?" Cindy asked.

More silence followed.

"I was thinking," another patient said. "Why don't we all just agree that no one will use the phone for more than fifteen minutes a day."

"Fifteen minutes?" an elderly man said. "Why not three minutes?"

"Are you going to tell me I can't use the phone more than once a day?" Cindy asked. "That's ridiculous."

"How about twice a day?" someone said.

"What is this—a communist country or something? It's a free country. I can call whomever I want."

"Yeah, but you'll be on the phone all day," someone said.

I tried reintroducing the issue of vacations.

"What about ten minutes a call?" a patient said, ignoring me.

"I still want to get my messages."

"Yeah, but why can't everyone just agree: no more than ten minutes a call?"

"I have a pad of paper in my room," another patient said. "I can put it by the phone and we can write down messages for each other."

The animated conversation continued. No one wanted to discuss the vacations. The patients were solving a problem among themselves, without the staff, who were leaving anyway.

After half an hour the negotiations were still heated.

"Excuse me," I interrupted, almost intruding. "The meeting time is over." The patients remained in their seats, looking at me, as if to ask who I was to say that. "We have to stop," I added. Everyone sat still. But in my newfound position of authority, I had to maintain limits and fight my inclination to let the meeting continue. I stood up. The other staff followed my example. They filed out behind me. The patients slowly followed in small clusters and packs, continuing to converse.

In the post-community meeting Todd spoke first. "They weren't dealing with the vacations!" he said, as if that were a problem.

"But they were problem-solving around the phone issue," Rhonda, the OT, said.

"It shouldn't be a problem-solving meeting," Todd said. "We should have discussed other issues, like vacations. The issue should have been brought up."

"It was," I said, "and patients tried to deal with it as best they could."

"They didn't want to discuss it," Rhonda added.

"Then the staff should have kept them on the topic."

"We can't tell them what to think about," Mark said.

"But that's one of our jobs," Todd continued, "to focus them on issues."

"But they were discussing an issue they felt was important," Valerie said, jumping at Todd.

"Look," I finally said, "I tried to reorient them and they didn't want to change the subject."

"How was the meeting?" Eliot Higgens asked me afterward.

"It was the most active discussion we've had so far, also the first time we had a real argument in the post-community meeting." I told him what had happened. "Valerie's going on vacation was one of the big issues. It was really about her leaving. Do you interpret something like that back to them during the meeting?"

"I see interpretations as something one only makes and uses in the context of an ongoing therapy," Eliot said. "But I find it helpful in situations like this to use the analogy of a puncture in a tire. If there's a hole, you don't have to announce there's a hole and make everyone nervous and aware of it. Just patch it up. At a meeting such as the one this morning, you can say something like, 'Well, who's going to be taking your place, Valerie?' Let everyone know that there's a chain of command, that someone else will be available for handling problems. I also wouldn't have used that moment to announce your own vacation time. But," he said, raising his eyebrows and rocking his head from side to side, "that's a judgment call." I was still learning.

Valerie left on vacation. "I hope nothing happens while I'm away," she said before going.

The following week I left as well.

A few weeks after my return, my rotation on the ward came to a close. Though having gotten to know the patients and the staff, I would be moving on, leaving behind these relationships and connections. A new resident would replace me. Strangely, everything on the ward would remain the same—except for Todd and me. But comings and goings are always hard for both staff and patients. At my last community meeting I announced my departure. Cindy had been elected patient representative and read the patient agenda. No mention was made of Todd and me leaving the ward and new doctors coming to take our places. I asked a few times if people had reactions to our leaving but no one commented. I also gave them the name of the doctor who would be replacing me and who would be visiting the floor on my last afternoon there. As we all sat in a circle for the last time, the patients giggled and made jokes. The conversation was energetic and didn't slow down at the end. "Our time is up," I announced after half an hour. The patients still sat tittering nervously. No one wanted the meeting to end. No one else had mentioned my leaving. As we were about to get up to go, one patient stopped. "Thank you, Cindy," he said, on behalf of the other patients, "for running the meeting." Everyone then shuffled out of the room.

Desserts

Not until the very end of our three years in the hospital did the faculty finally ask residents formally and explicitly for feedback on our education.

Every year, an annual farewell meeting was held where graduating residents talked candidly in public—for the first time—about how they felt. Though the Christmas Show allowed us to joke and make innuendos, explicit face-to-face discussion of the issues only occurred once—the week before we graduated.

A few days before this meeting the chief resident had met with us, telling us to begin to think about what to say and asking three of us—Anne, Sarah, and myself—to prepare some remarks in advance.

"Do we tell the truth?" Anne asked. "Should we be honest?"

"Yes," he answered. "You can talk about whatever problems you want . . . complaints about your fellow residents, or whatever . . ."

But of course none of us felt that our fellow residents were the problem.

I thought a lot about what to say.

I had first attended one of these meetings three years earlier, as an intern. Graduating residents complained that the faculty were cold and aloof. One woman said the hospital had "no *menschlichkeit*," Yiddish for heart, warmth, soul.

Another departing resident said, "Growing up I was told, 'If you don't have anything nice to say, don't say anything.' But you only go through life once, so here it is. . . . This department is vindictive, doesn't listen, is unfair and unsupportive, and I hesitate even to say these things because no one's going to listen. At the first of these meetings I went to, three years ago, people said the same things they're saying now. But it's what I feel so I say it anyhow."

The consensus at past meetings was that residents had been well trained as psychiatrists but felt the faculty were infantilizing and sadistic. Some of the junior faculty later admitted privately that they felt this way, too. When I was an intern, the residents complained about "the problem on the inpatient units."

"What problem is that?" Dr. Danziger finally asked.

A long silence ensued.

Finally, Dr. Robins, the director of education, spoke. "I think the problem being referred to is that of scapegoating of residents on the units by faculty. And the worst three perpetrators of this are: Dr. Swire, Dr. Nolan, and Dr. Kasdin, in that order." The three accused men were seated in the room and remained motionless and stone-faced as their names were mentioned in front of the entire faculty and resident body. But the problem disappeared the following year when I began on the wards. This act of public shaming and humiliation precipitated by a more senior faculty member had served to resolve the situation, which recurrent complaints to Dr. Robins by residents and discussions with faculty members individually over the years had failed to accomplish. On Dr. Swire's ward, residents had previously chalked onto the blackboard in the nursing station a box with the heading, "Goat Du Jour," and each day had written in the name of whichever resident they felt was being the most scapegoated at that particular time.

The farewell meeting finally arrived. The faculty squeezed onto the narrow chairs in tight concentric circles near the middle of the room, looking stranded with nothing around them. They sat with their arms and legs crossed tightly, awkward, uncomfortable, exposed. Most of the senior psychoanalysts, I noticed, wore the same eyeglasses—big lenses in horn rim frames, spanning their faces, making their eyes seem large, giving them an air of intelligence, as if they saw more from behind their big crystal lenses. The residents sat for the most part on the periphery, on the windowsill and atop radiators. Many stood up by the door, after all the seats were taken. Many came in late from finishing work on the wards or being paged to answer questions and address crises.

Anne spoke first and said that the most important things that had happened to her in the past four years had happened outside of the hospital—in her home life, getting married.

Sarah thanked several faculty members and then said, "This is the brightest group of people I have ever been around. But, hey—loosen up, huh?"

Then it was my turn. I was nervous. In the middle of residency, I had thought it would never end and feared never again being able to feel the kind of innocence that I felt before. I had lost a sense of ease, of all-encompassing hope about and for the future, the sense that time could stretch forever. Weekends and vacations had become edged with concerns in the back of my mind about my patients. My hopes were now constrained, no longer filling me altogether. Only now could I begin to gather up the pieces of my life and my new career and try to make sense of them. I decided to present points that the faculty might hear and act on for the benefit of future residents.

I remained seated, as the other speakers had been, though wedged tightly in the corner amidst other chairs. "Before I talk about the education here, I want to just comment for a moment on this meeting." I cited the comments made at these gatherings in the past and asked whether the purpose of this meeting was to improve the education here or to have criticism expressed before residents left, to appear to contain the discontent and to create a semblance of no hard feelings by hearing complaints and thus seeming to acknowledge them, but without there necessarily being any intention of acting on them. I said I hoped that the first goal would prevail, and I then urged that the faculty maintain a broad vision in teaching psychiatry. "There is a tendency to support a narrow range of approaches here, despite the fact that the department has wider strengths. As an example, when I wanted to do research on social issues in psychiatry that required the use of qualitative methodologies I was asked, 'But what are you going to measure?' I've assembled statistics that I'd like to present now about who gets full research time approved and who does not, based on data from the past few years.

"On the whole, two-thirds of residents get their research approved; however, despite our being encouraged to pursue our own interests, doing so will not get you research time. If you want to study psychiatric education there is a zero percent chance you will get full research time granted to you. If you have a prior higher degree or have completed training in another field before coming here, there is only a thirty-three percent chance you will get full time. If you are black or Hispanic there is a fifty percent chance you will not get your plan approved. If you wish to study psychiatric aspects of AIDS there is only a thirty-three percent chance you will be granted full time. If, on the other hand, you wish to study with one of two particular quantitative senior researchers here, there is a one hundred percent chance your proposal will be accepted.

"In short, it's okay to pursue your own interests in psychiatry here as long as they're certain other people's interests as well." I then proceeded to thank several faculty in particular who had taught me a lot.

Mike spoke next. "It's like a poker game here," he said. "You have all the right cards in your hand, but you can play them better."

Joe Tauber spoke next. "I'm not angry," he said, "I'm enraged. I wouldn't recommend this place to anyone."

"I didn't come here an angry person," someone else said. "But I'm told I'm angry now. And I am. I wanted this to be a good experience for me," she said, breaking down into tears, "and it hasn't been." She stood crying. No one moved. Finally Anne walked over to her and put her arm around her. The attendings, the room full of senior psychiatrists, sat in their chairs rigidly, looking unmoved. So much for sympathy or compassion.

"After a day here," another resident said, "I have to go home and take a shower to wash it off."

"It's that bad!" Nolan muttered.

In general, the people staying on after residency were far more polite than those who were leaving. Those remaining couldn't afford to be critical.

At the end, Dr. Farb turned to Dr. Robins. "This," he said curtly, "is the last one of these that we're ever going to have."

"The meeting was the same as every year," Betsy Coover said as she left the room. To lump this meeting with all those previous diluted what was said. Jane Pomeroy and other junior residents thought more pain was expressed than before. "I guess it's: toe the line," she concluded, "or be crushed."

Dr. Randolph Johnson's only comment was, "That was the first group I ever remember that seemed to have found mentors and praised certain people. I don't ever recall that happening," he said somewhat indifferently.

"The residents are just angry as usual," Dr. Swire said to another attending. The faculty dismissed the complaints as if they were those of a psychoanalytic patient, and did not change their behavior or the bureaucratic problem. The issues the residents were angry about weren't important, just their effect. Even in the end, residents were viewed as analogous to patients.

"Well," Anne said to me, smiling broadly and putting her hand on my shoulder, "looks like you finally measured something like they asked!"

A week later Dr. Leon Berman and another professor held parties for us. Only now were we invited into a few faculty homes.

"I can't believe we're graduating," Jessica said when she entered Dr. Berman's apartment behind me. That was to be the only mention of it at the party. "I'm setting up my new office for my private practice, buying all this furniture and renting a space. I'm busy getting carpeting and a sofa," she said. "Then I have to get billing slips printed up. It's so expensive. I'm just putting it all on my Gold Card and hoping I get enough patients. Some I'm bringing with me."

"You must be excited about starting psychoanalytic training."

"I just hope it works out—that I get enough private referrals to afford it all."

"I'm sure it will work out."

"I figured out exactly how many patient-hours I need per week."

Many residents' financial motivations became clear. Psychiatry was a business.

Everyone was impressed with Sarah's boyfriend, a clarinetist, getting a teaching post at a local university-affiliated music school.

"Leon courted me with Mozart operas recorded in Europe," Mrs. Rebecca Berman announced. Psychoanalysts liked to feel connected with the arts, which they saw as the highest endeavor one could pursue. After all, the goal of psychoanalysis was to free people's creative energies, rather than leaving them bound up in neuroses. Yet within the practice of psychoanalytic psychotherapy there were clearly limits on how creative a therapist himself could be. One had to conform to accepted, often rigid, theory.

"I might have been a scholar," Berman said, "but I didn't

know that back in college. Instead I planned to be a surgeon and work with my hands."

"How do you find it, trying to integrate intellectual interests and psychiatry?" I asked him.

"Medicine is too demanding a profession. I don't have the time. And the financial rewards aren't there, either."

Mike said, "Friends of mine in law earn more than I do and in a few years will earn even more. Friends of mine in academic fields like anthropology earn less," he added with glee.

Berman went on to talk to Anne's husband, Walter, an orthopedics resident at another hospital. "Is Bob Reynolds still down there?"

"He's no longer chairman, but I knew him." Dr. Berman prided himself on his continued connections with internists and surgeons.

Berman's apartment was spacious. Room after room afforded grand views of a park below. He owned a large modern art collection, mostly twangy and frail wire sculptures of hollow human figures. Yet he served us only Triscuits and inexpensive wine in gallon-sized jugs that had twist-off caps, not corks. I was surprised, because he liked to be seen as a connoisseur and gourmet, and since I'm sure he would have served senior psychiatrists far more expensive food and drink. It was nice of him to invite us over, although it still felt as if we weren't quite accepted as colleagues, but rather were still "only" residents.

We had never been in his apartment before. We might never be there again. Only now were we allowed to see him as human, as a person with a private life. Had he invited us before, it might have separated us less and diminished the distance between us and the power that he and other analysts seemed to treasure.

Graduation was held a week later. I had thought family or friends would be invited, as they had been to every other graduation of mine—high school, college, and medical school—but they were not. For the first time, it was just the graduates. The few who were married brought their spouses. I walked into the cocktail party behind Dr. Robins. As he ascended the three steps to the room, he pulled a comb out of his pocket and scraped it through his few strands of black hair before entering the party.

The evening started with an open bar. I was talking to Dr. Ostrow when Mike joined us, drink in hand.

"Don't you look pleased with yourself," Ostrow snapped at him.

"I'm glad to be done," he said, smiling.

"You have to say something more diplomatic than that!" Ostrow exclaimed. He then quickly walked away. Mike was left standing with me, astonished. After all, he was at his residency graduation party.

Everyone asked us what we were going to do next year. In the end there were only a handful of options: inpatient or out-patient jobs, psychoanalysis, child psychiatry, or fellowships in research or a few other areas. The faculty seemed to enjoy hearing how we, too, despite the seemingly wide possibilities and hopes that brought us into the field, were going to conform to a fairly narrow range of career choices and join the main-stream of the profession.

Dr. M. came over and grinned. "I agreed with what you said at the farewell meeting," he said to me. "During psychiatric residency, people become more consolidated. Those who come in with outside intellectual interests usually end up in one of the institutes," that is, psychoanalytic institutes, "turned inward upon themselves—much too inwardly in my opinion—instead of being interested in the world. And they're much less happy—and I mean happy in whatever way you want to define it. This program focuses people, though too narrowly I think."

Dinner was served and we all moved into the dining area. Afterward, desserts were laid on a buffet table—thin slivers of chocolate cake draped with curlicues of hardened white icing. I got up to get a piece. "Anyone want dessert?" I asked the others at my table.

"We'll go up later. Thanks anyway."

Standing at the buffet table was Dr. Farb.

"Very nice affair," I said. He nodded.

Dr. Danziger strolled up and took two pieces of cake.

"Two?" Dr. Farb asked him with raised eyebrows.

"For my table," Dr. Danziger tried to explain.

"I see," Farb responded, suspicious, as if to suggest, "That's what they all say." Danziger skulked away.

"He's appealing to a higher principle," I said after he left. "Altruism." Farb didn't comment. I offered him the plate in my hand with its portion of cake.

He pulled his head back and looked askance, as if to say, "All those calories? I wouldn't eat that if you paid me."

I walked away with my serving.

Dr. Robins walked up to the podium. "This was a highly talented group of residents," he said. "Though they were often angry, as residents frequently are, I think they'd all agree that they received excellent educations here." Dr. Robins proceeded to call each of us up alphabetically one at a time and say a few words about us. Anne was praised for her wonderful management of one particularly difficult patient whom Ostrow had referred to her—a "Sid Ostrow Special," as it was called around the clinic. Ostrow thought he could cure the patient, who ended up suicidal. Though stressful, Anne persevered nonetheless, and received personal supervision from Ostrow.

One resident whom, it was rumored, Robins almost didn't admit, was much praised as a star.

Dr. Robins, as he proceeded alphabetically, omitted one resident altogether. She was starting a child psychiatry fellowship at the hospital, but was officially graduating the residency. The two other residents also continuing as Child Fellows had been called up to the podium and praised. But she was not. She sat at her dinner table and started to cry. Robins realized he had forgotten her and included her at the last minute between two other residents.

When Robins spoke about me, I couldn't look at the audience, and glanced down, though seeing them out of the top of my field of vision.

Around the room of faces were a few to whom I felt close: Mike, Anne, Sarah, Dr. M., Roy, and Greg. Shelly Tarr sat chain-smoking. Henry Nolan stood up against the wall in the rear. They all had shaped my experience here. I felt closer to them than I would have thought—was fond of them and would miss them. Looking back now, I see that despite the frustration, they had taught me vital lessons and given me important skills. My apprenticeship had been difficult, but I was emerging well trained, aware of a wide range of issues in myself and others. But it was a shame that the faculty had to challenge us and take us apart to put us back together again. I had been fundamentally altered.

Dr. Farb soon replaced Robins at the podium. "Twenty-five years ago," he said, "I used to toast the residents' wives for their support and for making the residents less angry at me. Then, twenty years ago, I toasted the residents' significant others. Fifteen years ago, I toasted their husbands and wives and significant others. And now, I toast anyone who has spent a night with a resident." The faculty laughed heartily. I did too at the time. In retrospect, I feel his remarks were in poor taste and at our expense.

The residents presented a gift to Dr. Robins—an empty box decorated with inlaid woods.

After the speeches, we all got up and milled around. Robins smiled. "It's been a pleasure," he said to me. He looked down, bewildered, at his box. His eyebrows were raised, his eyes moist. Two years before, he had received from the graduates as a gift a letter opener shaped like a dagger. He now walked around with his box, hugging it and showing it off. He didn't hug any of the graduating residents, but he hugged his box. I was moving downtown to a neighborhood that I knew to be near his. Later in the evening, standing near him, I asked him, "Where do you live again?" I had happened to go to his house once. He eyed me quizzically though, analyzing why I was asking. He was assessing if I had some other motive or agenda, as if I were a patient asking him a personal question. Only with reluctance did he answer.

Henry Nolan came up to me. "Graduation isn't for the graduates, you know. By the way, I agree with everything you said at the farewell meeting. You know, I've made it a point to be in the chairman's office only once, and that was when I was hired. Not since, thank you. These men are in touch with very primitive sides of themselves"—presumably from being in psychoanalysis. "But you have to be very careful with them."

Anne was moving to Los Angeles to work in a hospital. A few days after graduation, we sat down together one last time. "The thing I'll always remember most is the four of us starting out, working together on the twelfth floor," she said, referring to Mike, Sarah, herself, and me. "That was the highlight of residency for me."

The four of us had remained special in my mind as well.

"There's only one way I survived here," she continued. "I decided that the best defense was a good offense. I started work at six-thirty each morning, often seeing patients then. It was pathological. Plus, I saw more patients in the beginning of the third year than anyone else. First impressions are everything. For the rest of the year I coasted. But what I did was sick." Yet it was adaptive. "I also realized that you can't let su-

pervisors know you're unhappy, or else you get labeled that
way. People don't care, they just don't. Do you know what it
was like being supervised by Ostrow for one year and not being able to say anything negative the whole year? It sucked.
When I worked on the fourteenth floor, if you revealed your
vulnerabilities, Dr. Swire"—the attending there—"went after
you like a leech. It took a year for my ego to recover. If you
opposed him—forget it. Swire interpreted your personality. He
was a bigot and a racist and an elitist. The faculty didn't have
to be sadistic. They're fragile little men with titanic egos and
aren't very pleasant people. Hysterics I can deal with. They get
emotional, but that's okay. But narcissists are out to kill. I remember seeing a T-shirt once in the 1960s that sums up their
attitude. The shirt said, 'America eats her young.' Well, at this
hospital, they eat their young. Many of them are self-hating
men who have to put others down to uphold themselves and
ignore the threat of their own obsolescence as psychoanalysts.
Just think: their evaluation forms on us are nine pages long,
have sixty questions on them, and are filled out on each of us
six to eight times a year. Inevitably all of us are found to have
problems. Ask enough questions on an evaluation form and
something will be found wrong with everyone. Their goal is to
feel better about themselves. I just learned to try to do the best
for my patients despite their criticisms. In the end, that's all I
could do.

"The other way I survived was to keep my life going separately outside here. I'm glad to leave. In the end, I learned
much more from my patients here and from other residents
than from my supervisors. I sometimes feel bad about going,"
she said. "I'm setting up new medical backup rosters for each
of the incoming residents, since the old listings were out of
date. Patients will know clearly who their new doctors are, and
doctors will all receive the same number of patients. No one
resident will be overburdened. I'm doing it for the whole
clinic. It should ease the changeover for everyone." She
seemed motivated by guilt and remorse about leaving but also
wanted to leave something helpful behind.

She was more open with me now than ever before. Now
that we were leaving, the competition between residents was at
last off.

"I think you and I will stay in touch," she said. "We have
similar backgrounds." We were both Jewish, had gone to Ivy
League schools—she to Brown, me to Princeton—and we

knew people in common. "My therapist called up to cancel my last two sessions. She said, 'I know this is bad timing, but a family emergency came up.' I think that because I haven't been able to say goodbye to her, I haven't been able to separate well from anybody else. It's crazy but true." She showed me an envelope of photos of her family. It was the first time I had seen her family, except for her husband. She also had photos from our graduation. One snapshot showed me, surprised by the photo, with Dr. M., who was smiling. "You've grown a lot, Bob. I've seen you become more confident." But in many ways I had felt more self-confident in the beginning than I did now.

Jessica and I passed each other in the hall and stopped. "Goodbye," I said.

"Goodbye. I'm glad it's over."

"I'll miss some of the people, though," I said.

"Me too. But not all. We've had our ups and downs, but with you it's been better in the past year and a half. Some of the residents in our group are *so* competitive. Plus, with some of the faculty it's another story. Some of these guys are just in their own little worlds. I'm glad to get out of here."

Back in my office, someone knocked on my door. I assumed it was a final patient five minutes early. I prepared to tell him, "Have a seat. I'll be with you in a minute." But it was Shelly Tarr, clasping her thick leatherbound combination calendar and notebook against her breast. She had never come into my office before. "I'm having people over for a picnic at my house on July Fourth," she said. She shifted her weight. "I'm bad at goodbyes," she added. "But try to come." She quickly disappeared down the hall.

"I'll try to make it," I said after her.

My patients and I had trouble with my leaving.

"Don't make any major elective changes in medication regimens immediately prior to leaving," Dr. Ostrow had told all of us. "Let a new doctor tangle with problems that may arise." I had thought it might be unfair to patients, but I now see the logic more clearly. The first patient with whom I terminated was a medication clinic patient I saw only once every month or two. I thought I might not ever see him again, I who for two years had been responsible for him and his functioning.

I had told Isabelle Dupree that a new doctor would be taking over but didn't yet have his or her name. Dr. Jane Pomeroy was assigned a week before I left. "What kind of notes do you write?" Jane asked me. "And what do you do if they're suicidal?"

"There's always an attending around."

"I'm afraid I won't know what questions to ask my patients," she said. Residents didn't voice these concerns to others in their same year, but she clearly felt them as much as I had. I introduced Jane and Isabelle but felt obliged to see Isabelle just one last time to say goodbye, rather than terminating too suddenly. I felt uneasy and tried to arrange as smooth a transition as possible.

I had gotten attached to many of my patients. Some accused me of not being as connected to them as they were connected to me. They wanted me to say, "Yes, you mean a lot to me. I'll miss you." To say this, at least explicitly, didn't sound professional. I could ask clever, suggestive questions like "What makes you think you aren't important to me and that I won't miss you?" But these fell short, certainly, of any display of affection. And I certainly couldn't say, "Of course I'll miss you—you helped teach me how to do psychotherapy and become a psychiatrist."

"I've had many doctors," one said, "but you were the best. You cared the most about me." I had once admitted her when she became psychotic and depressed, and had gotten to know her well over two years.

One patient gave me a gift certificate to Bloomingdale's. I told her it wasn't necessary, but she insisted and refused to take it back. I didn't spend it, as it didn't seem appropriate, but kept it, thinking at the time of perhaps waiting until I was no longer her doctor. I still have it.

Over the last few days I cleaned off my shelves, removing piles of journals—some obscure, others not yet read because of little free time—textbooks, copies of articles, memoranda to be filed. I put three years of accumulated possessions into boxes.

"So is this your last day?" people started asking a few days before I left.

"Not yet."

"Well I'll see you tomorrow then," they would say.

Finally, my last day arrived. A heavy rain fell over the city. What I had to do on this last day was mostly paperwork, and more goodbyes. A pile remained to be completed of insurance forms for patients, three-month summaries, questionnaires on the educational experience, questionnaires on the questionnaires, forms I had put off doing for as long as a year, notes on patients. Even on this final day, I had to be careful and felt anxious, on guard against any possible mistakes. I could never fully relax, too often having had to face unexpected problems from left field.

In my mailbox I received an almost apologetic note from Dr. Robins. "I know we haven't always shown you anything resembling appreciation, but you were terrific, nonetheless." I didn't know how to interpret this set of qualified qualifiers.

An annual departmental photograph was scheduled to be shot at ten o'clock. As a resident I had never had time to go and almost none of the residents in my year did. As I walked through the lobby of the main hospital now, Roy, Greg, and others spotted me and persuaded me to join them. The only residents there were a few who were also graduating. We crowded inside the lofty but narrow stone lobby. Outside, rain poured down and drenched the tall windows. Inside it was damp. Our feet had tracked sooty black mud over the marble tiled floor. We huddled together in rows, arranged by the photographer. Dr. Farb hadn't yet arrived, and we stood waiting for him. No one wanted to leave until he got there.

Randolph Johnson was talking to Kasdin, who was on my other side. "I'm planning to go fishing this weekend. I hope the weather improves." Kasdin nodded. Johnson looked at me.

"I see you have new glasses," I said to him.

"Do you like them?" I was surprised that he was, for the first time, having a personal conversation with me.

"They look very academic," Kasdin replied.

"Is that good?" Johnson asked, unsure, and again for the first time revealing insecurity.

"It means you'll be asked a lot of questions," I said.

"Is that good?" He didn't know.

"It depends if you want to answer them," I replied.

Finally, Dr. Farb showed up. The photographer loaded film and rearranged us.

"How much is this costing in our time?" Dr. Farb asked.

"Five thousand dollars," Robins was quick to reply.

The photographer took one shot, removed the film, put it away, and inserted another roll into the camera. "What is he doing?" I asked, "taking one picture of each of us?"

"Every year," Robins said, turning to the group in response, "one of my jobs is to pick the final picture. I always choose the one in which I look the best."

Another resident was moving into my office and booted me out at noon. A resident a year below him had occupied his office the day before. It wasn't until I lost my office that I realized the need to hurry up with last-minute tasks, finish saying goodbye to people in the halls, and leave. I completed my paperwork in a glass-windowed, partitioned office next to Gina's desk. Mike, who was staying on at the hospital, saw me and stopped and pawed at the window as a joke, dragging his fingernails down the glass wall several times.

My name was removed from my mailbox. Sarah, who was also staying behind, was promoted to the top row of mailboxes.

"So this is it!" people started to say to me in the hall. In the early afternoon of my last day, I was greeted in the hall not by continued hellos, but by "What are you still doing here?"

"I'm beginning to wonder," Roy said. "It's hard to leave, huh?"

"Would you start telling people that I'm not here," I told Gina.

I had come here filled with excitement and idealism and a sense of intellectual adventure. The experience had in many ways bruised me. Faculty had unraveled my self-confidence and doubted me, leading me to doubt myself. More than ever before, I questioned myself and what I took for granted about my own mind. I thought I knew myself in the past but was now more aware of unconscious defenses—some more adaptive than others—impulses, and emotional reactions such as anger and resentment when provoked. These basic elements of human nature that I had ignored and thought "bad" in myself I was now working to understand and deal with better. Yet this knowledge was extracted at a high price. Gone were the days of innocence, of acting unselfconsciously. I had trudged on. In part, I had been driven by ambition and the desire to bring closure to this experience. I had invested years of my life toward the goal of becoming a psychiatrist. But most important, the problems patients faced were ultimately still vital.

In the end, I had made it—had graduated and survived. At last, despite the pain and the torture, pressure and stress, I was a psychiatrist. And, I knew, a good one.

I was glad to have learned skills that could help others. Psychiatrists aid many individuals. I had been able to benefit Helen Beckett, Enrico Gómez, Harold Daniels, Gene Blango, and, to a more limited extent, Ronald Bransky and Anita Connors, had offered hope to Gary McClintock, set up treatment for Doris Perkins and Isabelle Dupree, and tried to for Timmy Maguire. I could provide them much that they needed and appreciated, helping them in many ways—expected and unexpected, large and small. I knew how to use both biological approaches—which helped many patients more than I would have thought—and psychological approaches, which at times disappointed me in their effectiveness. I had learned valuable lessons from faculty and from other residents, both in my year and a few years ahead of me, such as Greg and Roy. I had also gained confidence in my abilities by standing up to others at times and doing what was right.

I saw myself much differently now. Most simply, I was now a psychiatrist, having learned how to detect, diagnose, and treat mental disorders, and sharing the view that mental illness could and should be treated. But, more important, I had gone through critical rites of passage. Being a psychiatrist was now an integral part of my identity. I sniffed evidence of possible personality disorders, mental illness, and defenses in friends, family members, acquaintances, co-workers, neighbors, store clerks, bus drivers, street people, and others, as well as in myself. I liked belonging to a large international network of other psychiatrists with whom I shared experiences and expertise. When I met other mental health professionals at parties, we spoke the same language and knew the difficulties we each faced that the lay public didn't understand. We knew that we sometimes offered patients less than they wanted, yet believed that mental health workers generally tried their best and that these professionals' attempts were usually worth the effort. Many in the general public would disagree with these positions. Mental health professionals receive a lot of grief and criticism, and are the subject of sizable stigma and suspicion.

Other people now saw me in the light of my profession. "Shrink Bob," some friends jokingly called me. Some who met me assumed I possessed insight into dark secrets of the mind.

But these gains had come at a price. As the end of residency had drawn near, I felt increasingly embittered. A horrible taste lingered in my mouth, as if I had been punched in the stomach, beaten, and left gasping for breath, collapsed in some shadowed alley. This academic environment was the least tolerant, least intellectual, least inquiring of the several of which I had been a part. The oppressiveness of the institution disappointed me. I felt as if the most important parts of me, particularly creative and spontaneous responses to people, had been discouraged. There were pressures to conform and to accept various theories that, though often leaving out key aspects of patients' lives, were rigidly and unquestioningly followed. Failure to accept these assumptions was criticized. It has been assumed that the older image of psychiatry, with its state hospitals as "total institutions," represented errors of the past that could be forgotten in the current new era. But ghosts lingered on. The faculty never mentioned the oppressiveness of the institution. It was less than in earlier times and more implicit, but still present, even if not acknowledged.

Psychiatry was in many ways much more personally difficult than other medical specialties. In internal medicine and pediatrics, the battle lines were clearer—other doctors, patients, patients' families, nurses, the institution, and I all cooperated, united together *against* the disease. Not in psychiatry. Here, residents often found themselves pitted against nurses or patients' families or supervisors or the institution itself. The profession turned me against patients at times; I couldn't always align with them. The pressure was to place my allegiance with the institution first.

As a result of these stresses, I had at times seen the need to distance myself personally from the work, as other psychiatrists did. I didn't always like this response and fought to remain as warm and concerned and emotionally available to patients as possible, but I often had little choice and had to achieve a balance, incorporating both concern and detachment. We were forced to construct a professional self and muster whatever personal resources we could to maintain a cool demeanor at all times. To adopt a professional self disturbed and disappointed me. I sometimes felt like an actor playing a part. We often hid behind our white coats, as if behind a costume, a mask. Yet no one in the hospital commented on these tensions.

Some of my fellow residents became harried and hardened, more consistently removed from their patients and colleagues. Some residents began to dismiss more complicated aspects of patients' lives. "Oh, she's just acting up again," they'd say about a patient, rolling their eyes, as if to say, "What a pain in the neck." It was easy not to think about our patients' pain. Many psychiatrists erected a wall. They entered a professional mode each day, bustling about, and in many ways became less concerned with certain human elements of their patients' existence. I was saddened to see some colleagues lose part of their warmth and sensitivity. Some readily joined the most conservative of psychoanalytic institutes and unquestioningly followed the most conservative interpretations of Freud, which disheartened me, as I hoped that inquiry and advancement of these theories could occur.

Several areas of the profession gave me pause. Though many residents accepted the profession fully and unquestioningly, I found myself, partly as a result of studying medicine in other cultures, aware of problematic features of the discipline that needed to be further examined, researched, and improved. I couldn't blindly accept all of the institution's claims, and found relevant my meeting beforehand with Satuma, the witch doctor in Papua New Guinea, who believed he could cure kuru. His fellow villagers thought he understood the illness. Yet, in fact, his treatment was wholly ineffective against the virus, and his explanation was incorrect. I saw the need to try to maintain at least a glimpse of the social, cultural, and institutional contexts, issues, and assumptions underlying our work, to question ourselves rigorously, especially when we didn't succeed as we had expected, and to try to maintain an open-minded approach with patients.

Along with successes, I had seen limitations in psychiatry. Medications, even those much heralded, often had side effects that prompted patients to stop them. The role of psychoanalytic approaches was also problematic. Psychodynamic approaches often met with modest success at best. For example, with borderline personality disorder, as in Nancy and Anita, we sometimes ended up turning our backs on patients' cries for help.

I questioned analysts' use of power. Many psychoanalysts, feeling that they knew how troubled individuals used maladaptive defenses, assumed that they could use the same principles to run a large, complex social and financial organization. But compromise and politics are important in an institution, more so than in psychoanalysis with a single patient. Problems presented by residents to psychoanalytic faculty would commonly be interpreted rather than repaired. As a fourth-year resident, evaluating other residents, I saw how important it was to give helpful suggestions that weren't merely criticisms of one's personal character.

I was wary of many psychoanalysts' beliefs that they had a panacea. They had used their technique to treat schizophrenia, depression, panic attacks, drug abuse, homosexuality (which they had considered a disorder), and neurosis, and though they had gradually yielded to recognize other treatments for some of these, still clung to their principles when treating others. Psychoanalysts believed they possessed The Truth about human nature. Historically, such claims, when made, have usually later been found to have been incorrect. Psychoanalysts' approach was devoid of rigorous self-questioning, which the philosopher Karl Popper has argued is a defining element of a science—attempts to "falsify" itself, to disprove itself—in order to make itself stronger. Psychoanalysis avoided any such challenges. Even with the advent of new, more effective treatments, psychoanalysts have not all questioned their basic premises, or sifted through their theories, revising or rejecting selected ones to take account of new scientific findings. Among its practitioners, criticisms of psychoanalysis fall on many deaf ears. The lack of room for substantial query has become more apparent now that it is needed the most. Such problems result partly from limitations in knowledge about the mind and the brain that need to be redressed through further research. In the meantime, many psychoanalysts fear that admitting some flaws in their system challenges the whole.

"I don't know if psychoanalysis works," I told my psychoanalyst, Dr. Knoedler, at one point in the beginning of my treatment with him.

"It works," he declared.

"How do you know?"

"It does."

"But it's never been proven to work," I said, repeating Dr. Farb's comment.

"Why are you bringing this up now?" He didn't answer my question, and merely posed another question in reply.

"How do you think it will help me?" I asked.

"That's not for me to say."

"Why not?"

He laughed but didn't answer. What else could he say?

Among the mental health professions, questions as basic as who should receive psychoanalysis as opposed to psychotherapy, and what kind, aren't always clearly resolved in practice.

What patients get may depend on whom they happen to consult. People I've met usually find therapists through word of mouth. Whether someone ends up lying on a couch in psychoanalysis will probably depend on whether his therapist also happens to have been trained as a psychoanalyst. A general psychiatrist who is not also a trained psychoanalyst will almost never recommend psychoanalysis to a patient. Further public education about mental health problems and treatments is much needed.

The use of medication has been unclear at times, too. Many patients who might benefit from medications haven't received them because their therapists are opposed to them on theoretical grounds or do not have the training to prescribe them. Roy once saw a patient who had been in psychoanalysis for many years for depression. Roy thought the patient would benefit from an antidepressant, such as Prozac, possibly in addition to continuing to see the therapist. However, the therapist became irate at the suggestion, accused Roy of interfering with the treatment, and wrote a letter angrily complaining to Dr. Farb that Roy was implying that psychoanalysis was not the best treatment for the patient. Roy won out in the end and the patient was helped by the medication.

In recent years, fewer and fewer medical students in the United States have chosen psychiatry as a specialty, in part sensing these shortcomings. The profession, wanting to continue to attract medical students, and particularly good ones, has become concerned, and the decline is now discussed and analyzed with alarm and regret on the front pages of psychiatric magazines. The profession has been forced to examine itself more closely to try to alter this trend.

Several factors account for the decline. Medical students sense that the field is less personally satisfying, given persisting ambiguity about the mind and the brain, compared to the more established scientific bases of other branches of medicine. Moreover, other specialties have a larger number of effective treatments, and often more definitive cures, gratifying physicians who can then more readily solve the problems they face. The low demonstrated effectiveness of some psychiatric treatments, most notably outpatient psychotherapies, including psychoanalysis, has decreased the reimbursement rates for these activities both at present and in proposed health care reforms. As a result, psychiatrists earn on the average less than almost all other specialists. Many medical students also seek to engage personally with patients at a meaningful level and feel that the profession's increasing biological emphasis leads in the opposite direction. Many students have decided not to enter the field because of bad experiences with faculty, nurses, and other staff that the students felt were unjustified or inappropriate. The politics on wards contrasts sharply with the more scientific rationales behind many activities in other specialties.

The profession, in trying to understand its lessened appeal, has begun to recognize the importance of examining itself and the process of psychiatric education more closely. Psychiatry's leaders realize more and more that the field cannot afford complacency or presumption, but must carefully analyze its workings and assumptions. More effective medications will surely be developed over time. But meanwhile, broader systems issues need to be looked at, acknowledged, and taught. As part of that, the experiences of trainees must be understood, and appreciated, and seen through their eyes.

The field must produce psychiatrists who are as sensitive to their patients as possible. Some logistical changes in residencies have already been instituted. After my training was over it became state law to have attendings in the ER. At my hospital, a new residency training director changed the policy concerning selectives to distribute time equally to all residents. But having faculty more aware of and responsive to the situations encountered by residents would help as well. Residents were rarely given the benefit of the doubt. More understanding treatment of residents by faculty will produce psychiatrists who are, in turn, more sensitive to their patients. Empathy breeds empathy. Otherwise, a less feeling culture results.

Toward these ends, teaching in psychiatric hospitals needs to be further emphasized and respected, as well. Faculty tend to be rewarded for the quantity of research papers they produce, rather than for the quality of their teaching. Too often the complexities both in the art of clinical care and in ethical decisions that emerge are underappreciated and undertaught. Cultural, social, and moral conflicts continually arise but are virtually ignored in seminars and lectures.

The experiences in psychiatric hospitals described here have received little attention within the profession, and are rarely glimpsed outside. Patients in the clinics and wards of psychiatric hospitals are usually treated by residents, who quickly move on in their careers to treat higher-functioning patients, leaving these sicker and generally more difficult patients to in-coming residents. These patients are all but forgotten.

These problems result partly from society's shunning the mentally ill, and being unwilling to devote the necessary re-sources to care fully for them. Moreover, increasing social problems such as poverty, drug and alcohol abuse, homeless-ness, AIDS, and government and institutional cutbacks exacer-bate mental illness. More research is also needed to study the workings of the psyche and the brain.

Along with the inner core of the atom and the outer rim of the universe, the brain remains one of the last scientific fron-tiers here on earth. But overly rigid conclusions or ideolo-gies—be they reductionistically biological or Freudian—will not always assist patients. Rather, what is required is a human-istic open-mindedness tackling problems that have bewitched man from his start—understanding mental health and mental illness. We have learned much but there is still a long ways to go.

Clearly, the social, cultural, and human aspects of psychiatry need to be more acknowledged and better understood. The field would gain from looking at what it does not just from a narrow medical model of diagnosing and prescribing treat-ments but from a broader perspective. Patients require more than merely addressing their psychodynamic or pharmacologi-cal responses to situations. Biology, while helpful, sometimes threatens to make us psychiatrists deal less with our patients and be less sensitive to their needs. Again and again I saw the need to avoid lapsing into the ease and comfort of rigid struc-tures and theories, and—though much harder—to try to under-stand patients and their problems from a wider, more all-encompassing viewpoint, to see ourselves as actors in the dramas of our patients' lives, appreciating not merely issues of transference but also the influence and power we have in other ways as well. Adherence to theories and ideology often misses more subtle and nuanced aspects of patients' predicaments. Moral, social, and humanistic perspectives in the profession re-quire further exploration and research to enable the field to gain the most, and help the most patients in the future.

These thoughts flitted through my mind as I finished in the hospital. Finally, I exited the building for the last time. Just then, Shelly Tarr was entering the front door. "Goodbye," I said. "And thank you for everything."

"This is it?"

"This is it. But," I started, "I'm going to try to come to your July Fourth party."

"Do you need directions?"

"I'll get them from Roy"—who was then working part-time in the outpatient department—"or I'll call." My arms were full and I was running late.

"Yes. I suppose you can just call for them." She was holding the door open as she spoke. "You can call Gina, I guess, also."

"Or I may actually come with Roy." He had a car and had offered me a lift. "But I'm in a hurry at the moment." I had to be across town in twenty minutes.

"You may come with Roy?"

"Yes. But unfortunately, I have to run." I was standing in the driveway, clearly on the way out.

"Oh. Well," she said. How awkward many psychiatrists were socially. I think many of them became psychiatrists for that very reason: to increase their understanding of people with whom they had to interact and felt uncomfortable.

"Goodbye," I said.

"Goodbye." I offered her my hand to shake. She awkwardly lifted hers and put it into mine. It felt cold and limp.

I walked down the driveway and out onto the street, glad to be done. I turned around and looked one last time at the edifice that had contained and restrained me for three long years. The sun shone on the upper floors above the shadows of a few trees. The building seemed much smaller now. I could pick out windows where particular patients of mine had stayed—there was Nancy's old room, and Bransky's, and Jimmy Lentz's. There was my old office. I still felt very attached to what had gone on there.

The next day, I stayed at home, packing and moving my belongings out of the apartment where, a few blocks from the hospital, I had lived as a resident, slept when on call in the ER, and often talked to patients. Only now, as I moved from my home, did my residency feel over.

How much room there was in my apartment when emptied. How much space that I had been too busy as a resident to appreciate or use. The bedroom stretched to the window where my desk had sat. The living room was larger than I had thought. The foyer seemed longer. I had done push-ups and sit-ups every morning on a little blue throw rug that I had bought for the purpose and used as a mat. My bicycle had stood there, though I never had time to use it. My guitar had also remained in the corner, boxed in its black case throughout my residency, gathering dust. How little time I had had there just to relax during these years. The room, now empty, looked simpler. I had forgotten about the green marble-patterned linoleum on the floor of the closets.

As I was busy moving, Roy called. "I feel left behind," he said. "It won't be the same here without all of you who are graduating." I didn't know when I would again see the hospital, the neighborhood, my colleagues, patients, or friends.

I finished loading my belongings into a truck and finally slammed the doors shut. I glanced back toward the tall medical center building in the distance one final time, then climbed into the driver's seat and drove off.

Follow-ups

I have gone by the hospital occasionally since graduating. The building seems ever smaller with the increasing passage of time, and more harmless, such that I'm amazed how stressful the experience was then. Gradually, I look back more positively at it, through the veil of time.

Slowly, I have been able to reconnect with earlier parts of my life and return to earlier interests. I have been able to read the whole Sunday newspaper, including the Travel section, and have even been able to travel abroad. I was surprised when I returned to my former self, as if awakened from some bad dream. Never before had I felt as strongly the power of a social institution on me, affecting my experiences and view of the world. Once residency—the most intense period of professional change and growth in my life—ended, I was able to pick up the pieces and settle back into the world, shaky at first, but I suspect somehow wiser.

In my final year, I had applied for and was offered several jobs, and selected a fellowship in public psychiatry—that is, psychiatry in the public sector. I would soon see that it was possible, in fact, to use skills learned during my residency to research and work on some of the issues that interested me and seemed important. For example, as part of my fellowship program, I ended up working in an HIV mental health clinic. There, we helped patients with psychological and social issues they faced. I developed the area of my selective and began to investigate more fully cultural, psychological, and ethical aspects of the epidemic, conducting in-depth interviews on the meanings of the illness and on coping and adaptation.

It turned out that I didn't have to conform wholly to a single career path in the profession but could focus on areas that interested me. I had paid a price for the skills I learned in my residency but, as time passes, increasingly feel that it was worth it. I wish the process were different and see many areas for improvement in the field. But psychiatric training had got me where I am now and had become an important part of me.

The other residents in my year all followed different career paths.

Anne moved to Los Angeles and is doing research on anxiety disorders. Sarah paints in her newly discovered leisure time and hopes to have a gallery exhibit of her work. Mike plays a lot of softball and had been dating a sculptress for two years. Joe Tauber became enormously successful in mental health education, even though his selective in this area had been completely turned down. One evening, at the opera, I ran into Jessica, who was wearing pearls and a long mink coat.

It was difficult to get any kind of follow-up on my patients.

Eventually, Nancy Steele had been readmitted, though the staff is more wary of her actions now. I don't know whatever happened to Helen Beckett or the patients seen in the emergency room. This lack of follow-up ultimately removes residents from patients, ensuring that we meet them for only brief periods of time before they disappear from our lives.

But occasionally, I hear about patients or staff, and my mind returns instantly to the experiences we had together.

Just a few weeks ago, walking to the subway near my home, en route to the hospital where I am now doing research, I sensed someone following me and glanced back. A figure a few yards behind me strolled, huddled in an army surplus camouflage coat. I dropped my token in the subway turnstile and walked to the uptown platform to catch my train. While looking down the tracks, I suddenly heard a voice. "Hey, Doc." I turned around. Beneath a linted navy ski cap were familiar, though somewhat vacant, eyes. I couldn't immediately place the face but had a haunting feeling about the person. Then it hit me. It was Enrico Gómez, who had once tried to drown himself. He raised and then lowered his chin slightly as a greeting, his hands remaining buried in his pockets.

"Enrico!" I said—a smile spreading across my face— stepping toward him. But he was quickly gone, continuing down the stairs to get to the platform on the opposite side of the tracks. He didn't look ill or like a psychiatric patient. In my fleeting glance, he seemed okay overall. He had survived. A train immediately arrived at his platform. When it pulled away, the sooty concrete waiting area was bare. I looked at the silent, empty platform for a few moments, until my train arrived to take me to my new hospital for another day.

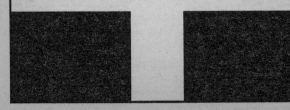

BEHIND THE SCENES AT *ER*
by Janine Pourroy

Television is a medium of shadow and light.

The flickering characters we watch from our living room sofas are not really playing out scenes from their lives; they are actors speaking lines they have memorized from a script someone else has written. They do not exist in any real place; they perform on sets made of breakaway walls and borrowed coffee tables. All too often, even the laughter is contrived.

There are, however, moments when truth filters through these illusory images. As an audience, we know the difference. We can tell when characters make connections, and when they miss. We *know* that life is flawed and messy and imprecise and fabulous—and it does us good when we see that reflected in the shows we watch. While being entertained, we discover that we are not alone, and television becomes what good theater has always been: a transcendent experience.

On *ER*, the reality is added in layers that begin with the writing. Characters are revealed in glimpses, not in heavy-handed declarations. As doctors they are heroes, but we discover behind their boldness, fragility. And humanity. Truth slips through the drama with such subtlety that it leaves us thinking about it the next day at work.

Creator Michael Crichton established this reality in the pilot, but in continuing the show as a weekly series, the producers faced daunting challenges. Crichton recalled, "None of us was entirely sure how to make the series work. John Wells's feeling was, 'We know the elements, we'll have to play with them and see what happens.' But the fragmentary storytelling techniques established in the pilot—the idea that you only saw intermittent glimpses of ongoing events and characters—were difficult to use on a weekly basis. Because there couldn't be a formula. There could be no obvious rules that tied the incidents in an episode together because if there were, the audience would quickly sense that and the show would lose its realism. No one had ever attempted a TV show like this, and there was a real possibility that it just couldn't be done. But ER's writers do it, week after week. Breathtakingly well."

It was also important to retain the medical sensibilities Crichton had insisted on for so many years. "One of the things we decided early on," said John Wells, "was not to pander to the viewer medically. Traditionally, medical shows have had the attitude that the viewer has to understand what's going on medically at all times. So you hear characters saying a lot of ridiculous things like 'It's time to do the laparotomy! Joe, get that tube so we can see if there's blood in his stomach!'—when, clearly, everybody in the scene would know what a laparotomy was. Instead, we allowed the audience to feel as if they'd stepped into a real hospital, and decided not to underestimate their intelligence. We knew it wasn't necessary for them to understand all the medicine to follow the story. It's sort of like watching a conversation in a foreign language. You depend on your other senses. You watch the body language between the characters. You see the gestures, you listen to the tone of voice, and you very clearly see what's going on. I think that takes you deeper into the drama of the scene, because you're not worried about the specifics medically, which aren't all that important, anyway. You get a sense of what's happening and what the stakes are for everyone involved."

Additionally, the producers felt it was essential to keep the focus on the doctors, not the patients. "Generally speaking, doctors in medical shows have been nice, earnest people who are very talented," said Wells. "They're either the Ben Casey kind of gruff or the Marcus Welby kind of warm and empathetic—and they stay with the patient throughout the course of an hour-long episode. But in reality, doctors' lives are not much like that. I've had a lot of doctors tell me, 'I can stand here and hold the patient's hand, or I can go help two or three other people.' In an emergency room setting, that's particularly true. The extra time a doctor spends with one person is time taken away from somebody else. Because we wanted to stay realistic in that way, we needed to focus on the emotional journey of the doctor, unlike the traditional medical story, which tended to focus on the emotional journey of the patient."

Such journeys begin with well-considered scripts, determined in part at lengthy writers meetings where Wells and the other writer/producers lay out the show's intricate multiple story lines. Working with Wells are co-executive producer Lydia Woodward; co-executive producer Carol Flint, who joined the production team the second season; coproducer Paul Manning; medical consultants Dr. Lance Gentile and fourth-year Harvard medical student Neal Baer; and staff writer Tracey Stern. (Robert Nathan, one of ER's original writer/producers, left the show after the first season to produce The Client.) In-house director Mimi Leder is also involved in the story process, as are Michael Crichton and Steven Spielberg, who regularly offer their ideas as well.

Plot issues are discussed, character motivation and growth are examined, and slowly, the writers begin to determine the specifics for each episode—and the overlapping, intertwining stories that will eventually make up a season's worth of episodes.

Until the early eighties, dramatic show[s] have one basic story line per show. Series [like] *Mannix* or *The Defenders*, for example, dealt w[ith] solving a single case within the confines of their allotted hour. That style of dramatic television changed in 1981 with the advent of Steven Bochco's *Hill Street Blues*, when a kind of Dickensian multiple story line was introduced. This style of storytelling was typically told using three or four different stories—an A, a B, and a C story, with a D story, or "comic runner"—woven together throughout the course of the program.

With *ER*, the producers decided to reinvent dramatic television once again. "We usually have anywhere from nine to eighteen stories running in any episode," said Wells. "We wanted the pace to move in a way that would hold the audience's interest. The joke around here was that *ER* is the show for the era of remote controls because there is no need to channel surf: all you have to do is hang around for a minute or two and you're going to see another story. People have called to tell us that they thought the show was only a half hour long because there was so much in it. It literally moved so fast that they weren't able to gauge the length compared to a normal hour of dramatic television. Well, even though those elements had worked in the pilot, there was still some concern about bringing them to the series. We had a lot of people warning us, 'The audience may enjoy going to see the movie *Speed*, but they don't want to see it every night.' To which I was always thinking, 'Why not?'"